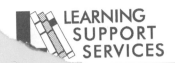

OXFORD MEDICAL PUBLICATIONS

The nervous system

The nervous system

Peter Nathan MD FRCP

SECOND EDITION

Oxford New York Toronto Melbourne

OXFORD UNIVERSITY PRESS

1982

Oxford University Press, Walton Street, Oxford OX2 6DP

London Glasgow New York Toronto
Delhi Bombay Calcutta Madras Karachi
Kuala Lumpur Singapore Hong Kong Tokyo
Nairobi Dar es Salaam Cape Town
Melbourne Auckland
and associate companies in
Beirut Berlin Ibadan Mexico City

First edition © Peter Nathan 1969
Second edition © Peter Nathan Charitable Trust 1982

First published by Penguin Books Ltd 1969
Second edition published by Oxford University Press 1982

British Library Cataloguing in Publication Data
Nathan, Peter
The nervous system. – 2nd ed.
1. Nervous system – Vertebrates
I. Title
596'.01'88   QL923
ISBN 0–19–261344–8

Set by Macmillan India Ltd.

Printed in Great Britain
at the University Press, Oxford
by Eric Buckley
Printer to the University

To Ursula, Nickie, Jennifer, and Brian

The quotations used at the beginning of
many of the sections of the book are from
Christopher Smart's poem, *My Cat Jeoffrey.*

Acknowledgements

I have much pleasure in thanking the following people for the drawings and photographs in this book: the late Mr Sidney Woods for Figures 3.1, 4.1, 5.1, 6.1, 7.1, 8.1, 9.1, 10.1, 12.1, 16.1, 16.2, 18.1, 19.1, 19.2, 19.3, 21.1, 22.1, 22.2, 22.3, and 24.2; Professor Peter Matthews, F.R.S. for Figure 8.2; Dr Juergen Tonnsdorf for Figure 4.2; Professor Norman Geschwind for Figure 21.1; Professor Ida Mann and Dr Antoinette Pirie for Figure 3.3; Professor H. Hydén for Plate 1; the late Professor E. W. Walls for Plate 2; Dr Alan Ridley for Plates 3 and 4; Dr David Landon for Plates 5 and 6; Dr Tony Pullen for Plates 7 and 8; and Mr Leslie Frampton for Plates 9, 10, 11, 12 and 13.

I am grateful to the following scientific workers who have allowed me to quote from their work: Dr Macdonald Critchley; Dr Dalle Ore; Dr Michael Espir; Professor Robert G. Heath; the late Professor Wilder Penfield, O. M., C.M.G., F.R.S.; Dr Curt Richter; the late Professor W. Ritchie Russell; Dr W. B. Scoville; and Dr H. Terzian.

I should like to take this opportunity of thanking the following editors of scientific journals and publishers of encyclopaedias, journals and books: Dr Russell de Jong, editor of *Neurology*; Dr Bruce Lindsay, editor of the *Journal of the Acoustical Society of America*; Dr Robert Mayor, editor of the *Journal of the American Medical Association*; the late Professor W. Ritchie Russell, editor of the *Journal of Neurology, Neurosurgery and Psychiatry*; Dr Victor Soriano, editor of the *International Journal of Neurology*; Harper and Row for permission to quote from *The Role of Pleasure in Behaviour*, edited by Robert G. Heath; Major C. W. Hume for permission to quote from material by myself in *The Assessment of Pain in Man and Animals* published by the University Federation for Animal Welfare; Professor Cyril Keele, editor, and Oxford University Press for permission to quote from *Applied Physiology* by Samson Wright; J. R. Newman, editor, and Thomas Nelson and Sons and Harper and Row for permission to quote from the *International Encyclopaedia of Science*; and Oxford University Press for permission to quote from *Traumatic Aphasia* by the late W. Ritchie Russell and Michael Espir.

I take this opportunity of thanking Sheridan Russell who criticized the book from the point of view of the interested non-medical reader. I am also grateful to Dr Catherine Storr, who went through the book with a toothcomb. Above all, I am grateful to Dr Marion Smith and Martin Starkie who read each chapter and criticized it in detail and whose advice in ways of improving the earlier versions was of great value.

P. N.

Contents

List of plates

Introduction

Neurology is the study of the nervous system. The nervous system is made up of the brain, the spinal cord and the nerves throughout the body. The structure of the nervous system is neuroanatomy and its functioning is neurophysiology. The disorders and diseases of the nervous system that bring patients to neurologists are paralyses, tremors, shingles, Parkinsonism, epilepsy, multiple or disseminated sclerosis and others, most of which are not yet satisfactorily treated.

Theoretically psychology is a part of neurology, for every sort of behaviour is the result of the functioning of the brain. But in practice, it is convenient to keep it as a separate subject. Psychologists are not usually doctors of medicine. They do mental testing, carry out tests for what is called intelligence, vocational guidance, and they do research on certain aspects of brain functioning, such as vision, sensation, reading, writing and topographical memory.

Psychiatrists are medically trained; they specialize in the diagnosis and treatment of psychotic patients and of neuroses and illnesses in which social and emotional features play an important role.

The boundaries between neurology, psychiatry and psychology are fluid and indistinct. If someone starts behaving oddly, he may need the help of a psychiatrist, a neurologist or a neurosurgeon; it depends whether he is suffering from depression, from senile dementia or a brain tumour. It is the neurologist who makes the diagnosis.

As the adjective 'nervous' has popularly come to mean anxious, apprehensive or frightened, it will be avoided in this book; the adjective 'neural' will be used instead, which is present practice in neurology.

A book on psychoanalysis, psychotherapy or psychology can be understood by anyone who has had no education in biology. But neurology, like the rest of medicine, requires some knowledge of physics, chemistry and anatomy.

This book is a new edition of the author's Pelican book *The Nervous System*. It has been altered in many ways; it is not for the author to say it has been improved. Some illustrations have been brought up-to-date, and some electron micrographs have been added. Some chapters needed to be re-written as advances in the subjects have been made by continuous research work. I have tried to make the account simpler without leaving out any information. These chapters are those on

Listening, of which the section on echo-location has been enlarged and to which a history of the subject has been added; Tasting and Smelling, each of which now has a chapter on its own; Smelling includes a section on pheromones; Touching and Feeling, which includes recent investigations on man, which allow us to omit investigations on other species; Balance and the Vestibular System. A chapter on pain has been added. Another new chapter is on chemical neurotransmitters and their targets; great advances have been made in this subject. The chapter on Nerves and Nerve Fibres has been re-done and a section added on the trophic activity of nerves and transport of substances within nerve fibres. The chapters on Communication within the Central Nervous System and Moving have also been totally re-done. Throughout, a little more about diseases of the nervous system has been given; although this book is about the normally functioning nervous system, so many people have asked me to explain where neurological diseases fit into this general account of the nervous system, that I have made comments on how things go worng. The chapter on being awake or asleep has been much enlarged; we now know more about sleep in human beings and about the sleeping habits of various animals. I have added a short account of some sleep disorders, such as sleep paralysis and narcolepsy. The chapter on the hypothalamus has been largely altered and the chapter on hormones has been entirely re-done; in this subject advances and retreats are made every day.

The first chapter of the book is introductory, starting with a concise explanation of what the nervous system does, followed by basic fats of its anatomy. The five senses are discussed in chapters 2–7. Following the five senses, there is a chapter on the senses unnoticed by the Greek philosophers, the senses of the body itself, muscle sense, the sense of balance, the sensations of the visceral organs. Chapter 9 is on the physics of the nerve impulse; for this chapter some knowledge of physics and chemistry is an advantage. How neural messages are sent around the central nervous system is discussed in chapters 10 and 11. What the brain decides to make the body do is nearly always some sort of activity; otherwise it is repose from activity. Activity means moving. Chapter 12 concerns moving, and that includes everything like building a nest, moving your eyes up and down, standing and running, breathing, or playing the violin. The chapter on pain is chapter 13. Pain is not only a sensation; it is a sensation accompanied by emotion. It is the same for every kind of sensation, though the strongly unpleasant emotion accompanying pain forms an obvious example of this.

Psychologists used to imagine that animals did not react or behave until they were stimulated; they were just blanks waiting to be stimulated; and they then reacted. That is exactly how it is not. Animals are inquisitive and go out to explore the world. They are seeking what is interesting to them. Curiosity, as we know, killed the cat. This exploration and seeking stimulation, and its opposite, lying resting at home and going to sleep, is discussed in chapter 14. How animals are motivated is the theme of chapter 15 and the anatomical bases of motivation are the subject of chapter 16. Chapter 17 is on the endocrine glands and hormones, the chemical messengers affecting the structure of tissues and the animal's total behaviour.

With chapter 18, we come to the higher levels of neural activity and the higher levels of the brain. What we have learned about the brain by the electrical stimulation of parts of the brain in conscious patients during operations is reported in chapter 19. Chapter 20 is about sensation. A section on what the visual cortex receives has been added; this is based on the work of Professors Hubel and Wiesel and subsequent investigations; a similar section on the auditory cortex has been added.

People tend to think of what the brain does only in relation to what are called the higher nervous activities: these are thinking, calculating, remembering, learning, reading and writing. This part of neurology is discussed in chapters 21, 22, and 23. The chapter on speech has been written at a more advanced level than before; it now includes an account of American psychologists' work on teaching chimpanzees to read and write. The short section on congenital dyslexia has been enlarged, as this trouble is now generally recognized to have a neural and anatomical basis. The ability of a unicellular animal, the paramoecium, to learn is now discussed, and how cockroaches' legs learn is also reported, as well as how human beings can learn to control the involuntary or autonomic nervous system. More has been added about phrenology, which was at first a real advance in our knowledge of the anatomy and physiology of the brain. The final chapter on some aspects of personality and the brain now reports another case of a man who had a bullet through his brain, which he introduced by shooting himself in the wrong way. The part on the results of leucotomy has been shortened, as this operation is no longer carried out.

Although the writer of any book imagines his ideal reader starting on page 1 and continuing absorbed to the hard-won words—'The End', I have tried to write this book so that any single chapter may be read on its own or left out.

1 Functions and structure of the nervous system of vertebrates

The function of a nervous system is to keep its possessor informed about the world. All animals need to have a continuous supply of information about what is happening; and things are happening in two worlds, the world outside the body and the world of the body itself. The actual state of affairs around the animal is not reported; the nervous system provides a selected representation of the environment which is meaningful to that animal. Anything changing is noticed with vigilance, for it could be desirable or dangerous. Particular notice is always given to the behaviour of other animals, especially those of one's own group. Adaptation to one's environment, and this includes one's fellows, is a first law of life. It requires, among other attributes, memory and the continual filling of the memory store.

The function of the nervous system is to provide its possessor with the ability to move, both move around the world and move its own body. It arranges the movements of the parts of the body, the limbs and tongue, and the unseen parts, such as the stomach and other viscera, the bladder and the rectum.

Nervous systems of vertebrates consist of the brain and spinal cord, called the central nervous system, and the nerves running to and from the central nervous system, called the peripheral nervous system. There is another part of the nervous system, the autonomic nervous system, sympathetic and parasympathetic. This is the nervous system of the viscera and blood vessels, the glands and the skin. It helps to adjust the animal to its environment, either in preparing for action or for relaxation and sleep.

In the earliest and simplest vertebrates the central nervous system was a tube running the length of the body; later it became encased in bone. During evolution the front end of this neural tube enlarged into three swellings which developed into the brain. As the central nervous system is buried inside the body, it has to be kept in touch with the world and with everything that is happening in the body. Peripheral nerves are cables of nerve fibres that bring messages to and from the central nervous system. The ones going to the central nervous system, called afferent nerves, report what is happening outside the body, things that can be seen or heard. The nerves coming away from the central nervous system called efferent nerves go to muscles, glands and viscera. The nerves are joined to the spinal cord and brain, passing through holes in the skull and vertebral column. Nerve fibres convey messages coded in pulses, like the morse code. These pulses are simply called, nerve impulses. When the nerve impulse reaches the end of the nerve fibre, it puts out a chemical substance that acts on the structure to which the nerve is running. Some nerve fibres are specialized in secreting this substance, so that the difference between this kind of nerve and a gland pouring out a chemical substance is a matter of degree.

The nervous system is made up of cells, like every other tissue of animals and plants. The principle cell is the nerve cell or neuron. There are two sorts, excitatory and inhibitory; the excitatory cell brings other cells into activity and inhibitory neurons cancel this out, tending to stop the activity of other neurons. Neurons of the central nervous system are collected together in layers and in small groups; these groups of cells are called nuclei and one is a nucleus. Both nuclei and layers of neurons are often called centres, particularly when their function is being thought of; and so one has visual centres, a vesical centre to work the bladder, and autonomic centres working the autonomic nervous system. To the naked eye, collections of neurons in nuclei or layers look grey and so they are called grey matter; nerve fibres are white and they make up the white matter.

A photograph of a living neuron is shown in Plate 1. This neuron was dissected out of the brain of a rabbit by Hydén of Göteborg University in Sweden. The neuron has been magnified 1800 times. The main mass of this cell is the cell-body; the arm-like structures streaming out of it are the dendrites, branching prolongations of the cell. One of the cord-like prolongations of the cell-body is the axon; this might be the tentacle in the bottom on the left. The axon is the long thin telegraph wire of the neuron, conveying the message from the neuron to muscles, glands or other neurons. The pale circular spot in the middle is the nucleus of the cell, and in the middle of the nucleus is the black nucleolus. The little black spots on the surface of the cell-body and the dendrites are the nerve-endings of other neurons, passing excitatory or inhibitory messages to this neuron. Between these nerve-endings and this neuron is a minute gap, called the synapse (Greek for grasp).

The brain is an enormously enlarged part of the spinal cord. Where this enlargement starts is a part of the brain that is obviously an enlarged spinal cord; this is called the medulla oblongata, having no name in English. It is shown in Plates 10, 11, and 12. This basic part of the brain organizes basic functions—the heartbeat, the blood pressure, breathing, swallowing.

The position of the central nervous system in the body of man is shown in Plate 2. The lowest part of the brain, the medulla oblongata, is seen to lie behind the hard palate and the upper part of the cavity of the mouth. The cerebral hemispheres, of which the left one is seen here from the midline, are by far the largest part of the brain and they fill most of the cavity of the skull. The hypothalamus is in the centre of the front part of the brain. Running forward from it, the stalk of the pituitary gland can be seen. The various structures shown in this photograph will often be referred to in the subsequent chapters of the book; and reference to it will show why we speak of the parts as being in front, behind, above, and below.

2 Examining the world

All living organisms since the beginnings of life on earth have passed their lives under the influence of certain permanent physical features of the world. Such are night and day, the increasing duration of daylight as spring follows winter in the Northern and Southern Hemispheres, various kinds of movement of the environment, winds, currents, waves, tides in the sea; there are sounds, usually made by other animals; there is the ambient temperature and barometric pressure; and, less obvious, there is gravity and the earth's magnetic field.

In some organisms these forces are felt by all the tissues of the body, in others they are felt by special cells; these cells and the tissues in which they are encased are called receptors. The receptors are either specialized cells connected to nerve fibres which take the information to the central nervous system; or they are the nerve fibres themselves without specialized cells. Not all species of animals are sensitive to all the physical characteristics of the world. Birds, snails and fish can sense the geomagnetic field and they use it to find their way around. Termites tend to orient themselves in an east-west direction; this is also based on the earth's magnetic field. Although we human beings think we know nothing of the earth's magnetic field, Dr Robin Baker of Manchester University has discovered that we make use of it for finding our way about. He blindfolded volunteers and then took them on journeys; then he took the bandage off their eyes and told them to point towards their homes. They were surprisingly accurate, pointing in the right direction. They were better at getting the direction right when they had been blindfolded. If they had the usual visual clues or noted the position of the sun or tried to work it out intellectually, they did not do so well. If he repeated these experiments, this time with magnets fixed against their heads so as to disrupt the sensing of the geomagnetic field, the people no longer knew in which direction their homes were. All living organisms have developed over millions of years with the forces of geomagnetism exerting a constant influence. It is nevertheless surprising that the electromagnetic field has an influence as it is very weak, far weaker than that produced by hair-dryers and television masts. But it is continuous and ubiquitous.

Man is insensitive to two aspects of light which some other animals can sample—polarized light and ultraviolet light. Man's hearing is rather limited in the upper range compared to that of small mammals and the larger mammals of the sea. In general, animals have no sensory receptors designed to respond to features of the environment that they do not normally meet. Animals that live in caves are mostly pale and blind. There would be no point in going to all the trouble of being pigmented if there were no one there to see you. These troglodytes concentrate on smell, taste and touch. The tick can neither see nor hear, but its sense of smell is attuned to the sour smell of the mammals on which it feeds. It is also sensitive to warmth so that it can tell when it has landed on a warm-blooded creature.

Of the many kinds of animals that are sensitive to the same sort of energy, each class of animal does not have the same sort of receptor, nor does it have the receptors in the same part of the body. Many fish, for instance, have taste receptors not only in their mouths but also scattered over the surface of the body. These are not so much to enjoy food with as to detect it, to find the particles of it suspended in the water. Fish with barbels, such as the sturgeon or the red mullet, have taste receptors on the barbels. The barbels are like the antennae of insects, on which there are olfactory receptors, the sense organs for smelling. Mosquitoes also feel radiant heat with their antennae. The receptors of those spiders who build webs are on their legs; they feel the vibration which is set up by the insect caught in the web with their feet and legs. Many sorts of butterflies and most flies taste with their feet. Flies have their olfactory receptors for smelling on their antennae and palps. When a fly finds some food, it steps into it so as to taste it. It then makes use of other taste receptors on the hairs surrounding its mouth. If the food tastes good, it sucks it up. When it is replete, it vomits a little and then defaecates. If we behaved in this way, we would find a restaurant by smell and not by sight. We would go in and stand in the food. We would give a preliminary opinion on the food, put our moustaches in it, and then give a definite opinion on it. If the food was good, we would suck it up until we felt full, vomit some back on the plate, defaecate on the floor and go. Clearly, it takes all sorts to make a world.

We all have our limits; man is able to sample only certain aspects of the world. Mammals on the whole are less limited in their sampling of the environment than insects. Simpler animals may be able to use only one kind of sensory information. Female crickets recognize the male of their own species only by the chirping sound it makes with its wing-covers. If male crickets are placed beneath a glass from which no sound escapes, the females take no notice of them, even though they can see them. Wasps recognize female wasps entirely by their sense of smell.

Blinded wasps can easily find the females. But wasps in which the antennae have been removed do not recognize female wasps; for on the antennae are the chemoreceptors sensitive to the smell of the female abdominal gland secretion. So important is the sense of smell that after the female's scent glands have been dissected out, many male insects attempt to copulate with the glands and not with the female herself.

Bees and ants can see ultraviolet light, but they cannot see into the red part of the spectrum as far as we can. Red appears black to them. Many insects can see the direction of polarized light. Man is so intelligent that he makes use of the receptors and sensory systems of other animals. He trains pigs and truffle-hounds to smell out truffles beneath the ground; he uses bloodhounds to smell out the trails of men he wants to track down and St Bernards to find men lost on the mountainside. As we have only recently learned about animals being sensitive to sounds of very high frequency and insects being sensitive to polarized light, we may well learn of further sensitivities of living organisms and through them come to appreciate other aspects of the world.

Receptors are used in the same way by all animals. Animals do not wait around until they are stimulated. They use the receptors of their sense organs to explore the world. Books usually say that the eye is for seeing. It is not, it is for looking; the ear is for listening, not hearing.

Receptors are usually classified as exteroceptive, those sampling the environment, interoceptive, those signalling what is going on within the body itself, and proprioceptive, used for controlling the position of the body and its parts. Exteroceptive receptors are for taste, smell, vision and hearing. The proprioceptive receptors or proprioceptors are receptors within the inner ear used to report the position of the body in space and those used for sampling the position and the movement of the head, the limbs, and parts of the limbs. The interoceptive receptors convey information about the bladder, the gut and the pressure the blood exerts against the walls of the heart, the blood vessels, and within the brain itself; others report on the amount of oxygen, carbon dioxide, and glucose in the blood, and others are sensitive to the osmotic pressure of the blood, others to the temperature of the circulating blood. There are receptors sensitive to stimuli that cause pain throughout most structures of the body. There are no receptors sensitive to painful stimulation in the brain itself. Patients carry on conversations unconcerned while needles are passed through their brains.

Receptors are also classified according to the sorts of stimuli to which they are sensitive. In this classification we have the chemoreceptors, for instance receptors sensitive to carbon dioxide or glucose; thermoreceptors, sensitive to changes in temperature; nociceptors, sensitive to stimulations that threaten to or actually do damage the body; and mechanoreceptors which are excited, by pressure on the skin, by pulling or stretching the skin or merely indenting it. Many mechanoreceptors are hairs of the skin or hairs on the cuticle of insects. Insects have mechano-sensitive hairs on the legs which tell them about vibration. One hardly knows whether to call these hairs tactile organs or hearing organs. For mammals use hairs in the skin to report low-pitched vibration and similar hairs in the inner ear to report high-pitched vibration; the first is called touch and the second is called hearing, yet the mechanism is similar in the two cases.

Receptors are also classified according to whether they report a constant state or a changing state. Constant state receptors continue to send in impulses to the central nervous system as long as a certain state, such as a temperature, remains constant. Changing state receptors signal a change in the stimulus. These are the commonest sort of receptors, for all animals need to know about new events. Whenever a stimulus first affects the body, that is something new and maybe important; so this kind of receptor sends in a volley of nerve impulses. It is of equal or almost equal importance to know when the stimulus goes; so that is signalled with equal intensity. The continued presence of the stimulus maybe less important, and so this is signalled with fewer and fewer impulses. In some cases there is a constant slow discharge of impulses; in others, they cease altogether.

There are two features of all kinds of stimulation: intensity of stimulation and localization. Intensity is reported to the central nervous system mainly by the number of impulses sent within a certain length of time. If the brain receives 500 nerve impulses a second, it concludes that stimulation is less intense than when it is receiving 2000 impulses a second. Localization in space, regarding both where stimulation is on the body and where the stimulus is in the environment around the body, is not a great problem; for the body itself and the brain are spread out in space. A cloud in the sky is at the top of the visual field and a worm on the ground at the bottom; they excite different parts of the retinae and are reported by different nerve fibres to different parts of the cortex of the cerebral hemispheres. It is the same with a thorn in the foot or in the finger. A different region in the brain is excited by the different regions of the body that have been pricked. Localization outside the body depends on having pairs of receptors, one on each side of the body. Tastes and smells are not clearly located in space; to do this well, one should have two noses and two tongues, one on each side of the head.

With two ears separated by the whole width of the head, we can tell where a sound is coming from. Two ears give us discrimination between sounds, allowing us to separate one voice out of a buzz of conversation or to hear it in a howling wind. Two eyes give a larger field of vision than one eye and they also provide stereoscopic vision or vision in depth. When our ancestors moved around among the branches of trees, stereoscopic vision must have been a great advantage. For in the forest, you need to tell which of two branches is nearer to or farther away from you. But having groups of receptors on the two sides of the head brings its own problems. We have to make a fusion of what we receive from each sensory organ. Two eyes do not tell us that there are two cats in the room; we interpret the information received by concluding that there is one cat. Our two ears tell us someone is talking to us, not that the sounds of his voice are coming to one ear at one time and to the other ear a fraction of a second later. We have to learn to make this interpretation in babyhood. In seeing, we learn to keep the visual axes of the two eyes parallel. When the young child does not do this, he is said to squint. This should be corrected as early as possible, in the hope that he grows up to use both eyes together.

There are some animals which have a third eye. This organ is on the top of the head; it functions in the reptile known by its Maori name of tuatara, and in some lizards, frogs, toads, in the inguana and lampreys. The third eye is believed to record the amount of sunlight. This information is necessary for the circadian rhythms of the body, which will be discussed in chapter 16. During the millions of years of evolution, plant and animal life has related itself to the cycle of dark and light of night and day. Many rhythms of the body depend on this alternation. In those animals with a third eye, the rhythms seem to depend on this eye; for the rest of us, the two eyes in the face supply the information.

3 Light receptors: looking

For he keeps the Lord's watch in the night against the adversary.
For he counteracts the powers of darkness by his electrical skin and glaring eyes.

Those bandwidths of the electromagnetic radiation that we experience as light have effects on the protoplasm of even the simplest single-celled organisms—in some cases light attracts, in others it repels. As animals evolved, it must have been an advantage to collect in one place all the receptor cells sensitive to light. To enable these cells to absorb the light effectively, a light-sensitive pigment developed in them. In the higher kinds of animal, this region became the retina.

The general arrangement of the eye remains the same throughout the animal kingdom. That is surprising. It appears to be that no better kind of eye could be formed during evolution. The simplest kinds of eye are pits in the skin lined with cells of light-absorbing pigment. These cells react to light and dark; they are the light detectors or photoreceptors. Light affects the molecules of pigment of these cells and this reaction sends off nerve impulses to the parts of the central nervous system developed to cope with reactions to light.

The eye is a ball, of which one can only see the front part. This part consists of a transparent conjunctiva, which gets inflamed in conjunctivitis, a transparent cornea, and behind that a transparent lens. Lining the eyeball is the retina. As has often been said, the eye is like a camera. In both eyes and cameras, there is a light-sensitive film, with black backing to absorb the light that has passed through the film. Both have an iris or diaphragm to adjust the amount of light, and both have a lens for focussing. The lens in the eye of the mammal is elastic; its curvature can be adjusted by muscles within the eye; and this changes its focal length. It is slightly yellow; this is like a yellow filter, and cuts out some of the violet light. As we become older, the lens becomes yellower and blue light is not seen so well. Colours appear more orange. It has been suggested that Turner's later pictures all have this orange tone and are lacking in blues on account of this change in his lens, of which he himself would not have been aware.

The human retina is amazingly sensitive to light; we can see a single candle at night five miles away. The range of light intensity to which the retina can respond is equally amazing, for between the slightest amount of light just visible in the dark and the brightest sunlight, there is a difference in intensity of about ten thousand million to one (10,000,000,000 to 1).

Both cameras and eyes work with an optimum amount of light, and modern automatic cameras and age-old eyes automatically adjust the size of the aperture to let in this correct amount. Both film and the retina absorb light; both react to a certain bandwidth out of all the possible frequencies of radiation. This selected bandwidth brings about a chemical reaction in both of them. In the retina, this bandwidth of radiation is absorbed by a pigment in the photoreceptors; in the film it is absorbed by the emulsion in the gelatin.

There are some obvious differences between cameras and eyes. The eye selects; it does not record everything in the indiscreet manner of the camera. The camera has to be kept quite still; the eye has to be kept moving; it carries out little invisible movements at a rate of 30 to 90 a second. If this were not done, the image on the retina would fade out; for it has to be transferred to different photoreceptors. Cameras work whether they are always in use or not; but eyes and the whole visual system have to learn in order to see. Chimpanzees brought up in darkness for sixteen months from birth are blind when they are first brought out into the light. It then takes them a long time to acquire sight and to learn to identify objects. Our vision has gone through a long period of learning when we were too young to remember how we were doing it. But some of our vision is innate and does not require learning or practice. Turning the eyes and the head towards a light or a sound is a reflex and does not need the higher parts•of the brain.

With photography, once the light has been taken in, it is fixed; and once it has been fixed, this chemical reaction is irreversible. This is not so for the eye. After receiving light, the retina is ready again almost immediately for the next picture. It is not quite immediate, as we learn if we go out of strong sunlight into a dark room. For the first second, we cannot see properly. During this time the photoreceptors are becoming re-adjusted by means of a chemical reaction so as to be ready to absorb light again.

Although the retina is as thin as a sheet of paper, it has three layers of cells. First are the photoreceptors, known as rods and cones, as that is what they look like down a microscope. The cones need more light than the rods, about a thousand times more. They are scattered throughout the retina, with a concentration at one spot in the centre, about the size of a pin's head; this is called the fovea. Cones are sensitive to colour and are also needed for fine discrimination. In any cone, there is one of three different pigments, each of which is sensitive to a different wavelength of light; and so there are cones sensitive to red, to blue, and to green. Rods are also scattered all over the retina but they are absent from the fovea. They are good at seeing movement but cannot see colour. With rods alone, we would see only shades of grey, like newspaper pictures.

The next layer consists of bipolar cells and horizontal cells, to which the rods and cones are connected. The bipolar cells take information to the third layer, the layer of ganglion cells. The amacrine cells are thought to play a role both in the spatial aspects of vision and in colour vision. The ganglion cells send back what they have received to the brain; their axons form the optic nerve.

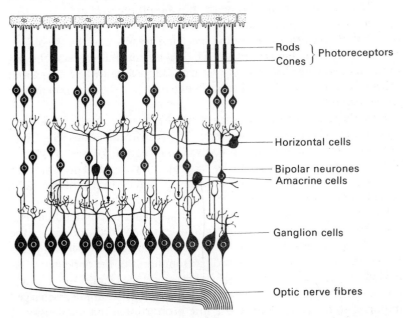

Rods ⎱ Photoreceptors
Cones ⎰

Horizontal cells

Bipolar neurones
Amacrine cells

Ganglion cells

Optic nerve fibres

Fig. 3.1. Diagram of the retina. The light rays come from the bottom of this diagram and run through the retina to the photoreceptors at the top.

At night and at twilight, only rods are useful, for there is not enough light to excite the cones. Many nocturnal animals have only or mainly rods. The Australian opossum avoids the light of day and stays in the attics of houses, protected by law; at twilight it saunters bravely out. The South American night ape or douroucouli possesses only rods and is nocturnal. The fish of the deepest seas also have only rods in their retinae; they have very large retinae to catch all the light that penetrates the ocean depths. The owl and the pussy-cat see better than man does in poor light.

If we see a nocturnal animal with small eyes, then we can presume that it does not make much use of vision. The common shrew has small eyes but it also has sensitive bristles on its snout; this is its feeler. It is also guided by smell and it sniffs the air continually; it hears, but it is not much interested in visual aspects of the world.

Birds have very good sight, for their lives depend on seeing. Their eyes make up a large proportion of their skulls. Some can keep objects in focus hundreds of metres away and also within a few centimetres of their eyes. Probably the winner is the great condor, which from a height of 5,000 metres can see small rodents moving on the ground.

The colour of objects comes from the reflection of certain bandwidths of radiation; the other parts of the spectrum are absorbed by the object. When we see something as red, the red light is being reflected and the rest of the light is being absorbed. We see it as red because we have cones and other cells able to react to red light. The redness, like beauty, is in the eye of the beholder.

How the retina works is more easily investigated in animals with a less complicated visual system than man. The very ancient horseshoe crab, left over from Silurian times 400 million years ago, has taught us about vision and about sensory systems in general. This crab has unusually long optic nerves, so it is not too difficult to record the traffic passing along them by means of electrodes. In this animal, the eye consists of many visual units called ommatidia. An ommatidium is a transparent crystalline cone ending in a lens; behind the cones are the photoreceptor cells. H. K. Hartline, in the United States, investigated the vision of this animal by recording from fibres of the optic nerve. He devised a narrow beam of light that could be shone on a single ommatidium at a time. He observed that each ommatidium discharged impulses along its nerve fibre at a rate proportional to the intensity of illumination it received. Having got an ommatidium steadily sending off impulses in response to a constant amount of illumination, he found he could change its rate of firing by illuminating the surrounding ommatidia. Although the central ommatidium was still receiving the same amount of light, it fired off far fewer impulses. When he stopped illuminating the surrounding ommatidia, the firing rate of the central ommatidium returned to its previous level. The brighter the light on the surrounding ommatidia, the feebler was the reporting of the central ommatidium. Every ommatidium was found to have a surrounding ring of ommatidia that could stop it firing.

This principle of antagonism between a centre of cells and the surrounding cells is called surround inhibition or lateral inhibition. It was first discovered in this crab's eye; but it is a general principle used for reception throughout the nervous system. In the monkey, all the receptive fields of the ganglion cells are organized on the basis of centre-surround contrast. It is the same in the human retina.

The eye is used for looking; and what makes us look is catching sight of something moving. If you are a carnivore, then you are wanting to see something moving, for it may be something to eat. If you are a herbivore, you need to see something moving, for it may be something intending to eat you. Preying animals behave as if they know that the slightest movement betrays them. They move slowly so that their movements do not excite the movement-detecting receptors of the retina of their prey.

The fovea of the retina is particularly good at seeing objects clearly and in detail, and so the animal needs to focus the light rays from an object on the fovea. To do this, there are reflexes from the eyes and the ears. Most of the retinal photoreceptors are particularly sensitive to movement. They detect the moving object and move the two eyes so that the rays of light from the object fall on the fovea. Once the object is focused there, movements of the head and eyes are arranged to keep it there. Keeping something constant is arranged in the body and in engineering by stabilizing servo-mechanisms. A general plan of such a self-regulating mechanism is shown by Fig. 3.2.

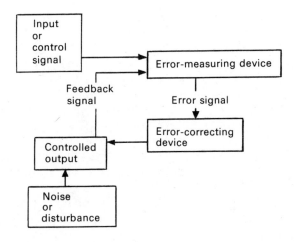

Fig. 3.2.

In order to keep the output constant, the difference between the actual output at any time and the control signal is continuously measured and corrected. The difference between the output and the input or control signal is referred to as the error; so a mechanism for measuring this difference is called an error-measuring device and the correcting mechanism is an error-correcting device. A part of the output is fed back, as the feedback signal, to the error-measuring device. Such a system is working by negative feedback; the effect of the feedback is to decrease the error. Positive feedback is when the feedback increases the error.

In the case we are considering, the output to be controlled and kept constant is the focusing of the rays of light on the fovea. The error that has continuously to be corrected is a deviation of the eyes that changes the angle at which the rays of light reach the fovea. The error-correcting devices are the muscles of the eyes, head, and neck.

Focusing the rays of light from the object depends on changing the focal point of the lens; this is done by a muscle within the iris. When this muscle relaxes, the lens becomes thicker and its front surface more curved. This brings the rays of light from a near object on to the fovea. To focus a distant object, the lens is made flatter by contraction of the muscle. If the rays of light from an object do not focus clearly at the fovea of both eyes, we see double.

For looking at far or at near objects, the size of the pupil also needs to be adjusted by the muscles of the iris. If you hand someone something and say 'Look at this!', you can see his eyes roll inwards and downwards and you will see his pupils contract. The accompanying change in the lens cannot be seen. The size of the pupil is altered to deal with the extremes of illumination. Where the light is poor, the pupil is dilated to let more light into the eye. If the light is very bright, the pupils are brought down to pinpoint size. This may seem to be as quick as a flash, but it is not. That is why photos taken by synchronized flash show pupils of normal size. The picture is taken before the light stimulating the retina sends nerve impulses to the centre of the brain and other impulses run along other nerve fibres to make the iris contract. But if you shine a light into the eyes of a friend, human, canine or feline, you will have time to see the pupils constricting. Start with someone young as the young have larger pupils than the elderly.

In the servo-mechanism of the pupil, the output that has to be continuously controlled is the amount of light reaching the retina. The error is the difference between the right amount and the actual amount of light. The error-measuring device is the retina itself. The servo-mechanism is made up of a part of the brain, the nerves to and from the eye, and the muscles of the pupil.

The conception of the nervous system and its various parts as examples of automatic control was the contribution of Professor Wiener of Boston. He got communication engineers, biologists, neurophysiologists and anatomists together and showed them that they were all dealing with the same problems, those of the communication of information and of servo-control. He called this subject cybernetics.

The total field of the environment that is seen is called the field of vision or visual field. A diagram of it is shown in Fig. 3.3 for man, bird and fish. Not all fish have this visual field; the flounder lying on the bottom of the sea has a panoramic visual field, taking in about 180° around his head. Dragon-flies have the same large visual fields, one for each eye. Most carnivores and birds of prey have their eyes in the fronts of their faces; they need to judge distance with accuracy once they have sighted their prey. Herbivores have very large fields of vision. They need to see both sides, in front, and behind, for they serve as food for other animals. Man has the eyes of a predator: set in the front of his face, with good distance judgment and a moderately wide field of vision. Eyes in the front of the face permit stereoscopic vision. As the eyes are a certain distance apart, each eye sees the world from a slightly different angle. The resulting vision in depth was probably developed by man's forbears as they lived in trees. Moving among the branches of trees demands accurate judging of distance. But of course binocular vision brings its own problems. When the two eyes need to look at the same object, both have to be focused to get the image of the object on the fovea of both retinae.

The image each eye receives is two-dimensional, The three-dimensional picture of the world to which we are accustomed is an interpretation, based on hours of learning throughout babyhood and childhood. This picture of the world has become so ingrained that when we lose the sight of one eye, we still see the world in three dimensions. Only when we have to do something needing the careful judgment of distance, such as pouring tea out of a narrow spout into a cup at arm's length, do we find that we have lost our ability to judge distance. If we need to rely on monocular vision, we can still do very well. We can judge the relative distance of two objects by seeing which appears to be the larger, by observing all the clues given by perspective, by judging the relative nearness of two objects to the horizon, by seeing whether one object overlaps another. If we move our heads, we can make use of parallax. If objects are moving, we observe that those seeming to move

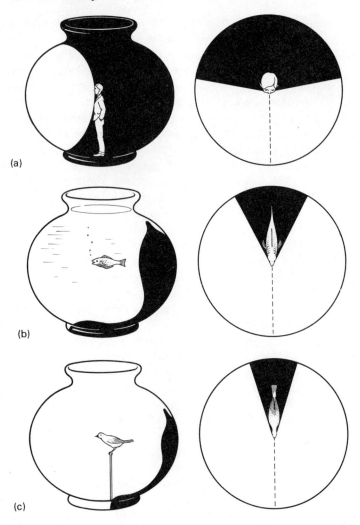

Fig. 3.3. If a man, a fish and a bird were placed in the middle of a goldfish bowl, each one could see everything white and nothing black. The white part is the visual field.

faster must be nearer than those appearing to move more slowly. Things nearer appear to be more brightly coloured and are seen in greater detail.

Man and other primates are good at seeing colour. Cats can see green and blue. Most mammals are monochromats; they cannot see colour. But reptiles, most fish, birds, butterflies and bees see colour. Bees cannot tell red from black but they see a colour in the ultraviolet that is hidden from us. von Frisch points out that scarlet flowers are very rare among the indigenous flowers of Europe, because the insects that pollinate flowers cannot see red. But in Africa and America scarlet flowers are common; this is because flowers there are pollinated by birds which can see red very well. In America this is done by humming birds and in Africa by the sunbirds. Interestingly enough the strelitzia is pollinated by the sunbird's feet, as it lands on the horizontal petals. Red European flowers, such as dianthus and daphne are pollinated by butter-flies which are the only insects able to see the colour red. Poppies which are bright red to us reflect ultraviolet light, and so bees can see them. Thus flowers and insects form good examples of symbiosis in evolution, the two developing together, each making use of the other.

On the whole, animals which are themselves brightly coloured are able to see colour, for usually colour is there for other members of the species to see. There would be no point in having colours to display if no one else could see them. Peacocks display for peahens, butterflies for butterflies. But certain animals are coloured especially for other species. Probably the wasp is indifferent to its own colours; they are there to warn birds to keep off.

Colour blindness in man is surprisingly common. Among Europeans, 7 per cent of men have it and 0.5 per cent of women, a distribution indicating that it is sex-linked. It is due to a lack of one or more of the three pigments of the cones. Most colour blind people cannot tell red from green; the red end of the spectrum is not seen as a colour; deep red looks black to them. Others see both red and green as yellow. In a much rarer form, there is yellow-blue colour-blindness. Most colour-blind people lack one of the three colour sensitive pigments and have to make out colours with a combination of the remaining two. There are some very rare people who have total colour blindness; they can see no colours. Everything appears grey to them, like pictures in the newspaper.

Eyes are not only for seeing and looking; the light they absorb has other effects on the body and on behaviour. In some animals, the effect of prolonged daylight is to suppress the activity of the pineal gland (*pineale*, Latin for a pine-cone.) In fish, reptiles, and amphibians, cells of this gland are photoreceptors. In mammals, the cells themselves are not sensitive to light but they have connections with the retinae, receiving their input of light from the eyes. As the pineal suppresses the pituitary, the increasing length of daylight has the effect of making the pituitary active. If you are able to detect the increasing length of day, you are getting information about the seasons; and this information may be what you need if you are raising a family, building a nest, or seeking and holding a territory. All of these activities need hormones secreted by the pituitary gland. The subject is discussed in detail in chapter 17.

If the duration of daylight is artificially altered, the whole rhythm of the reproductive cycle in birds can be altered. Professor Thorpe slowly decreased the amount of light of the environment of greenfinches and chaffinches; he found that not only did they stop singing but that their testes had regressed to an inactive state. Then he gradually increased their daily ration of light until they were receiving sixteen hours of light per day in the middle of September. These birds were in full song in the middle of November.

In simpler kinds of animals, light is received but not through the eyes. Some have photocells scattered over their bodies. If a shadow is cast over them, they reflexly withdraw. Such a reflex is inexorable and cannot be modified or altered by learning. Earthworms have no eyes but they have a light-sensitive receptor on each side of their front ends. They arrange their position and their movements so that the same amount of light falls on both these receptors. They avoid daylight and burrow back into the earth when they are brought to the surface by gardeners. But at night when it is dark everywhere, they come to the surface of the ground. This is the time when they meet for sexual intercourse. In their preference for the dark of the night for this activity, they resemble human beings.

4 Sound receptors: listening

For his ears are so acute that they sting again.

One might wonder why hearing was evolved. Living creatures have always been faced with all aspects of the world and so they have reacted to them. The world is full of sounds; and those animals that could hear them could make use of them in their struggle to keep alive. They could hear the approach of animals hunting them, they could hear the flow of streams which they often needed, and they could keep in touch with their friends and relations.

In physics, all aspects of a tone are described by its wavelength, its frequency, and its magnitude. Most animals are very sensitive to differences in frequency; we are more sensitive to some frequencies than to others, and so some notes appear louder to us than they really are. Sounds having too little intensity are below the threshold of audibility. We measure the intensity of sound in decibels (dB), a logarithmic scale. One decibel is the smallest change of intensity detectable by the human ear. A whisper $1\frac{1}{2}$ m from the ear is about 10 dB. Loud sounds reach the pain threshold at 140 dB. To hear speech we need to hear frequencies between 500 and 2500 cycles a second; to hear music we must hear frequencies between 40 and 16 000 cycles a second.

Every kind of animal hears only a certain range of frequencies, the range suitable for its purposes. There are limits of frequency and limits of intensity. Horses, rats, mice, cats and dogs all hear higher pitched sounds than human beings. Below frequencies of 18 cycles a second, man feels sounds, he does not hear them. The upper limit of hearing for the young is 20 000 cycles a second; at the age of sixty, the upper limit is only 8000 cycles a second, in Western societies. Man calls sounds with a frequency above 20 000 cycles a second ultrasonic, as he cannot hear them.

Sounds are detected by vibration receptors. In nearly all animals, these are movable hairs. They follow the frequency of the pressure waves and thus detect the note. Waves of pressure spread out from a source like ripples on a pond spreading out from the stone dropped into the pond. The hair is moved by the waves of alternating pressure like a water-lily being rocked by the ripples.

As the ear is developed out of the skin, it is interesting to examine the skin to find out if it has any similar properties; and it is quite easy to do this. Just get three tuning forks having frequencies of 128, 256, and 512 cycles a second. Then get a friend to set them vibrating and apply them separately to the hairs on your forearm or leg, taking care not to touch the skin itself. Keep your eyes shut and your ears blocked up, so that you do not see or hear the forks vibrating. You will find that you can tell if the fork is vibrating or merely touching the hairs without vibrating (the fork with a vibration of 512 cycles a second may cause some difficulty). You will find too that you can tell the pitch of the note from the vibration imparted to your hairs; that is to say, you will not hear a note, but you will be able to distinguish which fork it is that is vibrating; for the hairs of the skin are sensitive to the frequency of vibration of the three forks. This experiment also shows us how apt hairs are as receptors for the vibrations of sounds.

The mammalian ear is best thought of as consisting of three parts, the outer, middle, and inner ear. All three parts develop in the embryo out of the surface epithelium, the covering that later becomes the skin. And so it is not surprising to find that the receptors of the inner ear are a sort of receptor used in the skin; they are pressure and movement detectors, hairs embedded in a base.

The outer ear is the part of the ear you can see—in fact what people call the ear. It is separated by a drum from a little chamber, the middle ear, and this is separated by another drum from the inner ear, which is deep inside the bone of the skull. This is the part containing the sound receptors and the nerve fibres.

The pressure waves of sound pass down the funnel-shaped passage of the outer ear to affect the ear-drum. This drum, known to anatomists as the tympanic membrane, is a flattish cone, like the cone of a loudspeaker. This membrane is connected to another membrane, the oval window, by three little bones. The oval window seals the inner ear from the middle ear. The inner ear appeared so complicated to the early anatomists that they named it the labyrinth. It consists of the cochlear apparatus, the semicircular canals and the vestibular apparatus; it is the former that is used for hearing. Figure 4.1 shows the inner ear.

The middle ear is a chamber containing air, which is kept at atmospheric pressure by a tunnel connecting it to the throat. When the tunnel is blocked up, as occurs momentarily when we yawn or for some days when we get a cold, our hearing is impaired. It is not absolutely necessary for the pressure waves to pass through this air-filled chamber for hearing; vibration can be conducted directly to the inner ear.

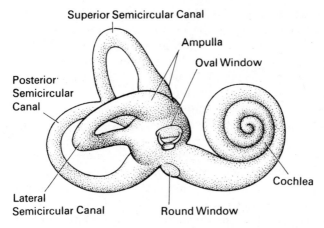

Superior Semicircular Canal

Ampulla

Oval Window

Posterior
Semicircular
Canal

Lateral
Semicircular Canal

Round Window

Cochlea

Fig. 4.1. The inner ear. The part on the right is for hearing and the parts on the left are for balancing and keeping the right way up.

You can examine the characteristics of air conduction and bone conduction of sound in yourself by listening to your own voice. Just read aloud from a book, and in the middle of reading, block up both your ears with your fingers. You will find that when your ears are blocked up and you are hearing by bone conduction, your voice sounds deeper; conversely it sounds higher when the sound is conducted through the air to your ears. Bone conduction damps the sound of higher frequency and so the low frequencies predominate. Now continue your reading, but whisper what you read; and again, block and unblock your ears. You will find that you can hardly hear your whispered voice when your ears are blocked. The reason is the same. Whispering makes use of the higher frequencies; there are so few low frequencies used that there is almost nothing to conduct, so you hear almost nothing.

In the outer ear, the waves of sound are conducted in air; in the middle ear, they are conducted in solids; and in the inner ear, in fluid. That the transmission of sound waves from air to fluid does not readily occur can be observed by anyone bathing on a noisy beach or in a swimming bath. The noise around you when your head is above water goes if you put your head under the water. The air–water interface forms an effective sound-barrier, most of the sound being reflected from the surface of the water.

When the sound waves have to pass from air to fluid (and this has to happen in all animals who live in the air), a great loss of energy occurs. The middle ear contains the mechanism for compensating for this loss.

This mechanism consists of the tympanic membrane, three little bones hinged together to form a system of levers, and the oval window which seals off the fluid of the inner ear. The compensation is achieved by the great area of the tympanic membrane compared to the small area of the flat footplate of little bone (the stapes) up against the oval window, and by the lever action of the three bones.

In man, the tympanic membrane is about twenty times the area of the footplate of the stapes. But as the membrane is firmly fixed all round its circumference, this whole area is not available to move. The effective difference in areas of the membrane and the stapes footplate is about 14:1. The lever system of the three bones collects the pressure from the tympanic membrane and concentrates it down to the footplate of the stapes; it increases the energy by about 1.3:1.

The lever action of the three little bones is controlled by the small muscles of the middle ear. They can reduce the intensity of sound reaching the cochlea when the source of the sound is near and allow the full intensity of sound to reach it when the source is far away. In experiments on cats, it was found that the muscles became active when the intensity of sound was 80 dB above the human hearing threshold. These muscles seem to be used to reduce the intensity of sound reaching the inner ear when we ourselves make the sound; for their action is linked with that of the larynx.

There is an ear disease called otosclerosis in which the stapes gets fixed onto the oval window. Hearing is much impaired. If the person loses more than 30 dB, quiet speech is not heard. These people can be helped by surgical removal of the stapes and having a hearing aid.

The sound waves pass from the middle ear, through the oval window into the inner ear. Here they pass along one narrow passage, called the scala vestibuli, round a very small corner into another passage, called the scala tympani, on to the round window, where the pressure is dispersed into the middle ear.

In the scala vestibuli there is a membrane, called the basilar membrane, which in man is 30 to 35 millimetres long. This membrane supports hair-cells of two kinds, globular ones along the inner part and slender tubular ones along its outer part. The hairs of the hair-cells are adherent to a membrane above them, called the tectorial or covering membrane.

When the sound waves are transmitted to the fluids of the inner ear, they send a ripple along the basilar membrane. This wave can be imagined if one thinks of the basilar membrane as a long narrow sheet, fixed at both ends and also along both sides; but fixed loosely, so that a

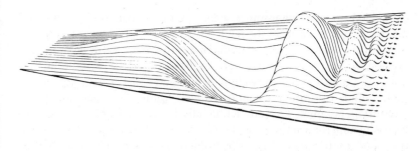

Fig. 4.2. A wave pattern in the basilar membrane of the inner ear.

shake given it at one end sends a wave of movement along its whole length. This wave is complicated, for the membrane is of different thickness and consistency in its different parts and it is also coiled round the snail-like cochlea. The kind of wave pattern it probably makes in this membrane is shown in a spread out membrane in Fig. 4.2. When the membrane is raised into folds and ripples like this, the hair-cells in it are rocked about. As the basilar and tectorial membranes have different mechanical properties, being different in stiffness, tautness, thickness, and elasticity, the wave of pressure causes a different form of ripple in the two membranes. This difference in the movement of the two membranes displaces and twists the hairs of the hair-cells, causing a shearing movement between them and the tectorial membrane in which their tips are embedded. As the hairs are minute levers, their movements affect the hair-cells themselves. The hair-cells convert mechanical energy into nerve impulses, which are pulses of electric current.

The basilar membrane, thrown into ripples by the sound waves, analyses and transmits to the brain two features of the sound, its frequency or pitch and its amplitude or loudness. The long axis of the basilar membrane is mainly concerned with its frequency and the side to side axis is concerned with its intensity. Intensity is analysed mainly by the following mechanism. The hair-cells of the basilar membrane are arranged in two groups, the inner and the outer hair-cells. The inner hair-cells are along the inner edge of the basilar membrane, just at the point where the membrane becomes free from a supporting ledge of bone. They are not very mobile and so they need a sound of large intensity to move them. The outer hair-cells are more freely mobile and so they are moved by sounds of lesser intensity.

Different notes cause waves of different shape in the basilar membrane; thus no two notes cause the same effects on all the hair-cells embedded in the membrane. Each auditory nerve fibre fires off maximally when a note of the pitch it is sensitive to is sounded. It is fired by a rather narrow range of frequencies; this bandwidth is about 100 cycles a second for every nerve fibre, in the cat's auditory system. But it is not only a question of a nerve fibre being fired by a certain frequency in each sound. For when a sound is much louder, a larger number of auditory nerve fibres are conducting; all of these nerve fibres would not be conducting for a single note played quietly. This disposes of any simple theory of conduction of sounds by firing of a few nerve fibres, each being related to a certain place in the basilar membrane. For it means that an element in the central nervous system tuned to fire to a certain note when that note is quiet responds to notes up to three octaves lower and half an octave higher and all the notes in between when the sound is loud. As in other sensory systems, there is surround inhibition: nerve fibres fired by a certain frequency are inhibited by those fibres fired by the adjacent frequencies.

There are other mechanisms necessary for hearing, but they are not yet fully understood. For one thing, when a note of constant pitch and constant intensity is kept on for a long time, the nerve fibres reporting it send in fewer and fewer impulses to the cochlear nucleus; and fewer impulses are sent on to other parts of the brain. And yet we hear the note steadily and at constant intensity.

The receptors of the basilar membrane can be damaged by a lot of noise going on for years. The noise made by everyone speaking at a cocktail party reaches 80 to 85 dB, 'not quite enough' as the two Canadian research workers who looked into the matter wrote 'to cause permanent impairment of hearing'. But there is no doubt that the noise of civilized countries damages the receptors. In 1961, an expedition went out to a remote tribe living in Sudan near the western borders of Ethiopia. The purpose of the expedition was to examine the hearing of these tribal people, who live in the quiet of a stone age culture. They were found to have far less deafness with old age than is usual in America and Europe and infinitely less than those who work in noisy factories. The music made by rock and roll musicians is so loud that it damages the auditory receptors of those in the band. The noise level up among the musicians reaches 105–120 dB; this is the same as the noisiest industry, a boiler shop.

Animals note both the direction from which the sound is coming and the distance of the source of the sound. We learn to do this in childhood just as we learn to estimate the position and distance of everything we see. We learn that a loud clear sound comes from a source that is near and that the same sound when it is softer is likely to be coming from something further away.

Most animals, including man, which live in that mere millimetre of the universe, the surface of the earth, are only good at localizing sound horizontally. Birds who enjoy a three-dimensional life localize sounds as well vertically as horizontally.

Animals which are around at night either have large eyes or they live by using their ears or, like the owl, they make use of both. The owl has its ears set far apart on its head; it is unique in that the structure of its two ears is different. These two anatomical features are used for localizing the little sound made by the scuttering mouse. The mouse does not hear the owl, which has special feathers to render its flight silent. Fish-eating owls are not so silent for the sound of flight is not carried into the water.

We localize sounds by being aware of differences in the intensity and in the time of arrival at the two ears. Small mammals with small heads cannot use a difference in time of arrival of a sound at the two tympanic membranes as a good way of locating sound; for if a sound is coming from a source in front of or behind them, it will arrive at the two ears at the same time. Most mammals can move their ears so as to point the incoming sound waves towards the passage of the external ear. Dogs are better than man at localizing sounds, pricking up their ears and using them as direction indicators; man has to turn his head to help himself localize the source of a sound. Deaf people tend to turn their ears to the mouth of the speaker so as to get the sound into the funnel of the ear; they need to hear the higher frequencies of the overtones to hear speech distinctly. The old-fashioned ear-trumpet was good in this respect and it may well have been better than electric amplifiers which magnify all wavelengths. The best position of the head for sound-localizing is to have the sound source coming straight towards one ear, the waves of greater wave-length meeting the nose-neck axis of the head like a wave against a cliff. When this happens, the further ear will be in the very worst position for hearing the sound. And so, when we are receiving a sound so that we get maximal stimulation of one ear and minimal stimulation of the other, we know from past experience that the source of the sound is at right angles to the antero-posterior axis of the head. These are not the only mechanisms for sound-localization by only one ear. The quality of a sound changes as things move off or come near. As a sound gets nearer, the bass notes get relatively louder than the treble.

The shape of the external ear is partly a matter of its possessor's need to localize sound, partly a matter of having a flap of skin from which to lose heat, and also a means of signalling to its fellows. From the inner ear, the auditory nerve goes to the cochlear nucleus; and from the cochlear nucleus, impulses are sent to many parts of the brain. One kind of neuron has all nerve fibres coming from the left ear ending on a dendrite on the left and all those from the right ear on a dendrite on the right. This neuron can appreciate differences in the input from the two ears coming in at an interval of a ten thousandth of a second. But this is not the only way in which accurate timing and hence localization of sound is done. Some neurons of this nucleus are excited only when inputs from the two ears arrive simultaneously; and others are inhibited by inputs from one ear and excited by inputs from the other.

If sound waves reach both ears at exactly the same time, the person will localize the source of the sound somewhere in the middle and not in either ear. Stereo recording and reproducing of music is based on this fact. When we are sitting in the right position between the two loudspeakers, the sound appears to come out of the wall in the middle. This is so, even though most people are right-eared; they prefer the right ear and hear more accurately with it; though they make more use of the left ear for music.

Compared with many other animals, man is not particularly good at hearing. Birds are far better at distinguishing a lot of notes packed into a short period of time. The lives of most varieties of birds are much shorter than ours, and everything about them takes place more rapidly. All animals are good at hearing the kinds of sounds important for them. Chicks of penguins on their islands in Antarctica can recognize their parents from the sounds they make, and so can the guillemots on our coasts. In neither case can the human ear detect any differences in the sounds made by the parent birds. Large ranges of sounds cannot be heard by animals for which they have no meaning. There is an advantage in having only a restricted hearing for sounds of importance. These sounds alone will be heard, unsullied by the surrounding din.

Most fish communicate by sound. They serenade each other, like crickets and man. Their different calls of alarm and of aggression can now be recognized, since research work has been done on underwater recording of their repertoire of sounds. Shrimps make a great deal of noise for their small size. Fish cannot hear the high-pitched sounds made by the porpoises and whales that feed on them. In this respect, they resemble the fly whose composite eyes cannot detect the silk of the spider's web, but they are unlike the moths which hear the shrill cries of the bats that are searching for them.

To find out the source of a sound, fish have developed a way of feeling the movement of water particles. For sound in fluid is transmitted by similar waves of pressure as in air and it also displaces fluid particles. Fish can feel the movement of these particles by means of a row of receptors, concentrated in a line running along their sides, from head to tail. The receptors of this lateral line are just like the hair-cells of the rest of the vestibular system. In many sorts of fish these receptors are within a canal, sunk beneath the skin. As the fish has two rows of these receptors, one on each side of its body, it is able to tell the direction of disturbances in the water.

While on the subject of fish, we may mention electric fish. Some kinds of electric fish do not use their electricity generating organs as weapons, but as a sort of sonar. The discharge of the electric organ produces an electric field around the fish; objects of greater or lesser conductivities than the surrounding water can be detected within the field. Experiments on the gymnotid fish of tropical South America demonstrate that these fish can tell distilled water from ordinary water as it does not conduct electricity. They have electro-receptors in the lateral line organ which can detect a change in the current density distribution of the electric field. These receptors are incredibly sensitive; changes in the field of one-millionth of a volt per foot can be detected.

When the first amphibia left the Silurian seas two or three hundred million years ago, they relied entirely on bone conduction of vibration for hearing; they were not equipped to hear vibration in air, having just come out of the water. It seems that vibrations in the earth were transmitted from the bones of their lower jaws to the bone surrounding the inner ear. In order to hear, they probably kept their lower jaws touching the ground. As animals evolved, they first raised their heads in the air and then their whole bodies. As long as these first terrestrial animals, the reptiles, kept their lower jaws to the ground, they heard by bone conduction. Once they raised their heads from the ground, other mechanisms for hearing were evolved; for hearing now meant sensing the vibrations in the air.

The first hearing organ of amphibia and reptiles was the saccule. As animals raised their heads into the air, the saccule got more receptors in it with more nerve fibres connecting them to the brain. Then a tubular outgrowth developed out of it; this was the beginning of the cochlea. With the evolution of the cochlea, there was an increased sensitivity to vibrations of higher wavelengths, in other words, to the sounds that are propagated in air.

When we follow the development of hearing among the vertebrates, we see that an improvement in hearing occurred when the change from cold-blooded to warm-blooded species took place. The constant higher temperature allowed all neural events to be speeded up. And speed is an advantage in the struggle for living; it gets you away from a predator, it gets you more quickly on to your prey, it allows you to beat your adversary whoever he may be. At higher temperatures nerve fibres conduct impulses more quickly and muscles contract and relax more quickly. Each nerve fibre also recovers more quickly after the passage of a nerve impulse, and so it is ready to conduct another impulse sooner. This fact permitted the range of hearing to increase upwards: more rapid vibrations could be conducted by nerve fibres able to conduct faster. In fish, the auditory nerve fibres can follow the vibrating receptors only at very low rates of vibration; in frogs the nerve fibres can follow up to rates of 500 vibrations/sec, in turtles up to 1000 vibrations/sec, in mammals up to 4000–5000/sec.

It seems to be that the earlier, more primitive inner ear detected the pitch of a sound according to the principle of resonators. The individual receptors were turned to vibrate at certain frequencies. They vibrated at the rate of the frequency of the sound, and the nerve fibres from these receptors conducted impulses at this rate. When the cochlea developed, the pitch of a sound was signalled by the movements of the membranes in which the receptors were embedded. In mammals both mechanisms are used. For low frequency sounds, volleys of nerve impulses pass to the brain in time with the pressure waves of the vibration. There is also a displacement of the basilar membrane as the sound wave passes along it. For high frequency sounds, signalling to the brain is only by the mechanism of displacement of the basilar membrane.

Whether snakes hear only by keeping their jaws touching the ground or whether they can also hear when their heads are in the air has not been agreed upon by zoologists. It seems certain that they do not hear the music played to them by snake-charmers. The real purpose of this music is to charm money out of the pockets of tourists. What elephants hear of the soothing songs from the lips of the mahouts who tend them, we do not yet know. Interestingly enough, African elephants can hear the same songs, for the negroes of the Congo learned them from Indian mahouts brought over by the Belgians to train them before the First World War. The elephant does not use his big external ears only for hearing. He uses them to communicate, to warn us that he is threatening and will charge if we do not go away. They are also used as vanes from which to lose heat. The skin is relatively thin and it contains dilatable blood-vessels from which heat can be dissipated into the surrounding air.

Bees are able to hear by feeling the vibration in solids. Their buzzing, which to us is so characteristic of bees, is something they do not hear;

they feel it. When they are standing on something solid, the vibration of the buzz is transmitted through the solid to other bees, and they feel it with their legs. As well as with their legs, they hear with their antennae, on which there are receptors specialized for certain vibrations. When a bee arrives back in the hive, other bees come up to it and touch its thorax with their antennae; in this way the foraging bee can tell the others where food is to be found. This way of communicating a message allows the bees to speak to a few individuals in a crowd alive with buzzing, where another additional buzz would be lost among the noise. In addition to this, bees have a way of screaming out the urgent news. If a bee discovers a rich source of nectar when the whole hive is short of food, it opens a scent gland in its abdomen, and flying off to the flowers, it leaves a scent trail behind it for all workers to follow. The queen bee has her own royal speech; its fundamental note is about 300 to 380 cycles a second, and its harmonics go up to 1,500 cycles a second. The other way in which bees communicate is by dancing the message, the language discovered and interpreted by von Frisch in Munich.

Echo-location

How bats are able to fly in the dark and avoid all obstacles was first examined in a series of experiments by the great naturalist Lazzaro Spallanzani in Italy. One night in 1793, in company with his brother and a cousin, he hung from the ceiling of his room a lot of 'threads provided with little bells. There was no moon and the shutters of he windows were closed so as to 'exclude even the faintest beam of light.' The bat flew around the room without touching the threads or the walls. It was able to fly around the room in complete darkness, as Spallanzani reported 'with the same abilities in complete darkness as with the light of a candle.' To try and find out how bats could fly and avoid obstacles in the dark, Spallanzani next covered bats' heads with opaque hoods. This did prevent them flying efficiently; they bumped against the walls and fell to the floor. He then took the hoods off their heads and covered their eyes with disks. He was amazed to find that these bats flew about quite happily. He then removed the eyeballs of a bat; this bat flew perfectly.

When these observations were communicated to the Natural History Society of Geneva, a surgeon, ornithologist and botanist, Dr Charles Jurine confirmed the truth of these observations. He thought of plugging the ears of bats with wax. He then saw that these bats were unwilling to fly and when they did fly, they bumped into things and were unable to navigate. He concluded that bats are able to use their ears for navigation in the dark.

When Spallanzani heard about these experiments, he repeated them and confirmed the fact that bats 'collide and fall down if they have their ears plugged. Moreover, they behave in this way not only when blinded but even when they have their eyes.' He came to the conclusion that hearing 'replaces vision in these winged quadrupeds.' He let blinded bats fly around the campanile of the cathedral of Pavia and found that they could catch insects. He finally deduced that bats use echo-ranging or echo-location. 'Thus I think that the organ of hearing of bats is delicate to such a degree that they hear the noise of their wings and body when they are flying, and that they judge the distances from the quality of the sound, like Sanderson (a famous blind man of the time) who determined the size of a room on the basis of sounds reflected from the walls. In this way the sound of the wings reflected from the walls may cause them to know the distances and therefore to avoid them.' Like modern investigators of echo-location, he also thought of trying to jam their radar by making a noise. He beat a drum and got a lot of people to shout and clap in a room where bats were flying. To his disappointment it had no effect.

This early research work that answered the question correctly was forgotten. It was rediscovered by D. Dijkgraaf who went to Pavia to look into the eighteenth century scientist's notebooks. There he also found Spallanzani's discoveries about swallows and eels.

The rest of the story was guessed correctly by Professor Hartridge in England in 1920. He proposed that 'bats during flight emit a short wavelength note' and this sound is reflected from objects in the vicinity. Twenty-one years later, the navigation of bats by echo-location was rediscovered in the United States by Griffin and Galambos.

Nowadays we are all familiar with sounds reflected from large objects. We hear it when we drive in a car past a row of trees or parked cars with gaps between them. The car we are sitting in produces the sound and it is reflected back from the objects along the side of the road. As trees and cars are separated by gaps that do not reflect sound, we hear a changing pattern of sound, a kind of rushing sound when there is reflection of the sound and a quieter sound when the sound is not being reflected. Auditory clues like these can be useful to blind people; with practice they can gather a lot of information about gaps in walls or doorways. They listen to the sound made by their own footsteps or to the taps they make with a walking-stick and they can hear when the sound is no longer reflected off the walls. A well-trained blind man can walk down a passage and avoid screens thrown half-way across the passage by listening to the sound of his own footsteps reflected by the screens.

The bat's ear has been changed from the usual mammalian pattern to make use of echo-location. The little bones of the middle ear are smaller, lighter, and more tightly bound together so that there is less movement between them; this probably reduces transmission losses. Another development is the increase in size of the muscles working this system of bones. The cochlea is relatively large in relation to the small size of the animal's head. Also it is acoustically isolated from the other bones of the skull; this reduces bone conduction of the noises generated in the animal's own body. The auditory parts of the brain are much larger than in other animals.

Objects as small as wires or insects will cause only extremely faint echoes, yet these are what the bat hears. Bats are very good at hearing the differences in frequencies and intensities of these faint sounds. When we look into the physics of this situation, we find that there is quite a lot of time to do this; for sound travels in air at a speed of 34.4 cm/millisecond (344 m/sec.). The problem for the bat is how to hear a faint echo of high frequency very soon after hearing its own emission of the orientation cry, and how to tell the one from the other. The bat copes with the problem by making its orientation cry very short so that it will not overlap its own echo. It also uses the muscles that work the bones of the middle ear to damp down the emission sound as it makes it but it does not use them to damp down the echo.

The various species of bats make use of a large variety of sounds. All are very high-pitched with short wavelengths. To bounce sound waves off objects, the wavelengths must be short. If the wavelength were much longer than the object it meets, it would not be bounced back; a wave of one metre length would not be interrupted by a wire stretched in its way. This high-frequency sound must be given out in a narrow beam, like the light from a pencil-torch, so that it can be focused accurately enough to be reflected off an insect of 1 to 3 mm long. They achieve this so well that they can tell if an insect of this size is flying towards them or away from them.

The common European horseshoe bat makes use of the Doppler effect. When either the source of a sound or the hearer of the sound, or both, are moving, the number of vibrations a second changes. If a whistling train comes nearer when you are standing on a platform, the number of vibrations a second increases, and it decreases as the train goes off. The result of this is that the whistle sounds higher as the train comes towards you and lower as it goes away. The horseshoe bat uses fairly long bursts of a few pure tones, and guides itself by this effect. It hears the note becoming higher as it approaches an object and lower as the object recedes. It is obvious that for echo-locating the actual pitch of a note is unimportant; whether it is rising or falling is what the animal needs to know. Those bats that make use of the Doppler effect increase this effect by moving their ears. If one stops them moving their ears, they are lost; but within three weeks they learn to move their heads backwards and forwards instead, and are then almost as good at echo-location as they had been before.

The horseshoe bat emits its sound through its nose. The horseshoe is made up of folded skin around the nose which acts as a sort of trumpet, narrowing the sound down to a beam. To locate the echoed sound well, this bat makes much use of movements of the ears and head. All bats do this to a fair extent, and one can interfere with a bat's ability to carry out echo-location if one prevents these movements.

Bats have a sense of smell; they use this for finding their mates and not for finding food. Many bats have eyes well adapted for seeing at twilight, but even these do not use sight for finding their way about or for catching insects. Most bats live in caves into which no light penetrates and so sight is impossible.

How successful this manner of hunting by echo-location is, is made clear to us when we find that bats can catch mosquitoes at a rate of two per second. The final proof that bats do find their way about by this system of radar was obtained by Griffin and Grinnell. They jammed the bats' echo-location by high frequency noise. The result was that the bats preferred to stay at home and did not venture out.

It has been suggested by naturalists that the furry bodies and wings of moths and some other insects form a protection against echo-location. For unlike shiny bodies and wings, furry bodies absorb the sound of the bat's radar.

In the balance of nature, those preyed upon and their hunters wage an equal battle. Whenever this was not so in the past, either the one or the other species passed away. The noctuid moths that are preyed upon by some bats have evolved auditory systems to deal with their enemy. The total auditory world of these moths is now known to us through the marvellous work of K. D. Roeder and E. A. Treat of Tufts University in the United States. The moth's ears consist of two tympanic membranes; they are connected to two tympanic organs, each of which has only two neurons, an acoustic and a non-acoustic neuron. This animal's whole world of hearing, which is ultrasonic, is brought to its central nervous system by four nerve fibres. As Roeder and Treat realised: 'The small number of receptor cells in the tympanic organ makes it possible to define with some precision the total amount of impulse-coded information available to the moth.' They showed that with this simple apparatus the moth can distinguish the loudness of sounds, their duration, and the direction from which they are coming. The bat is first heard when it is 35 to 40 metres away. At this distance, the moth hears a warning sound of low intensity. This sound makes the moth fly away from the source of the sound. At this time, the moth tends to win, for the bat's echo-locating system does not work at this distance. When the moth hears a sound of high intensity, it has two alternatives. It either folds its wings and falls to the ground, or it goes into a power dive. When the sound heard by the moth is loud, the bat may be able to find it by echo-location, but it probably does not pick it off the ground. The design of this moth has evolved to aid it escape from its enemy. Its ears are in the middle of its body, just behind the attachment of the second pair of wings; and the auditory nerves are closely connected to the neurons that work the flight-muscles. The distance between these nerve-cells is very short and so the impulses from the ears reach the flight-muscles very quickly.

Not all kinds of bats live on insects; some live on fruit, a very few live on fish, and even fewer live on the blood of men and horses. Fruit-eating bats rely on vision to find their way about and not on echo-location; they are around during the daytime. One sort of fruit-eating bat flies both by day and night. It uses its eyes when there is enough daylight; and when the sun goes down, it listens to the echoes of the clicking noises it makes with its tongue.

Instead of saying 'as blind as a bat', it would be better to say 'as careless as a bat'. Bats, it has been found, often pay no attention to their echo-location systems. If a new obstacle is put into a tower in which bats live, many of the bats fly into it and hurt themselves. Their echo-location systems are working perfectly; they do not bother to listen in once they have got used to the location of the objects in their accustomed environments.

Bats have existed for more than fifty million years. As complete skeletons of that age have been found which are the same as bats' skeletons today, we may safely assume that they were using echo-location fifty million years ago. This is confirmed by the fact that the shape of their skulls indicates that the part of the brain used in hearing was very well developed. At this time, the horse was the size of a present-day wire-haired terrier.

Some other small mammals, such as certain kinds of mice and shrews, also use echo-location; for some of them are active both by night and day.

Vertebrates which live in the ground specialize in hearing the lower frequencies of sound, for higher frequencies do not penetrate the ground. They probably make more use of conduction via the bones of their skulls. Dr Douglas Webster of New York University has studied the gerbil of Central Asia, the jerboa of North Africa and the kangaroo rat of the southern United States, and he found out that these little mammals of the desert from quite different parts of the world deal with their acoustic problems in the same way. The range of hearing of the kangaroo rat is from 1,000 to 3,000 cycles a second, and in accordance with this selective sensitivity, its basilar membrane is most developed in the apical part of the cochlea. Dr Webster has shown that the sounds made by rattlesnakes sliding heavily over the ground that prey on kangaroo rats come within this frequency range.

Baron von Humboldt in his wonderful book *Voyage aux Régions Équinoxiales du Nouveau Continent* published early in the nineteenth century tells us about the nocturnal birds of Peru. These birds live in complete darkness in caverns, coming out only at night to feed on fruit. The bird, called by the Peruvians the guacharo, is about as big as a hen and has blue eyes. Von Humboldt relates how the local Peruvians are afraid to go into the caves where these blue-black birds are living, and they speak of dying as 'going to join the guacharos'. Unfortunately they are not frightened enough. For once a year during the summer they enter the largest cave with long poles and destroy the birds' nests. These birds are very fat; they have probably evolved the fat as a protection against cold, for it is cool in the caves where they live. The Indians killed the birds to obtain their abdominal fat, which they used for cooking.

Professor Griffin, literally following in von Humboldt's footsteps, proved that these birds fly in darkness, though not in silence. He reported 'Our ears were bombarded almost constantly by a variety of squawks, screeches, clucks, clicks and shrieks'. For echo-location these birds used very short clicking sounds, averaging about 7000 cycles per second, within the range of human hearing. Outside the caves, the birds use their eyes.

However, these Stygian birds are not the only ones that fly in total darkness. The little swifts of the East Indies whose nests are stolen for bird's nest soup live in similar caves. Although they catch insects by day, they return at night to nest in caves. They also make clicking sounds for echo-location. There is some satisfaction in noting that the men who kill the guacharos and those who take the swiftlets' nests sometimes fall a hundred feet or more to the ground and either kill themselves or linger on with broken backs and limbs.

Echo-location in the sea is used by whales, seals, dolphins, porpoises and sea-lions. Blind sea-lions get along quite satisfactorily. The sounds they make for echo-location are not the barking we hear at the zoo; they make a kind of ringing sound. The echo-location system of this group of animals that has been most investigated is that of the dolphin. This animal has no sense of smell, it has good sight, a sense of taste, and above all a marvellous sense of hearing. The dolphin, like the bat, lives by echo-location. These mammals can avoid transparent plastic obstacles in their tanks, they detect fish in muddy water so turbid that sight is impossible, and they can do it with their eyes covered so well that they can distinguish between red mullet and other kinds of fish, and between fish 6 inches and 12 inches long. The dolphin emits a beep-beep sound at a rate of about five per second when it is not particularly interested in its environment. When it realizes that there is something interesting around, it speeds up its exploratory sound to a rate of several hundred beeps a second, the rate becoming faster as it gets nearer the object. The part of the sound made by the dolphin that man is able to hear sounds, according to Professor Kellogg, like a canary. And if you whistle to it, it whistles back.

How whales communicate and hear has been investigated since the war; though their voices were first heard, it seems, by Mr Fisher, who mentions it in his *Journal of a Voyage for the Discovery of the North West Passage* published in 1821. He describes the sound made by the white whale as 'a shrill ringing sound, not unlike that of musical glasses badly played'. Mr Fisher and his fellow explorers heard it by keeping their ears under water. Actually they must have missed most of the sound, for most of it is in the frequency range of 50,000 to 100,000 cycles a second.

These mammals that have returned to the water do not have the problems of air-fluid interface barriers which mammals living in air have. Arriving back in the sea after millions of years' evolution on land, they start off with the land-living ways of amplifying sound. Most mammalian systems amplify the sound twenty times before it is transmitted to the inner ear. Starting off with this advantage, one can see that they were in a good position to develop communication by echo-location.

5 Olfactory receptors: smelling

Our world is so visual that even our way of expressing ourselves is visual. When we understand something, we say 'Yes, I see', not 'Yes, I smell'.

Chemoreceptors have a very long history, for these receptors are probably the oldest of all. They are of most use to animals living in the sea where everything of interest is dissolved in sea water. This means not only everything of positive interest, such as food to be found and swallowed. It means also food to be avoided; for the reactions of vomiting and expelling food are laid down in the same basal parts of the brain as those of sucking and swallowing.

If we watch the behaviour of animals who have keen noses, we can see how all sense organs are used. A wind laden with odours passes by. The dog or the deer turns and faces the wind, pauses and sniffs. They are getting more of the odours into contact with their olfactory receptors so as to examine them in detail, to classify them, so as to know how to behave to all that the odour implies.

Ancestral fish of the ancient seas had already developed a good sense of smell; though in the case of fish one cannot separate smelling from tasting. The fish shows the basic pattern of vertebrates. The organs for sampling the environment are in the front, the power pack is behind. The front end of the fish houses the eyes and the nasal sac for tasting and smelling, for detecting particles or molecules in the water. There may be barbels for feeling the ground or the weeds streaming in the current. The result of receiving this news about the environment is some sort of behaviour. That is carried out by the rest of the fish; for most of the fish consists of the power pack, muscles encased in a streamlined lubricated envelope; they bring the fish nearer the interesting object or whisk it away from danger. Some fish hunt entirely by smell; these include the dog-fish, familiar to all biology students, and those fish that hunt by night when there is no light to see by. One of the schemes tried to keep sharks off bathing beaches is to put unpleasant smells in the sea; apparently the smell of man is not revolting enough.

Some fish have such a keen sense of smell that they can detect a substance when there are only a few molecules of it in the water. Although water spreads the molecules around just as air does, some mammals who have returned to the sea from the land, such as the porpoises and the dolphins, have no sense of smell. This sense, which their ancestors used on land, has lapsed to such an extent that these marine mammals no longer have olfactory bulbs; they have lost the very nerve tracts concerned with smelling.

Snakes have a good sense of smell. After they have bitten and injected venom into their prey, they do not always swallow it straight away. The poor frightened animal goes off and hides while it dies within an hour. The snake has to go and find it and it does so by smelling it out.

The sense of smell is so important to the mouse that the female, if she is deprived of her sense of smell by an operation, no longer shows maternal behaviour and will eat her litter of young. Sheep, goats, and rats recognize their young by smell. Our ability to recognize someone is so visual that we can hardly conceive of recognizing ones own baby by its smell.

Dogs as we all know are very good at smelling; though they make mistakes in recognizing human identical twins, just as we do when we use visual cues.

Human babies can smell the female breast, distinguishing it from other parts of the body. If a breast is put under a sleeping baby's nose, it makes sucking movements in its sleep. By six weeks, the baby can distinguish the smell of the breast of its own mother from that of other women.

It is surprising, insects being so different from us, to find that wasps and bees like the same flowers as we do. The smell of flowers developed just with the purpose of attracting insect pollinators and not to please us, though our noses may do a little pollinating as well. Insects have their olfactory organs on their antennae. In ourselves this would be equivalent to us having long mobile noses, a little like an elephant's trunk; we could then push our noses right up against the source of the smell. von Frisch and his colleagues have discovered that some flowers have different smells in their different parts. Our crude noses note only one general smell. But insects with their little olfactory organs on their antennae can push these sense organs up against the various parts of a flower and thus can locate the different parts according to their different smells. von Frisch has found out that in a narcissus the yellow ring is not only a different colour from the white corolla but has also a different smell. Having found that bees could easily distinguish these two parts by their smell, he then found that if the yellow and the white parts of the flower were separated, humans could also distinguish two different smells. The bee can follow the scent of the flower according to the strength of the smell; and so the flower has arranged matters that when

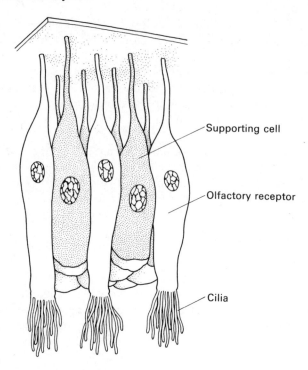

Supporting cell

Olfactory receptor

Cilia

Fig. 5.1. The olfactory receptors.

the bee is smelling the strongest smell, it is most likely to pollinate the flower.

Those animals that make more use of smell than of vision have more olfactory receptor cells than photoreceptors. In vertebrates, the olfactory receptors are in a special region of the nasal mucous membrane, right at the top of the nose. Odours reach them by two routes; they come in with the air and they pass up the back of the nose from the throat. The smells of the outer world arrive mainly through the nostrils. The smells of our food and drink pass up the back of the nose.

There are some people with congenital anosmia, people who cannot smell, like people born blind or deaf. The only abnormal feature of their olfactory systems is an absence of cilia, which are described below. There are also people who cannot smell certain fatty acids but can smell everything else.

A diagrammatic drawing of the olfactory receptors is shown in Fig. 5.

The receptor cells are packed among supporting cells. Each of the cells ends in hair-like processes, the cilia. They are the essential organ of smell; without them, there is no possibility of being able to smell. They are long hairs, forming a mat embedded in mucus. They are made of proteins, and these proteins unite with the molecules of the odoriferous substance. In the cilia there are enzymes which act on the combined protein of the membrane and the arriving substance, and this action starts off a nerve impulse in the olfactory nerve fibres. There are 50 million olfactory receptor cells in each nostril of man. The olfactory nerves pass up to the brain through small holes in the base of the skull.

Substances that can be smelled by vertebrates have to be transferred from air into the mucus of the olfactory membrane and from there to the surface of the cilia. This means that anything that we can smell must be volatile, so as to get into the air, and soluble in water so as to get into the mucus and reach the ciliary membrane. Whether the substance will be smelled or not depends on the shape, size and polarity of its molecules; and they determine what smell it will have. The protein membrane of the cilia can accept thousands of different molecules. The molecule of a substance we can smell must be able to fit into the protein molecules of the membrane of the cilia. Polarity is a feature of the arrangement of the molecule in space. One might imagine a molecule as having the shape of a butterfly's wing. There are two wings, one fitting the insect's body on the right and the other on the left. Although each wing is just like the other one, each one can fit the body only on its own side. It is the same with the molecules of many substances. Two molecules have exactly the same arrangement of atoms but they are arranged in the opposite way in space. In this case, one substance may smell and the other not, for one will fit the protein of the ciliary membrane and the other will not. It is like fitting a key into a lock.

The substance that can be smelled united to the protein of the cilia is acted upon by an enzyme, and that starts ions passing through the membrane of the olfactory cell; this process sends off nerve impulses along the olfactory nerves. All of these nerves are not resting inactive waiting for a smell to come along; many of them are active all the time. When a new smell arrives, some nerve fibres are excited, others are quietened down, and others are left inactive. These three ways of affecting the nerve fibres allows one to smell a vast number of smells, far more than would have been possible had smell depended merely on exciting or not exciting one lot of nerve fibres.

The olfactory nerve fibres are the smallest nerve fibres outside the central nervous system. They are connected to an outgrowth of the brain called the olfactory bulb, which can be seen in the photographs on Plates 10 and 11. An animal's ability to smell may be judged on the size of its olfactory bulbs, just as its use of vision can be judged on the size of its eyes. Among birds we conclude that the sparrow and the crow use smell to a minimal degree, whereas the kiwi or birds that live in marshes like the sandpiper or those that fish at sea like the storm petrel use smell for finding their food.

External communication by chemical substances: pheromones

Pheromones (derived from the Greek words for 'carry' and 'excite') are substances that excite the sense of smell. An animal sensitive to a certain pheromone performs a particular act on receiving the smell signal. Pheromones tell others that a territory is occupied, they are used to signal dominance in a social group, some are used to spread alarm, others to induce sexual behaviour, to lay a trail, or as a warning that an animal is likely to attack.

One of the advantages of pheromones is that the signal itself, the scent, is left to transmit the information while the animal that gave the signal goes off to do something else.

One pheromone is well-known to all Americans and to others by repute: the stink made by the skunk to protect itself. The skunk first threatens by turning its back, raising its hind-quarters and its tail. Its anal glands are aimed at its foe. If the foe does not beat a retreat, a strong solution of butylmercaptan is squirted at it. Any animal receiving this once would avoid a second encounter.

Zoologists first became interested in pheromones when they realized that there were alarm substances put out by a damaged member of a group in order to warn the others. Bees make a substance in their salivary glands that keeps other bees away. If this substance, of which the chemical composition has been worked out, is spread around, bees flee from the spot. When the skin of many varieties of fish is damaged, alarm substances spread in the water: fish flee from the area, except for predators who are attracted by the substance. When the alarm substance of the skin of the toad is dropped into water, it alarms toads, tadpoles and any fish that smell it. The dilution of the substance that is effective is infinitesimally small; a few molecules suffice. Alarm substances do not travel as far as sex attractants and they do not linger. This is nice to know. It would be a sadder world if the call to sex were brief and passing and the warning of danger were long-lasting and present everywhere.

Sex pheromones are probably the commonest kind of pheromone;

they are used by insects, crustacea, fish, salamanders, snakes and other reptiles, amphibia, and mammals. They linger in the air or water and spread over long distances. There are two sorts of sex pheromone, one used by the female to bring the male to her side and one used by the male to encourage the female to copulate. Pheromones in moths and butterflies is contained in scent-scales or scent-plumes. Many varieties of insect and of mammal have special glands to make these chemical substances. Fabre, the nineteenth century naturalist of Provence, one day found his house full of peacock emperor moths. He had put some females of this species under wire netting in his house. He then spent months trying to answer the question how these females had signalled to the males. Although he finally came to the right conclusion, that the sense of smell was involved, he concluded that this could not be the ordinary sense of smell, as he himself could smell nothing. It did not occur to him that there could be a smell that the male moths could smell and that he could not. This was an unfortunate moth to catch, for had he captured many other moths, he himself would have smelled something, for we can smell some of them; some smell like caramels, some like raspberries and some smell of vanilla.

The queen-bee produces a pheromone that has two effects. It makes the eggs develop into non-developing females, the worker bees. And it also acts as a sex attractant to the males during swarming.

The male moth is able to tell the direction from which a smell is coming. It does this by having two antennae and by estimating which of the two is receiving most stimulus. This is a similar mechanism to that by which one can tell the direction from which a sound is coming by having two ears.

There is a moth that was brought to New England from Europe and which has become a pest, denuding trees. The sexual attractant pheromone has been synthesized and is now used to trap the males; thus the lure of sex, not for the first time, leads eager males to their deaths.

The silkworm, being domesticated and available, has been studied more than other species with regard to sex pheromones. The male can smell the female up to 2000 metres away. When he receives this exciting odour, he always behaves in the same way. He flutters his wings, waves the antennae which receive the odour, and flies off to try and find the female. The antennae of the male have 34,000 sensory organs, called sensilla, and these have 50,000 olfactory receptors, sensitive only to bombykol. This is the name of the pheromone, the Latin for a silkworm being bombyx mori. Bombykol is absorbed by these receptors, which then fire off nerve impulses to the brain. It has been calculated that 200–

300 molecules of bombykol acting for 4/5 of a second suffice to bring out the typical pattern of behaviour of the male moth. The female silkworm can smell a lot of odours but she cannot smell bombykol; the male, on the other hand, responds only to this and related substances. Some male moths respond to odours in different ways, depending on an innate circadian rhythm.

For monkeys, the attraction of the female for the male depends entirely on smell. The pheromone concerned is in the vagina. If a male rhesus monkey is deprived of the sense of smell he is no longer interested in the female. The literature of monkeys, if it existed, would be a literature of smell. But it is not only the female that attracts the male by means of a pheromone; the male emits an odour attractive to the female. There is a pheromone in the urine of the male mouse that brings the female on to heat. The pheromone emitted by the female rat is attractive to the adult male rat but pre-pubertal and castrated rats pay no attention to it. The smell she emits depends on her sexual state, and so she makes use of a pheromone to broadcast her readiness to receive the male. The pheromone given out by the male pig, together with some other stimuli, induce an immobilization reflex in the sow so that she stands still during copulation.

The male hormone, testosterone, can be smelled by women far more easily than by men. Its smell is musky, similar to that produced by musk deer and the civet cat. But women who have had their ovaries removed become rather insensitive to this smell. When these women were given the female hormone, oestrogen, they could smell the subtance again. Women can smell the most diluted solutions of musky substances about 10 days before the period; at this time, the secretion of oestrogen is maximal. After the menopause when little or no oestrogen is secreted, women can no longer smell testosterone.

It has been suggested that the earlier age at which menstruation starts nowadays compared to fifty and a hundred years ago is due to the fact that boys and girls mix far more now than they used to do. The odour of the opposite sex causes the secretion of hormones that induces puberty.

Sexual pheromones bring couples together. There are also aggregation substances that bring all the animals of a kind together. Then there are dispersal pheromones, used for instance by millipedes to chase animals of the same kind away. It is surprising to note that insects use insect repellants. These substances have not yet been chemically isolated and manufactured.

Mosquitoes detect human beings by their smell; they prefer the smell of some people to that of others. Women become more attractive targets to mosquitoes at certain period of their menstrual cycles; but not only to mosquitoes: also to dogs, stags, goats, monkeys and bulls. It may be that women misunderstand the intentions of bulls approaching them in lonely fields.

Hediger first realized that animals use pheromones for marking out their territories and home ranges. These pheromones may be excreted in the urine, as in the case of the dog, or with the faeces, as in the case of the bear. The substances are produced by various glands around the body, on the forehead, near the eyes, on the breast, inside the rectum. Male mammals mark objects with the secretion of these glands as acts of aggression; and if two males try to spread these secretions on each other, it is a prelude to a fight.

There are pheromones which when left in the home range of an animal act as warnings to others to keep off or they may act as trails left for others to follow. The male bumble-bee leaves trails in the air as he flies and he deposits the same substance on the plants he visits. Trail laying has been studied in many different kinds of ants. Each substance is specific to the kind of ant producing it. Bees release a pheromone when they find a good source of nectar. They also take the smell of the flower back to the hive so that the other workers can search for that particular smell. von Frisch found that this substance is sucked up with the nectar of the flower and that it also clings to the body of the bee. When the other workers in the hive learn about the source of food by observing the dance, they learn about the amount of pollen and nectar, about its distance from the hive and the direction in which to fly; from the smell brought in by the foraging bee, they learn which is the actual flower they have to seek.

Bees, ants and termites recognize the members of their own colonies by their smell. If any other insect gets into a bee hive long enough to acquire the right smell, it will not be evicted or killed but will be tolerated even if it spends its time raiding the eggs and honey. This recognition of one's own colony or family by smell is very common. No doubt that when the mother of many of the mammals we know best licks her young after birth, she covers it with a smell which she then recognizes as her own.

Ants live in a world of smells and produce several pheromones. Their alarm pheromone diffuses for about 3 to 5 cm, and fades out in about half a minute. Ants leave trails for others to follow, using this way of signalling a good food supply. This pheromone in the fire ant fades in about 2 minutes. It has meaning only for ants of the same species. E. O. Wilson, who has studied the communication systems of ants, considers that ants convey as much information in their chemical trail laying as bees do with their communication by dancing. Ants respond to the alarm pheromone put out by aphids, trans-β-farnescene. They are called to the scene by this chemical substance, and then attack any insect preying on their aphids.

6 Gustatory receptors: tasting

The working of the alimentary canal is largely controlled by receptors scattered along its lining. They organize the production of enzymes needed for the digestion of the various sorts of food we take in. Most of them work without evidence of this activity reaching our conscious awareness; but when the tension receptors are strongly stimulated, their messages protrude into consciousness and we suffer the pain of abdominal colic. In addition to the tension receptors, there are chemoreceptors of all kinds; and receptors for sampling the pH or acid–alkaline balance of the alimentary contents.

The chemoreceptors in the front end of the alimentary canal, the end that takes in food, send messages finally to parts of the brain to cause sensation; this is necessary to adjust behaviour according to the message received. Among our early ancestors, the fish in the sea, these chemoreceptors were in the mouth; for the world flowed into the mouth, as seawater. When vertebrates left the sea, some chemoreceptors remained in the mouth and their messages were interpreted as taste; others moved to the top of the nose and their messages were smells. Our taste or gustatory receptors are on the top and edges of the tongue, on the epiglottis, the soft palate and scattered around the throat. They are arranged in little goblets, called taste-buds. The actual chemoreceptors of taste are narrow cells ending in a fringe. These receptors wear away after about 10 days and they are then replaced by epithelial cells, which metamorphose into taste receptor cells. Every taste bud has about 50 of these cells. Man has about 10 000 in all. They are drawn in Fig. 6.1. The function of the supporting cells is unknown; it may be that they serve to keep the environment right for the receptor cells.

The substance to be tasted has to be adsorbed onto the fringes of the taste cells. To enter the cells, the substance must be water-soluble. It also has to be lipid-soluble and not too large a molecule in order to pass through the membrane.

Man has an even less developed sense of taste than sense of smell, for a larger number of molecules of a substance have to be dissolved in fluid for it to be tasted than for it to be smelt.

A detailed investigation has been carried out in the United States on the gustatory apparatus of the blow-fly. This achievement of great technical difficulty was done by Hodgson, Lettvin and Roeder in 1955.

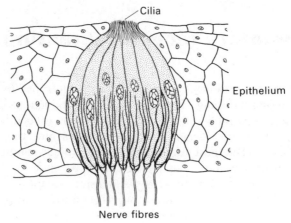

Fig. 6.1. The taste receptors within a taste-bud.

In this fly there are within the hairs around the proboscis two kinds of taste-receptors, one sensitive to many compounds including salts, acids and alcohols, and the other sensitive to sugars. Another finding of these workers was that the sugar receptors exist to make the animal suck up the substance and the other receptors to make it avoid those other substances. The sugar-sensitive receptors may be sensitive to the stereochemical properties of the substance, similar to the olfactory receptors described above. Hodgson also discovered that the crayfish, living as it does on decaying meat, has taste-receptors sensitive to amino-acids.

Cats are indifferent to sweetness and have no receptors for sweet tastes. One of my cats likes chocolate, so presumably it is not the sweet taste that it prefers. Most animals do taste and like sweetness; this is so for flies, butterflies, rats, mice, dogs, bears and horses.

Professor Pfaffman in the United States has spent most of his life investigating taste. Recording the messages in single nerve fibres coming from taste-receptors, he found that most of the nerve fibres were activated by more than one taste. Acids activated most nerve fibres; others activated by two sorts of taste; some were activated only by bitter tastes. It is thought that the polarity of the molecule of the substance to be tasted plays an important role, for some substances have different tastes depending on the polarity. Dextro-phenyl alanine tastes sweet and laevo-phenyl alanine is bitter.

It is usually stated that man possesses four primary tastes, bitter, sweet, sour or acid, and salty. What this means, I do not know. For man can taste many other things that are in no way a combination of these tastes. Experiments on gustatory nerves of cats and dogs show that the nerve fibres are activated by putting many different substances on the tongue. Substances, such as meat extracts, fish extracts, peptides and amino-acids all stimulate the taste-buds and send in impulses to the brain.

Man is most sensitive to the taste of bitter substances; far fewer molecules of bitter substance give us a taste than molecules of sweet, salt or sour substances. The taste of sourness is related to the pH of the substance, though not all acids taste sour or acid. All the salts of chemistry taste salty if they are soluble in saliva and if they dissociate at least to some extent into ions; both the cation and the anion contribute to the taste of the salt. For instance, sodium bromide tastes different from sodium chloride, and sodium chloride tastes different from potassium and from ammonium chloride. But there are some exceptions to the rule that salts taste salty. Lead acetates, for instance, taste sweetish. Some metallic salts must be described as tasting metallic rather than salty. And Epsom Salts, which is sodium sulphate, tastes bitter rather than salty.

The importance of smell is made clear to us when we have a cold. At a certain stage the mucous membrane of the nose is swollen with fluid or covered with mucus or pus; then the molecules of odoriferous substances cannot get at the receptors to excite them; and so we cannot taste our food properly.

As we get older we probably lose some of the sensitivity of all our receptors. This is so for hearing and smell; and it is very marked for tasting; many of our taste-buds disappear. The acuteness of the sense of taste in children may be one of the causes for their hatred of nasty-tasting medicines.

7 Cutaneous receptors: touching and feeling

For eighthly he rubs himself against a post.

The skin is not only the covering of the body; it is also a large area of receptors, constantly examining the world and sending information to the central nervous system. A part of its information is used for the automatic adjustment of the body which goes on without causing any sensation. It is used to control the temperature; some is used to aid in the control of the muscles; and some goes to alert the brain, telling it that more information is about to come in and to get ready to receive it.

What we feel and what afferent nerves bring to the central nervous system are two different things. The general principles of cutaneous or skin sensation were first studied early in the nineteenth century before anything was known about receptors and the central nervous system. Weber concluded from experiments on man that the senses are organized to take notice of differences between two stimuli rather than the absolute intensity of a stimulus; they are tuned to comparison and contrasts. Later in the century, Fechner used the concept of 'just noticeable differences' in investigating sensation in man. He proposed the hypothesis that the intensity of a sensation increased proportionally with the logarithm of stimulus intensity. Since his time, this has been shown to be true, and it is now known as the Weber–Fechner law.

The sensory apparatus of the skin has to report three sorts of information. It reports the nature of the stimulus, saying: 'You have been touched', or 'you are being tickled', or 'you are being burnt'. It reports the intensity of the stimulation, saying: 'This stimulus is slightly warm: this one is very cold.' And it reports the position of the stimulus, saying: 'You have been stimulated on the tip of the left little toe'.

Some receptors of the body are the nerve fibres themselves; others are nerve fibres joined to a non-neural cell, which is needed to start off the sensory message. There are both kinds in the skin. A simple nerve fibre receptor is shown in Plate 3. The dark-staining cells are the layers of the skin. The nerve fibre is the dark wire entering this layer from the deeper regions of the skin. This photograph was made from a small piece of skin punched out of the finger tip of a man. The specimen has been killed and stained especially to show nerve fibres. Although the photograph gives a good idea of a twig of a nerve fibre running through the superficial layers of the skin it does not show the dense network of nerve fibres there is throughout the skin. In reality, the close intertwining of nerve fibres is such that any natural stimulus must always excite a large number of receptors and nerve fibres. A receptor for signalling deformation of the skin due to something pressing on it or just touching it is shown in Plate 4. This receptor belongs to the class of mechanoreceptors; they respond to mechanical stimulation of the body surface.

For fifty years much research was done on animals to find out which nerve fibres of the peripheral nerves were activated by the various kinds of environmental stimulation. Now these questions are being answered for the case of man. In Sweden, Hagbarth, Vallbo, Hallin, and Torebjörk have developed a technique of recording the impulses in the nerve fibres of man. Very fine needle electrodes are put into the peripheral nerves; surprisingly, this is not painful.

The nerve fibres from the skin clearly fall into two categories, large and small. The large ones are the mechanoreceptors; they are excited by bending of the hairs, stretching or deforming the skin, by anything touching or moving along the skin. The small fibres are thermoreceptors and nociceptors: they report warmth and cold and any dangerous or noxious stimulation that causes pain.

Mechanoreceptors are divided into two groups, those with a low threshold to stimulation and those with a high threshold. The former are activated by the lightest kinds of touch or stroking of the skin, the latter only by heavy pressure or pinching. Mechanoreceptors are also of two kinds, rapidly and slowly adapting. The rapidly adapting receptors respond only briefly to stimulation; they soon adapt to the stimulus, ceasing to respond although the stimulus is still on the skin. They are good for reporting a moving stimulus and any changing conditions. Slowly adapting receptors give a sustained response to stimulation, continuing to send off impulses as long as the stimulus is indenting the skin. The receptor with little disks illustrated in Plate 4 is a slowly adapting receptor.

In the finger-tips, which are very sensitive to tactile stimuli, a single impulse in one or just a few nerve fibres can cause a perceptible sensation. In the palm, many more impulses are needed. In real life, there is never just one impulse and one nerve fibre is never excited alone. This is because the density of nerve-endings in any region of the skin is so great that no object could excite just one nerve fibre.

Warm thermoreceptors fire off impulses when the skin is warmed and stop firing when it is cooled; cold receptors do the opposite, firing on cooling and stopping firing when the skin is warmed. The names of warm and cold are rather vague for at a skin temperature of 33°C, which is comfortably warm, many cold receptors are firing. Warm and cold fibres are among the steady-state receptors, firing off constantly with different skin temperatures. Warm fibres fire between 33° and 45° and cold fibres from about 34° down to 18°. Within these ranges various fibres fire off constantly at different temperatures. Feeling cold in the hands depends more on the activity of these steady-state cold fibres than on the cold fibres that fire only when the temperature is dropped. This information about the temperature of the surface of the body is provided not only for conscious awareness; a lot of it is used for the automatic and unconscious control of body temperature.

Cats sample the temperature of the air with their noses; one can see them deciding on this evidence whether to go out or not. Hibernating hamsters have cold receptors in their noses that fire off when the temperature goes down to minus 5°.

Although one may speak of tactile fibres and of warm and cold fibres, one does not speak of pain fibres, but of nociceptors, receptors that report damaging or noxious stimuli. The reason is that these fibres do not necessarily cause pain and that one can have pain without exciting these fibres. Pain is different according to whether it is a sudden new pain as when one sits on a drawing-pin or when it is a chronic pain continuing, as after sunburn.

Mechano-sensitive fibres, mechano-thermo-sensitive receptors, mechano-sensitive nociceptors and polymodal nociceptors are all used to report damage or potential damage to tissues. Damaging chemical substances, both those caused by damage to tissues and those introduced into the skin by stinging nettles and poison ivy, stimulate the smallest polymodal nociceptors. The sensation we experience does not depend only on which kind of receptor or fibre is firing off. Although the firing of a nociceptor almost always causes pain, firing of other receptors can cause pain, if they fire rapidly and often enough. This effect of the summation of impulses probably underlies something we all must have noticed. You may be leaning against the sharp edge of a desk. At first all you feel is the pressure against your thigh. But suddenly the region which is pressed upon becomes painful, and you have to move. The effect of impulses arriving repeatedly from mechano-receptors has been to cause pain.

All impulses that come into the spinal cord are not necessarily relayed on to the higher levels of the nervous system. There are nerve fibres coming from the brain that can block the passage of the impulses just before they reach the posterior horn neurons. This is a form of inhibition; as it occurs before the first synapse, it is called pre-synaptic inhibition. It will be discussed further in chapter 13.

The arriving nerve fibres of the posterior roots mostly end in the grey matter of the spinal cord; the region where they end is called the posterior horn. The nerve fibres of the posterior roots penetrate to different layers of the posterior horns. There is one layer mainly devoted to mechanoreceptors; impulses from stroking or pressing or touching the skin go to the neurons of this layer. There are two layers most concerned with noxious events, which finally cause us to experience pain. Neurons in one of these layers recieve impulses from the skin, from muscles and from the viscera. These neurons are those that give us referred pain. Referred pain is pain felt in the skin or the body though it comes from a viscus; it is thus referred from the viscus to the wall of the body. The reason for the reference is that impulses from viscera, muscles and skin come to the same lot of neurons. As the brain more often receives impulses from parts of the body of which we are aware, such as the skin, the chest wall or the arm, it interprets the arriving impulses as coming from these parts of the body and not from the viscera.

Intensity of stimulation, as was said in chapter 2, is signalled to the central nervous system by the rate of sending off impulses: the stronger the stimulus, the larger the number of impulses that are sent within a certain time; and also the larger the number of nerve fibres used to send in the impulses to the central nervous system.

There may be a change in the quality of sensation when more impulses a second arrive and when the sensation becomes more intense. This is the case for sensation from the viscera. The very same nerve fibres from the bladder signal all the sensations we can get from that organ. When these nerve fibres are sending a few impulses per second, we have the feeling that we need to pass urine. When more impulses come in, we get an urgent need to do so. When a great many impulses come in, we get pain in the bladder.

How we can tell whereabouts in the skin we have been touched or picked depends finally on the representation in the cerebral hemisphere of the skin of the body. Putting it rather crudely, we can say that touches on the left big toe are felt in one part of the cortex, and touches on the back of the neck in another part. Different parts of the cerebral hemisphere are related to different parts of the body. And so when nerve impulses come to one part, we know that they originated in the big toe; and when they come to another part, they must have come from the little finger. Our knowledge that the little finger has been touched is only a part of the information received. Many parts of the central nervous system have received the same information, parts having nothing to do with our consciousness, with sensation.

How we localize the point of stimulation does not depend only on the nerves of the skin itself. For most touches or pricks, pinches or shoves excite the nerves deep to the skin as well. If some of the nerves of the skin have been cut through by accident, say by a knife or jagged glass, touch or pressure can still be localized fairly accurately, even though the skin itself is insensitive to very light touch, warmth, cold or burning. This is because the nerves of structures deep to the skin, of muscles, tendons and bones, may be uncut; and their information is adequate to tell us whereabouts we have been stimulated.

Any point in the skin is supplied by very many nerve fibres. When a point on the skin is stimulated, the nerve fibres beneath this point are stimulated unequally. For no two points on the skin come equally within the territory of all the same nerve fibres. This can best be shown in a diagram. In Fig. 7.1. each nerve fibre A, B, and C, supplies a little area of

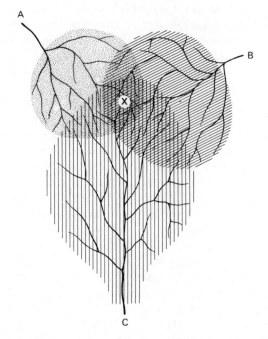

Fig. 7.1. Diagram to illustrate how any point in the skin has a particular relation to a minimum of three nerve fibres and no other point in the body has that same relation.

skin measuring a few square millimetres; and these areas partially overlap. If the skin is touched at point X, it is in the receptive areas of nerve fibres A, B, and C. No other point in the whole body is exactly in that position in the fields of these three nerve fibres. The number of branches of these three nerve fibres it might excite might be 10 per cent of A, 20 per cent of B, and 15 per cent of C. In reality, it is much more complicated than this; for any point on the skin is supplied by a great many nerve fibres. For instance the small region of pulp of a human front tooth contains 500–600 nerve fibres. The amount of overlap of the terminals of nerve fibres differs in different tissues and in one tissue it varies according to position. There are for instance, more nerve fibres in any area of skin of the hands and feet than in the upper parts of the limb.

The mechanism of surround inhibition is used to localize a point stimulated in the skin. When one small group of nerve fibres coming from one point in the skin is excited, the neighbouring neurons are inhibited. This interaction takes place at the first synapse, where the arriving nerve fibres enter the spinal cord. The same mechanism occurs at many higher synapses as the input is taken up through the central nervous system. The effect of this surround inhibition is to make the most active group of neurons stand out clearly against a background of relative silence, and this enhances the contrast between the point of the skin stimulated and the surrounding skin.

Throughout the animal kingdom, one sees how a general pattern of structure or of function can become specialized in certain directions. In one species, a certain structure is particularly well developed; in another, a certain kind of behaviour is developed, and this necessitates the development of certain kinds of receptors. In vipers and rattlesnakes of America and in Australian pythons and boas, receptors for warm have become specialized detectors. In the New World snakes, they are collected together in a pit between the eye and the nostril and in the Australian snakes they are in scales along the upper and lower jaws. Being sensitive to radiant energy, they detect the prey by the heat it gives out. The warmth given out by a rat is easily detected. As the snake has two pits, it gets a stereoscopic perception of the warm object; this allows it to estimate the distance of its prey with accuracy. A blindfolded viper will strike at a lighted electric bulb and not at a cold one; but if the facial pits are covered, it does not strike at all. The warmth of a human hand in front of the facial pit will excite the receptors in it, but if the hand strokes or touches the skin of the pit-organ, nothing happens. The pit viper has as many thermal receptors in about $\frac{1}{2}$ a sq. cm area as we have in 200 sq. cm of skin. These receptors are spontaneously active all the time and always sending off nerve impulses. When there is a change in the radiant energy reaching them, all that has to happen is for this spontaneous discharge to be changed in amount and in rhythm.

The sensation of pins and needles comes from depriving a nerve of its blood circulation. If a nerve is pressed on so that a length of it cannot get enough blood, the area of skin supplied by the nerve 'goes to sleep' and feels numb. When the pressure is removed, the nerve fibres fire off impulses spontaneously. The sensation of pins and needles is due to these spontaneous showers of impulses in the nerve fibres from the skin.

When a peripheral nerve is cut through either by accident or by disease, the effects appear in the muscles and skin. All the muscles supplied by that nerve are paralysed and they atrophy. There is no feeling in the denervated area. Owing to the division of the sympathetic nerves which accompany the peripheral nerves, the skin becomes dry; for it can no longer sweat. The little muscles that erect the hairs of the skin are paralysed and so, even when the skin is cold, these muscles cannot be contracted to make the skin hairs stand up and conserve a layer of warm air; also the blood-vessels are paralysed. At first they are dilated and the denervated area of skin is pinker than the surrounding region. Later, blood-vessels deprived of their controlling nerve fibres constrict, and the area becomes pale and cold. Eventually the skin becomes smooth and inelastic and the nails have white stripes and become ridged.

8 Receptors for the inside world

The receptors we have so far been reviewing keep the animal in touch with the outside world. There are also receptors to keep the central nervous system informed about what is happening in the inside world of the animal's own body.

All receptors are sensitive to those forces they are likely to meet and to no others. The receptors of the eye react only to light and those of the cochlea only to sound. It is the same with the receptors evolved to control the body. The receptors within the bladder do not respond to temperature, but they do respond to contraction and stretching of the muscle of the bladder wall. The receptors of the intestines are insensitive to temperature and to gentle touches; intestines can be torn or cut through in conscious patients without them feeling anything. But they are sensitive to stretching, to contraction and to certain chemical substances.

Equilibrium receptors: keeping the right way up

For he can set up with gravity which is patience upon approbation.

That we stand upright with our heads above our necks and our necks straight above the trunk seems so obvious that we do not realize that this position has to be automatically maintained. Gravity is constantly acting to pull us down and so we have mechanisms designed to counteract gravity.

The inner ear is not only for hearing. It is also the organ of equilibrium. In it are receptors sensitive to movement, to acceleration and deceleration, to rotation and vibration. The part of the labyrinth concerned with posture and balance is called the vestibule. It consists of three structures, the utricle, the saccule, and the semicircular canals, of which there are three on each side, in the three planes of space. They are shown in Fig. 4.1. The three semicircular canals can be seen, but the saccule and the utricle are on the far side and so are not seen in this view. In all vertebrates, one of these canals is in the horizontal plane; its angle varies with the usual head position of the animal. In fish, the head is in the same plane as the body and both are horizontal; in the giraffe, the head is usually tilted forwards and downwards, and so the position of the horizontal canal is arranged accordingly.

Balance is maintained by the eyes, the receptors of the vestibular system, the receptors of the joints of the neck and of muscles and ligaments. This input is co-ordinated to form a self-stabilizing control system. As the evolutionary scale of animals is ascended, the vestibular system becomes less and the eyes more important for the maintenance of balance. In fact, we pay so much more attention to what we are seeing that when we are sitting in a stationary train and we see the train alongside moving off, we have the impression that we are moving in the opposite direction. If we relied only on the accelerometers of our vestibular receptors, we would not get this false sensation.

Every movement alters the centre of gravity and tends to upset our equilibrium. The utricle and the semicircular canals contain the receptors that measure the changes that occur when we move. To compensate for this upset in our balance, muscles have to be contracted and relaxed; the head has to be kept up straight, then the neck, then the trunk, and the limbs moved a little, these adducted, those pulled away from the trunk. The computing device that determines the correct amount of muscular re-adjustment consists of large masses of neurons within the cerebral hemispheres, called the basal ganglia.

In mammals, the utricle is a position-registering organ. It sends in information about the position of the head in space and it is also sensitive to linear acceleration. The semicircular canals are sensitive to rotational acceleration; they act like three spirit levels, set at right angles to each other. Unlike man-made spirit levels, they are curved not straight, and the fluid is not spirits but endolymph, made from the fluids of the body. Incidentally, some aquatic insects actually do use an air bubble, exactly as in a spirit level. Around the bubble are hair-detectors, which are displaced by the movements of the bubble. In vertebrates, the semicircular canals report on angular acceleration and deceleration and rotation of the head. Every movement of the head stimulates at least one of these canals on each side of the head. When an acceleration becomes a constant speed, nothing more is reported than when the animal is still. If we keep our eyes shut when we are in a lift or an aeroplane, we do not feel that we are moving, once the speed has become constant.

All the receptor cells throughout the labyrinth are built on a similar pattern; they are hair-cells, the hairs being embedded in different sorts of jelly in the various receptor organs. In the semicircular canals, the hairs are embedded in firm jelly, which almost fills the canal. The receptor cells with their hairs or cilia are illustrated in Fig. 8.1. The cilia are arranged with one very long and stiff cilium on one side and with the shorter ones sloping away from it. The cilia differ in length and also in bending strength.

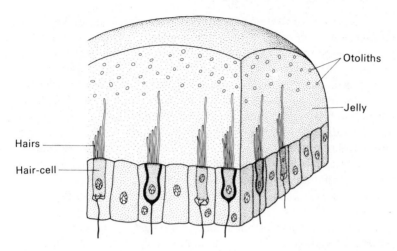

Fig. 8.1. The receptors used throughout the vestibular system.

In the utricle and saccule, the jelly contains crystals of calcite; these are called otoliths. The jelly with the otoliths in it has the consistency of stiff toothpaste. The tips of the hairs of the hair-cells penetrate the jelly and lie among the otoliths.

In 1893 a physiologist in Vienna, called Kreidl, put prawns in an aquarium in which the ground consisted of nickel filings. Animals like prawns and lobsters moult as they grow. During the moulting they normally replace their otoliths with grains of sands from the bed where they are living. Kreidl's prawns unwittingly put nickel filings in. In this way, gravity could be artificially supplied by means of an electromagnet. Much of the physiology of the gravity receptor was thus studied. It was discovered that under usual conditions, gravity excites hair-cells by pulling the otoliths down on to them. When the head is upright, the receptors of the utricles on each side of the head will be equally stimulated. When the head is tilted to one side, different groups of receptors on the two sides of the head will be stimulated. These receptors go on signalling as an animal is turned through 360°. They are position detectors. Other receptors of the saccule and utricle respond only at the beginning and the end of the tilting of the head. They are movement detectors. The effects of the input from the two utricles is to adjust the position of the head with regard to gravity and to the movements of the animal. The head then pulls the neck; afferent nerve fibres from the joints of the neck cause contractions of the muscles of the trunk, and so the posture of the whole body is suitably arranged to follow the new position of the head.

The receptors of the semicircular canals work in a similar way, though they have no otoliths. The canals are filled by two kinds of fluid, a rather viscous endolymph below and a covering jelly above. When the head is moved in any direction, this jelly remains relatively stationary, having more inertia than the endolymph. The difference in flow between these two substances bends the hairs and this movement excites the hair-cell receptors. The nerve fibres from these receptors are discharging nerve impulses all the time, whether the receptors are being excited or not. When the receptors are excited, they can alter this basic discharge of nerve impulses in two ways, either by increasing or else by diminishing the rate of discharge. When the head is moved in one direction, the rate of discharge is increased, and when it is moved in the opposite direction, it is decreased.

The function of the semicircular canals and the utricles is tested in patients by syringing the ears with hot and cold water and by means of a rotating chair. Hot water causes currents in the endolymph of the lateral semicircular canal towards the ear being syringed, and cold water to currents away from that ear. The effects of normal acceleration and deceleration are imitated by the rotating chair. These ways of stimulating the vestibule cause a movement of the eyes called nystagmus. When the left ear is syringed with hot water, the stimulation of the lateral semicircular canal causes the eyes to move slowly away from the left; the patient compensates for this and moves the eyes rapidly back to the left. Stimulation of the left ear with cold water produces the opposite movement of the eyes. If the semicircular canal or the nerves connecting it to the brain are not working properly, this nystagmus will not be normal.

You can see nystagmus any day by looking at the person opposite in the underground, when the train slows down as it arrives in the station; this is called train nystagmus. As he looks at something on the wall of the station and the train goes by, his eyes keep flicking sideways, while the train takes him past what he is gazing at.

Provided equal and opposite inputs from the vestibule of each side come to the brain, we maintain balance and stability without being aware that any of this system is working. But if there is any sudden disturbance of the balance of the two inputs, we get vertigo and nausea and we may walk as if we were drunk. In sea-sickness, there is a conflict between inputs from the eyes, the vestibular system and other proprioceptors; and above all, between the stimulation of these receptors by being moved passively and by moving actively. Deaf-mutes, who have not got connections from the vestibular apparatus to the central nervous system, lack the main component of conflict; and so they do not get sea-sick. In Cinerama, one may get sea-sickness. Here one is sitting still and one's vestibular apparatus is not being stimulated. But if you watch an air plane flying up and down or from side to side, you may get nausea and a headache. Your eyes tell you that you are moving up and down and from side to side and your vestibular apparatus tells you that you are sitting motionless.

Your eyes alone cannot inform you if you are moving or the environment is moving past you. You have to deduce this by taking note of other inputs and drawing a conclusion. As you sit in a train and the train just outside the windows starts moving off slowly, you cannot tell from your eyes whether you are moving or the other train is moving. You find out by taking note of your vestibular apparatus. If either you or the other train is moving slowly, the cues may be inadequate; but if either speeds up, it becomes easier to tell. You become aware of which is happening by making use of the accelerometers of your inner ears. They tell you whether you are being accelerated or not; and you fit this knowledge in with the input from your eyes. This examination of your position in the environment by comparing the inputs from different receptors is a particular example of a general principle: our knowledge of the environment is worked out: it is a hypothesis, which we are continually testing.

At least half the astronauts get motion-sickness in space. There is no stimulation of the otolith receptors because gravity, their usual stimulator, has been removed. But their semicircular canals are reporting acceleration. There is thus a conflict between the lack of otolithic information and the information reaching the brain from the canals. This strange combination of inputs has never been experienced before and it conflicts with the stored physiological memories of consistent inputs from the whole vestibular apparatus. That situation tends to cause nausea, sickness, headaches, and cold sweating.

Man manages surprisingly well when he is deprived of the vestibular receptors. There is a disorder of the labyrinths called Menière's disease. If all other treatment has failed, the vestibular nerves are cut, and no more impulses from the disordered organ reach the brain. Most of the patients who have had these nerves cut are able to compensate for the loss of this input. One of the difficulties they have comes from an inco-ordination of the input from their eyes and the movements of their heads. Normally, as we walk and our heads go up and down, what we see keeps jumping up and down; but we are unaware of this. But these patients find that what they look at when they are walking goes up and down, and they have to stop in order to see things clearly in the distance. We would probably never have realized that there is a problem here if these patients with the vestibular nerves cut had not found it. When these patients shut their eyes, they have some difficulty with balance, and this is made far worse if they have to walk on an uneven surface. With their eyes shut, the patients are relying on the receptors of joints, muscles, and ligaments. They then find it difficult to walk downhill or downstairs. Once they start falling, they have a lot of difficulty in correcting.

Proprioceptors of muscles, tendons, and joints

Posture and movement depend on proprioceptors of muscles, tendons, and joints and on the vestibular apparatus and the eyes. The proprioceptors of muscles are called muscle spindles, named after the spindle formerly used in spinning. Within each spindle are two kinds of receptor, named primary and secondary; they are drawn in Fig. 8.2. The primary receptor consists of a thick nerve fibre coiled around a thin muscle fibre and the secondary is similar, the nerve fibre not being so thick. There are about 10 of these modified muscle fibres in a spindle. They are thinner than ordinary muscle fibres and in the middle are a lot of nuclei. The nerve fibre from the primary receptor is the fastest conducting fibre in the body. The two receptors send different messages to the spinal cord. Both of them send in impulses when the muscle in which they are embedded is stretched and when the stretch has stopped.

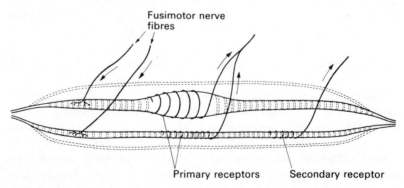

Fig. 8.2. Diagram of a muscle spindle. Two muscle fibres are drawn, surrounded by a capsule of connective tissue. The primary receptors are in the middle of the thin muscle fibres of the spindle and the secondary receptors at the ends. For the sake of simplicity, the secondary receptor is shown only at one end, on the right; all afferent fibres from the spindle are shown on the right and efferent fibres to the muscle fibres of the spindle are shown on the left.

The primary receptor is more sensitive to the rate of the stretch and so it fires only slightly when the stretch has reached a constant level. It therefore acts as a reporter of the start and end of a movement. The secondary receptor reports a steady state of stretch; it fires off impulses steadily as long as the muscle is being pulled.

The sensitivity of these receptors depends on the tautness of the muscle fibres of the spindles. When the main muscle fibres are completely relaxed, there is no pull on the spindles and the spindle receptors stop sending off impulses. Also when the main muscle fibres are fully contracted, the spindle is not being stretched and it stops sending off impulses or sends off only very few. But the spindles have to be kept tense in order that they can report the tension of the main muscle and the rate of change of its length. This is done by making the little muscle fibres of the spindles contract. The nerve fibres from the spinal cord to these muscles are called fusimotor (fusus is Latin for a spindle) nerve fibres. When muscles are ordered to contract, orders are sent at the same time to the fusimotor neurons, so that the spindle muscles contract; that tightens up the spindles, so that they can still act as measuring and reporting devices.

Some people who are psychologically tense keep their muscles contracted most of the time. This gives them aches and pains and they may feel tired and exhausted. Further, they feel their own physical tension and that makes them feel tense and anxious. These people may be making their spindles contract too much and continually or else they may be activating their main muscles. This constant contraction can be in most or in only some particular muscles. If the muscles of the jaw are kept contracted, pain in the face results or pain in or around the jaw-joint, which is just in front of the ear. Many headaches are due to constant contraction of the scalp muscles or the muscles of the neck. This muscular overactivity may be relieved by making the person aware of the fact that he is contracting his muscles and then training him not to do it. It can also be stopped by injecting local anaesthetic or just saline into the tender muscle, or by acupuncture.

When a doctor examines your knee-jerk, he is suddenly stretching the quadriceps muscle. This simple test is examining the primary receptors of this muscle, the afferent nerves to the spinal cord, the integrity and excitement of the local region of the spinal cord, the fusimotor neurons and the motoneurons of the quadriceps, the ability of the quadriceps to contract and relax, and the spread of excitability within the spinal cord which causes relaxation of the hamstring group of muscles, those that antagonise the action of the quadriceps.

There are also proprioceptors in the tendinous parts of the muscles called tendon organs; they report passive tension put on the muscle and active contraction of the muscles. And there are joint proprioceptors. They report the velocity of the movement of the joint and also the angle taken up by the joint. All of these receptors are constantly firing volleys of impulses which are used to maintain posture and movement.

If all the afferent nerves from the limb are cut, the person does not use the limb. The limb lies inert, just as if it is paralysed. Yet the efferent nerves are intact and so the limb could be moved. The continuous information coming in from the muscles, tendons and joints is so important that the spinal cord and the brain do not move the limb unless this input arrives constantly. Eventually, and with much difficulty, the patient may learn to use the limb again; he then uses his eyes to monitor the position and movements of the limb. If he is blindfolded, his movements are wild and unco-ordinated. Not only are our purposive movements disrupted by cutting the afferent nerves but all the more automatic parts of posture and movements are equally disturbed. This cutting of afferent nerves not only may occur with accidents and with gun-shot wounds, it can also occur with certain neurological disorders. The most typical example of this is the third stage of syphilis. In this disorder, afferent nerves from the skin are cut through by the disease process, and the patient can burn himself and stick pins into his skin without feeling it.

Receptors for controlling the internal environment
Other variables of the body have to be kept within certain limits; they are monitored by receptors connected to the central nervous system by nerve fibres. These are the blood pressure, the temperature, breathing, the turgidity of the cells of the body, the chemical constitution of the blood and of the alimentary canal, the amount of glucose and amount of hormones in the blood.

The first and main way of controlling the body's temperature, however, is the way used by all cold-blooded animals: the seeking of an environment that is comfortable so that the body neither gains nor loses heat. We are always doing this, whether we notice it or not; our newspapers are full of advertisements suggesting to us ways of keeping warm or cool.

The second way of controlling temperature is by having thermorecep-tors in the skin which send off impulses with constant temperatures and with changing temperature. These receptors cause local reflex alter-ations in the local blood-supply and adjust the hairs of the skin to conserve or to get rid of heat. They also cause distant similar effects via sympathetic nerves.

Breathing is a fundamental activity which is arranged automatically and which we can also influence when we pay attention to it. There are four main controls influencing automatic breathing. It is partly controlled by stretch receptors in the lungs and in the bronchial tree. It is controlled also by the feedback mechanisms and reflexes used for the control of all muscles. The depth and rate of breathing is under the influence of chemoreceptors in the medulla oblongata which are sensitive to the carbon dioxide and the pH of the blood; and they are influenced by baroreceptors in the large blood vessels and heart.

Much of the control of the internal environment of the body depends on chemoreceptors, receptors sensitive to chemical substances. Chemoreceptors for sampling aspects of the environment, those used for smelling and tasting, have been described in chapters 5 and 6. There are other chemoreceptors in the gut. One kind is sensitive to acids and another kind to alkalis; they are used to control the digestive ferments or enzymes needed to digest the food. More important are the pH-sensitive receptors in the brain and the great blood vessels, which are necessary to keep the acidity–alkalinity of the blood plasma between narrow limits. To keep this pH constant, there are three mechanisms. In the blood plasma there are buffers; these are salts which are partly ionized and partly non-ionized, the two forms of the salt being in equilibrium. If an acid or an alkali is added to such buffered solutions, the equilibrium is shifted; but the pH of the total solution remains unchanged, as the added acid or alkali is neutralized. The second method of controlling the pH of the blood is to excrete carbon dioxide in the breath. If carbon dioxide is retained, the pH will be lowered, as this gas goes into solution in water, forming a weak acid—carbonic acid. The third method is to excrete acid or alkaline salts in solution in the urine.

Chemoreceptors in the large blood-vessels are sensitive to the amount of oxygen and of carbon dioxide present in the passing blood. If the amount of oxygen is reduced or the amount of carbon dioxide is increased, these receptors discharge nerve impulses at a greater rate. The brain responds by increasing breathing to take more oxygen into the lungs and to get rid of more carbon dioxide; it also increases the heart rate and constricts the smaller blood-vessels.

In the hypothalamus there are chemoreceptors which monitor the amount of glucose in the blood; there are others sensitive to the amount of the various hormones that circulate in the bloodstream. These receptors are situated close to the neurons that control the secretion of each particular hormone. The receptors sample the amount of the hormone that reaches them; and the future amount of hormone to be secreted and passed into the bloodstream is then adjusted accordingly.

9 Nerves and nerve fibres

General features

The nerves connect the receptors with the central nervous system and the central nervous system with the muscles and glands. The brain and spinal cord control the body. They receive information from the world and from the body itself; they organize the animal's activity in relation to that information.

All nerve fibres have two functions. The surface of the fibre acts as a wire, transmitting messages as electrical pulses. There is also a tube along which materials conveying information pass in both directions. If we were to copy these two functions in the communication systems made by man, we would have pipes delivering gas and we would use the outside of the pipe like a telephone or telegraph wire. Yet the nerve fibre is more efficient than that; for this pipe passes not one but many substances along, moreover passing some in one direction and some in the other.

The peripheral nerves consist of bundles of thousands of nerve fibres. Some convey impulses away from the spinal cord towards the muscles and others in the opposite direction. Some of the fibres leaving the spinal cord are sympathetic fibres going to blood vessels, sweat glands, and to the hairs of the skin; they make these hairs stand upright with fear or when the body is cold and needs a protective layer of warm air around it. The fibres conveying impulses to the central nervous system come from the muscles, tendons and joints; most of them come from the skin, reporting everything that touches the body, burns it, cools it, or affects it in any way.

Transmitting the message along the surface of the nerve fibre: conduction

> For by stroaking of him I have found out electricity.

The nerve fibre is usually likened to a telephone wire; and the analogy is excellent. Both nerve fibres and telephone wires are electric conduction systems designed to conduct messages rapidly over long distances. In both of these systems, the message is sent as a code, formed of pulses of activity spaced in time; and in both systems the pulses are of constant size and are conducted along the wire at a constant speed. In both systems, the wires have to be insulated; if the insulation gets damaged, the carrying of the impulses breaks down. Here the analogy ends, for the nerve fibre is more complicated than the telegraph wire. It is not just a passive conductor of electrical events; it is both the accumulator and the wire. In telegraphy, the current is carried in a solid wire made of metal; in the living conducting system, the current is carried by ions in a fluid. In telegraphy the electricity is supplied to the wire and then transmitted along it; in the living system, the nerve fibre itself generates the electrical signal; it is a self-generating system.

What actually happens when the nerve fibre is transmitting impulses is a problem that scientists have been examining for over a hundred years. Before the First World War, Nernst suggested that the nerve impulse consisted of an electric current carried by ions through the membrane of the axon. In 1936, Hodgkin and Huxley at Cambridge working on the giant nerve fibres of the squid proved that this was right.

One of the main constituents of our bodies is a solution of common salt, sodium chloride. This solution surrounds all cells of the body and so it is called extra-cellular fluid. The solution inside cells is different, for it contains far less sodium and far more potassium. These two different solutions are separated by the cell-wall or cell-membrane. This membrane is selectively permeable to ions: potassium ions pass through with ease, chloride ions less easily, and sodium ions only with difficulty. The balance of ions outside and inside the axoplasm is maintained by the continual ejection of sodium ions from within the axonic membrane and by the continuous intake of potassium ions. Owing to the different concentration of ions on the two sides of the membrane, there is a difference in electrical potential across the membrane, the inside being negative and the outside positive. This difference of potential is called the resting potential. When the nerve is excited and is carrying the nerve impulse, this negative potential is reversed; the change from negative to positive difference of potential is called the action potential. The action potential is due to a sudden, transient increase in the membrane's permeability to sodium ions. Sodium ions pass through the membrane into the axon and they reverse the potential, making the inside of the axon positive with respect to the extra-cellular fluid. This increased permeability to sodium ions allows more sodium ions to pass, which reduces the resting potential still further. However, the process is stopped by an increase in the membrane's permeability to potassium ions; this reverses the potential across the membrane, bringing back the state before the passage of the action potential. The physics of these events has been worked out, and it is even known how much current is carried by a single ion. After many action potentials have passed along a nerve fibre, sodium is expelled from within the membrane and potassium is brought back.

The reduction of the resting potential by influx of sodium ions is referred to as depolarizing the membrane and bringing it back to its resting state is repolarizing the membrane. The membrane can also be made less permeable to all the smaller ions; this is called hyperpolarizing the membrane.

The action potential is also called a spike. This is because the trace it makes on a cathode ray oscilloscope has the shape of a spike. A group of spikes, one after another is called a volley of impulses, or more often, a volley.

The action potential does not start spontaneously in the nerve fibre; it starts in the receptor (or if you bang your funny-bone, it starts at the place where you bang it). The function of the receptor is to change the energy it receives into electrical energy. It does this by producing a difference in potential, called the generator potential; the amount of the generator potential is proportional to the strength of the stimulation of the receptor. Thus a stimulus excites the receptor, the receptor makes the generator potential, the generator potential reaches the nerve fibre and is changed into the action potential. How the action potential spreads along the nerve fibre is the next question. The events occurring when the nerve fibre is excited occur at an infinitely small point on the membrane. When the events occur at this point, current flows between this small point and the adjacent regions of membrane. This local passage of current allows cations to pass through the membrane at these adjacent regions. Thus the cycle of events starting with an increase in permeability of the axonic membrane then occurs at the adjacent region of membrane. And so, by infinitely small but rapid steps, an ionic current spreads along the axonic membrane. The spreading depolarization takes place in one direction only—ahead of the region of the membrane where these events have just taken place. The reason for this is that the membrane cannot be depolarized until it has been repolarized; the electrochemical events cannot be repeated until they have finished taking place and the resting state has been re-established. And so the little patch of electrochemical activity finds membrane in front of it free to be affected and membrane behind it not free to be affected, as the events have not quite finished taking place there. This ensures that the spreading electrochemical activity will pass along the membrane only ahead of the change in electrical potential to the part of the nerve fibre that has not yet been affected by these events.

These electrical events are always of the same extent, producing the same amount of current whenever they occur in one and the same fibre. A strong stimulus does not set up a big nerve impulse and a small one a small impulse; in any nerve fibre the size or amount of the nerve impulse is always the same. This is due to the size and physical make-up of the nerve fibre. But what can be altered is the number of impulses sent along the nerve fibre per second. Events are transmitted in the nerve as a frequency code.

Once the electrochemical changes taking place at the membrane of the nerve fibre have started, they spread along the fibre to its endings; they are self-propagating. This fact—that the nerve impulse is conducted throughout the length of a nerve fibre without being altered on the way—is an example of the all or none principle. The all or none principle states that an event either takes place or it does not; it is the same on all occasions and it cannot be altered in amount. One consequence of the all or none principle of impulse conduction is that when an alteration has to be made to a message, it cannot be made during its passage along the nerve fibre. Changes to messages have to be made at the places where the neurons meet, where the message is passed from one neuron to the next. A corollary of this is that when it is important to take a message from one place to another unchanged, one nerve fibre is used. When it is important to influence the message, to let messages interact, then chains of nerve fibres are used, so that at each junction or link in the chain, modifying influences can be introduced.

As we have seen, one of the characteristics of a nerve fibre is the number of impulses it can send in a certain time; another is the rate at which it transmits the nerve impulse. The manner of conducting nerve impulses we have described so far is slow; in mammalian nerve fibres the rates are from a half to two metres a second. This way of conducting nerve impulses is used when rapid messages are not needed; it is probably used when continual impulse transmission is needed, as for giving a background of excitation or its opposite, inhibition.

Faster nerve conduction was not achieved by making larger nerve fibres with larger diameters. A new step in evolution occurred; the covering of nerve fibres with a myelin sheath. A diagram of a neuron with a myelinated fibre is shown in Fig. 9.1. The neuron must be thought of as being in three dimensions and the nerve fibre must be imagined as being far longer than is shown here. The myelin sheath is not continuous; it stops at regular gaps called nodes. One of these is shown at immense magnification in Plate 5. The myelin sheath is an insulator, like the plastic covering of a wire. In a myelinated fibre the action potential occurs only at the nodes. Depolarization jumps from node to node; and so this is called saltatory conduction. A nerve fibre with longer

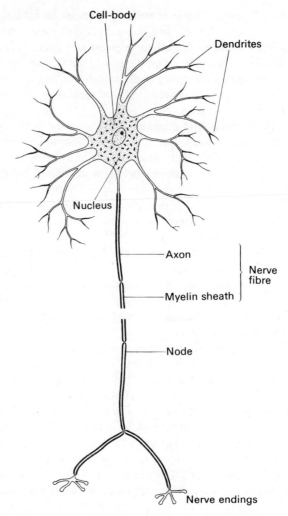

Fig. 9.1. Diagram of a neuron with its myelinated nerve fibre. Surrounding the axon is the myelin sheath, which is interrupted regularly at the nodes. The gap in the diagram is to indicate that the nerve fibre is longer than can be shown on the page.

internodal lengths will conduct impulses faster than one with short internodal lengths. In large nerve fibres with long lengths between nodes, the rate of impulse conduction goes up to 100 metres a second (225 miles per hour).

One might compare a nerve fibre with short internodal lengths and one with long lengths to a local train stopping at all stations and a fast train that stops at only a few main stations. It is obvious that the train stopping at many stations will be slower than the train covering large distances between only a few stations.

Nerve fibres used for conveying sensory information to the brain and spinal cord cover the whole range of conduction rates, with non-myelinated fibres conducting as slowly as half a metre a second and myelinated fibres conducting by saltatory conduction at 100 metres a second. The nerve fibres of the autonomic system and all nerve fibres to and from the viscera are small and slowly conducting. When we blush, we do not do so as suddenly as we jump, when we step on a sharp stone. It is unnecessary to signal to our fellows our embarrassment or humiliation with speed, but it is important to get our foot rapidly off the cutting edge of a stone. So fast conducting nerve fibres are used for this and slow conducting ones to dilate the blood vessels of our cheeks.

The amount of electricity used in nerve conduction is very small. Electricity is used in the body for signalling and not for power and work. The muscles provide the power. When they have received the small electrical signal, their molecules of protein contract and the whole body can be lifted by the muscles of one arm.

Local anaesthetics are solutions of various chemicals that prevent the passage of ions through membranes. In this way they block the conduction of nerve impulses and so the impulses that would eventually cause pain can no longer pass along the peripheral nerve fibres and so never reach the brain.

The electrochemical events that constitute the nerve impulse take a certain amount of time to take place; as one nerve impulse cannot follow another until these events have occurred, the number of impulses a nerve fibre can transmit is limited. This is one of the factors setting limits to the capabilities of nervous systems. Within such limits, the number of impulses transmitted within a certain time is very varied; one nerve fibre might transmit 500 impulses a second and another 10 impulses.

The only sort of message carried by the nerve, so far as we know, is the electrochemical change just described. All dealings with the world and with the body itself have to be translated into this coinage; there is no other sort of tender. This is similar to a computer. All the data fed into a computer have to be translated into its code and when the machine has finished its calculation, they have to be translated back from its code into the language of statistics, mathematics or everyday speech.

An analogy here is the taximeter. All the passenger is interested in is the amount of money the journey is costing. The taximeter automatically translates all events into these terms. Whatever transpires on the journey, rushing along here, stopping twenty minutes in a block there, slowing down for your driver to exchange a few well-chosen words with the driver of another vehicle is all presented to the passenger in terms of money. So it is with the nervous system and its journey through the world. Whatever happens both inside and outside the body, the nervous system is presented with a record of electrochemical pulses and from this it must construct the world.

The disease of disseminated sclerosis or multiple sclerosis (D.S. or M.S.) is a disorder in which there is damage to the myelin sheaths of nerve fibres within the central nervous system. Over a distance of a few centimetres, the sheath of myelin is ruined. These nerve fibres are left like wires that have lost their coating of insulation. At first impulses can be conducted slowly through the short length of demyelinated fibre, but eventually conduction fails. The manifestations of multiple sclerosis depend on whereabouts the demyelination has occurred. If it is in the optic pathway, then vision is upset; though complete blindness is rare in this disorder. If it is in the spinal cord, there may be some paralysis or numbness or other kinds of disturbance of sensation.

Transporting substances inside the nerve fibre: trophic activity

It would be a waste of space if nerve fibres were empty. The conduction of impulses just needs the outside of the nerve fibre; so the inside is used to carry substances in both directions. The outside is a telegraph line; the inside is a road carrying traffic both ways. This traffic within a nerve fibre is called axonal or axoplasmic transport.

If this transport of substances along the nerve fibre to its endings is stopped, the nerve fibre disintegrates. And what is more interesting is that the cells supplied by that nerve fibre are also badly affected. They do not disintegrate or die but they turn into fibrous tissue.

The main substance made by the neuron is protein. It is formed in the cell-body, then passed along the axon. This transport within the axon is probably also electrical. Within the axon are microtubules and neurofilaments. The material passes along the outside of the tubules; this mode of transport seems to be used to take things up to the cell body. The neurofilaments are protein threads that move along by contracting; substances become attached to them and thus get taken along. Various substances are transported at different rates: the slowest is a mm a day and the fastest is about 30 cm a day. Actual particles are transported at the fast rate and molecules at the slow rate.

One of the ways in which transport of trophic substances necessary for the target cells has been studied is to cut the nerves to the limbs of embryos of newts and amphibians. If the nerve is prevented from growing into the developing limb, the limb does not develop. A great number of experiments on these embryos have shown that the nerve controls the rate of protein synthesis of the target tissue. The correct proteins are made without the controlling nerve but so slowly that they fail to produce a limb. It is not yet known what this trophic substance is. It is a protein, made in both afferent and efferent nerve fibres. There is also a substance, called nerve growth factor, in afferent and sympathetic target tissues. It entices nerve fibres to grow towards it.

There is also retrograde transport, substances passing from the tissue supplied by the nerve fibre back along the axon to the cell-body. Perhaps some of these substances act as signals to control the manufacture of protein and other substances by the cell body.

10 Communication within the central nervous system

Neurons

The investigation of the nervous system by means of the microscope began about a hundred years ago. When the anatomists looked down their microscopes, what they saw was a thick tangled mass of fibres. As they made thinner sections and teased nerve fibres out until only a few were there at a time, they came to realize that they were dealing with two sorts of cells: there were neurons; and there were other cells, the function of which is to look after, feed and repair the neurons. Once all workers had come to this conclusion, a controversy arose whether neurons were continuous throughout the central nervous system, forming a vast and complicated network, or whether every neuron was separated from every other one, with a gap between them where they met. This latter view is now recognized as being the correct one. It was the view of Cajal, the founder of the Spanish school of histologists. One of the ironies of history is that the contrary and erroneous view was supported by Golgi who invented the method of staining the nervous system for microscopical investigation, which Cajal used to establish the correct view, a view Golgi bitterly opposed. And in 1906, Cajal and Golgi shared the Nobel Prize for their respective contributions to knowledge of the nervous system.

An electron micrograph of a living neuron is shown in Plate 6. This neuron has been grown in tissue culture. A small piece of embryonic tissue is cut out from a living embryo and grown in physiological and germ-free conditions. Often the embryo used is the chicken in the egg as it is so easily available. The advantage of using tissue culture is that the neuron appears isolated and separated from a mass of nerve fibres and other surrounding matter. This neuron has to be thought of as being in three dimensions.

Neurons of vertebrates belong to one of two categories, named as Golgi type I and Golgi type II, after the histologist who described them and realized that all neurons could be categorized in this way. Golgi type I neurons have long axons; these are the neurons with nerve fibres. A large neuron with its axon might measure a metre in a man and even more in a giraffe or a whale. Golgi type II neurons have short axons and make only local connections; the axon might be no longer than the dendrites of the cell, and could measure as little as 2 or 3 μm. A typical Golgi type II neuron is the amacrine-cell shown in the retina in Fig. 3.1

The cell body of a large type I neuron, cut through and photographed is shown in Plate 7. When the cell body is cut through, some of the nerve-endings of other neurons on the membrance surrounding the cell body can be seen. This neuron is a motoneuron of a cat, stained, and shown by electron microscopy. In this photograph, one sees three circles: the central dark one is the nucleolus, the next one is the nucleus, and the largest and most exterior one is the membrane of the cell body. Outside the cell body, dark staining ovoids and circles are seen; they are small nerve fibres passing by the cell body. The nerve-endings, measuring about 1 μm across, are shown by the arrow.

One of the most beautiful neurons, called a Purkinyĕ cell, is drawn in Fig. 10.1. It is called after the Czech anatomist who discovered it early in the nineteenth century. The branching dendrites, covered with spines, look like a flat fern. The drawing shows it in its widest extent; in the plane at right angles to this, the dendrites are slim, like a Lombardy poplar. On the dendrites of each Purkinyĕ cell, there are reckoned to be 120 000

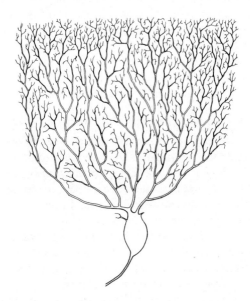

Fig. 10.1. A neuron from the cerebellum, named after its discoverer, Purkinyĕ.

spines. Continuing to think of resemblances between neurons and plants, we might see the dendrites with spines on them as the branches and the spiky leaves of a gorse-bush. Each spine receives one nerve-ending. Passing through these dendrites are hundreds of thousands of nerve fibres, forming synapses as they pass. Other nerve fibres also connect to these cells; they spread around the branches before reaching the dendrites, like a vine. That is what the Purkinyĕ cell receives. A neuron that connects to Purkinyĕ cells sends its axons and branches to 300–450 Purkinyĕ cells.

One should think of the surface of the cell body, dendrites and spines as looking like a mosaic. The little blocks of glass and stone of the mosaic would be the knobs of the nerve-endings on the surface of the neuron, and the cracks between the blocks would be narrow lines on the surface that are not covered by nerve-endings of connecting nerve fibres. The area of a cell-body with its dendrites offering an anchorage to nerve-endings is very large. It has been worked out that on every motoneuron supplying muscles of the cat's hindlimb, there are 33 000 nerve-endings.

Neurons, being such long cells, are always accompanied by supporting cells. In the central nervous system these cells are called the neuroglia; in the peripheral nervous system they are called Schwann cells, after the nineteenth-century anatomist who first described them. Nerve fibres are wrapped round and round by layers of these cells, and every nook and cranny between the neurons and nerve fibres in the central nervous system is filled with neuroglia. In the peripheral nervous system the Schwann cells make the myelin sheath; this sheath provides the insulating layers around myelinated nerve fibres.

Passing the message from neuron to neuron: the synapse

In the central nervous system, every neuron sends out numbers of branches that end on other neurons. As was mentioned above, the place where a nerve-ending affects another neuron is the synapse. There, the message is passed on; and there it can be influenced, reduced, increased, or obliterated. The synapse is sometimes called a relay, for the message is relayed there to the next neurons. Between the nerve-ending and the cell body or dendrite, there is a gap; this is the gap of the synapse; it is usually about 200 Å wide and is called the synaptic cleft or gap. Events and structures are named in relation to the synaptic gap: those before it are pre-synaptic and those after it are post-synaptic.

Neurons conduct impulses in one direction only. Afferent nerves take impulses to the central nervous system and efferent nerves take them out to the viscera, glands and muscles. Within the central nervous system, impulses are sent away from the cell body along the nerve fibre to the nerve-endings on the next neuron. The nerve fibre breaks up into many branches and the branches finally end as twigs, connecting to one neuron or to thousands of neurons.

There are two general patterns of connection between neurons: divergence where a neuron receives from a few other neurons and connects to thousands of other neurons; convergence where a neuron receives nerve-endings from thousands of other neurons and sends its connecting axon to only a few neurons. The synapse is an arrangement for spreading messages far and wide or for channelling them down into a few or only one pathway. The more synapses there are on a pathway, the more modifications can be brought into the responses to stimulation and into behaviour. A similar situation would arise if there were only one road between Manchester and London with no possibility of turning off, or if there were a road with many crossings. If there is only one road the journey is quicker as there is no stopping at the cross-roads; but it is also unmodifiable. Once on the road, you have to continue to the destination. If there are cross-roads, the journey is slower; but all sorts of modifications and ways round can be made.

How the message is passed across the synaptic gap from one neuron to another will be discussed in the rest of this chapter. When the nerve impulse in an excitatory nerve fibre reaches the synapse, it delivers a standard amount of excitations. An inhibitory neuron does the same, in this case a standard amount of inhibition. In most places in the central nervous system, a single impulse does not fire the post-synaptic neuron, though a single impulse in a nerve fibre coming from the skin can fire the post-synaptic neuron in the grey matter of the spinal cord; and this single impulse can finally cause a minimal sensation of being touched. Whether a volley of impulses fires the post-synaptic neuron or not depends on the kind of neuron it is and on its state of excitability at the time. This is a changing state, depending ultimately on the chemical environment of the cell. Some neurons go through rhythmical phases of increasing and decreasing excitability; the neurons that work the respiratory muscles are an obvious example.

The inpulses arriving at a neuron add up: the inhibitory impulses cancel out the excitatory impulses. If a neuron is firing off impulses at a constant rate, the rate of firing will be increased by excitatory impulses and decreased by inhibitory impulses reaching the neuron. The excitability of many neurons rapidly decreases if no excitatory impulses arrive; for instance, motoneurons of the cat have to receive 20 impulses a second to keep them firing. The summation of inhibitory and excitatory impulses is the same for inhibitory and excitatory neurons. An excitatory neuron is fired by excitatory nerve-endings on its dendrites and cell body or stopped firing by inhibitory endings; an inhibitory neuron is silenced by inhibitory nerve-endings and excited by excitatory endings. Inhibiting an inhibitory neuron is referred to as disinhibition. When two inhibitory neurons are linked together, the post-synaptic neuron's behaviour is the opposite of the pre-synaptic neuron's.

Some neurons seem to be firing most of the time; they do so to keep an adequate excitability at the synapses where their nerve fibres end. In such a case the neurons on which these nerve fibres end are ready to fire off and they can easily be triggered by the arrival of volleys of impulses. This is so with regard to neurons of the spinal cord that organize movement. There is an ever-present background of impulses coming in from the brain, keeping this system ready to respond to orders to move.

The excitation and inhibition described so far are called post-synaptic, as they take place on the neuron immediately after the synaptic gap. There is also another kind of inhibition, pre-synaptic inhibition. With pre-synaptic inhibition, the nerve fibre running to the post-synaptic neuron is inhibited before the synaptic gap, so that it cannot deliver its full quota of excitation. As far as is known, this occurs only on excitatory neurons; there is no pre-synaptic inhibition of inhibitory neurons. Pre-synaptic inhibition can be so effective that it blocks all the impulses in the axon and thus blocks the message. It may be, too, that it is a mechanism for directing impulses along one pathway rather than another. Most nerve fibres end up as many small branches, like the branches and twigs of a tree. Some of these twigs could be blocked by pre-synaptic inhibition, leaving the impulses to pass along other branches and twigs. This would be a mechanism for directing the excitation to one neuron and not another or to the dendrites of a neuron and not the cell body.

One might think of a synapse in the following way. Suppose someone is trying to lift a weight with his outstretched hand. The weight is the post-synaptic neuron and his hand is the exciting neuron. If you help him by adding your lifting power to his, together you might succeed in lifting the weight, whereas alone he could not have done it. In this case, you are an excitatory nerve-ending adding your quota of excitation to his. But suppose you push the weight down as he tries to lift it. Then you are an inhibitory nerve-ending. Whether the weight is lifted or not depends on the relative power of his lifting and your pushing it down. Now, say instead of pushing the weight down, you pushed his wrist down, so that he could not lift the weight up; this would be pre-synaptic inhibition.

The cell body, like the human body, is not equally excitable all over. The peripheral parts of the dendrites are relatively inexcitable. It seems that excitation delivered far out on a dendrite may be insufficient to fire the neuron but it may just be enough to increase its excitability momentarily. In this way continually arriving impulses could keep the neuron sufficiently excited to be triggered off when volleys of impulses arrive nearer the cell body. Thus the nerve-endings on far out dendrites may provide a background excitability that is needed to make a neuron fire off. The spines on the dendrites are thought to be excitatory regions kept separate from the rest of the surface of a dendrite. This synaptic region has a privileged position, there being no interference from other arriving nerve-endings.

Some nerve fibres travel a long distance and then have just one or two nerve-endings; the nerve fibres supplying muscles are of this type. Others have nerve-endings throughout the course of the fibre. This is the common pattern of sympathetic nerve fibres. The railway analogy would be a train taking goods just from London to Glasgow for the first type, and a train dropping off goods at every halt and station along the line for the second type. The actual number of endings along the line for a sympathetic fibre is 330 000 nerve-endings per cubic millimetre of fibre. This means that such a nerve fibre influences the structure it is supplying along the whole length of the nerve fibre. Thus a sympathetic fibre supplying the wall of an artery affects every muscle fibre it touches.

11 Minipackets of information: transmitters, modulators, and their targets

As was said in the preceding chapter, there was a controversy at the end of the previous century and the early years of this, whether the nervous system consists of a continuous network of neurons or of single, individual neurons, somehow connected together. When it was finally confirmed that the latter view was the right one, the question of how one neuron is connected to another had to be answered. In chapter 9, it was explained that the nerve impulse is actually an electro-chemical event that passes along nerve fibres from their cell bodies to their nerve-endings. Whether the nerve impulse excites or inhibits the cell to which it is connected depends on the nature of the two neurons concerned: the neuron transmitting the nerve impulse can be either an excitatory or an inhibitory neuron; and the membrane of the neuron receiving the nerve impulse can be excitatory or inhibitory.

The nerve-endings of any nerve fibre cover only a very small area of the post-synaptic membrane, for the nerve cell body is much bigger than a nerve-ending. This means that the amount of current a nerve-ending delivers is small. In synapses of crustaceans and fish, this current is enough to fire off or inhibit the next neuron. But in reptiles and mammals, a different mechanism has been evolved to increase the effectiveness of the nerve-ending. Substances are made within the presynaptic neuron that are designed to alter the characteristics of the membrane of the post-synaptic neuron. When this membrane has been affected, hydrated ions can pass through, thus causing depolarization (usually excitation) or hyperpolarization (usually inhibition.)

Early in this century, physiologists had come to the conclusion that nerve fibres probably have effects on post-synaptic neurons by putting out chemical substances at their endings. They saw that the effects of injecting adrenalin on certain tissues was the same as stimulating the sympathetic nerves. And so they thought it likely that the sympathetic system works by the local injection of these substances. Much research work has gone to prove that this is so. That the parasympathetic system works by secreting a chemical substance was shown by Loewi in 1921. The crucial experiment came to him in the middle of the night. He jotted it down, but in the morning he could not read his writing. Fortunately the idea returned during the following night. It was known at that time that stimulation of the parasympathetic nerve to the heart slowed down the heart beat and could finally stop the heart. Loewi stimulated the parasympathetic nerve to the heart of a frog and collected the fluid from this heart. He then transferred this fluid to the heart of another frog. The result was that this heart began to beat more slowly. Thus he showed that the parasympathetic nerve had released some chemical substance into the heart and that this substance had the same effect there as stimulation of the parasympathetic nerve. He later identified this substance as acetylcholine. In subsequent experiments he showed that stimulating the sympathetic nerves to the frog's heart released adrenalin. In the mammalian heart, it is noradrenalin.

These exciting discoveries opened up a new world in physiology and the treatment of disease. The next important event was finding that the motor nerves to skeletal muscles work by putting out acetylcholine. It is the same for the nerves working the bladder and the alimentary canal.

From the first experiments it was learned that there were two kinds of transmitter chemicals, cholinergic, making use of acetylcholine, and adrenergic, using adrenaline. Since then more than twenty transmitters have been found in the alimentary canal, the sympathetic nervous system and the brain and spinal cord.

A neurotransmitter is a chemical substance made within a neuron to be released into the synaptic cleft when nerve impulses arrive. It is stored in microscopical vesicles or granules – one cannot tell which as one has only the appearance on electronmicroscopy to go on. They are shown in immense magnification in Plate 8. One of them can be seen actually uniting with the pre-synaptic membrane, thus releasing its contents into the synaptic cleft. In the photograph, the synaptic cleft is so narrow that is difficult to see. Of the four layers of membrane below the vesicles, the uppermost layer, which is nearest to the vesicles, is the membrane of the nerve-ending; this is pre-synaptic membrane. The other three layers of membrane are on the target cell; they are post-synaptic membrane. The synapse is between the uppermost layer and the next layer of membrane below it.

When the nerve impulse arrives at the nerve-endings, calcium ions pass into the axon from its surface and this causes the release of the vesicles into the synaptic cleft. This transmitter then diffuses across the infinitesimally small distance of the synaptic gap to the post-synaptic membrane. The tissue of the cell that is being acted upon by the transmitter is called the target and the membrane that combines with the transmitter is called the receptor or receptor membrane. This receptor consists of large protein molecules. The shape of this protein molecule fits the shape of the transmitter molecule like a key fitting a lock. This reaction alters the shape of the pores in the post-synaptic membrane. If positively charged sodium ions pass from the extra-cellular fluid into the neurone, excitation results; if negatively charged chloride ions pass in, there is inhibition. In the case of some transmitters, this mechanism is more complicated; it includes an enzyme that is needed for the transmitter to be able to unite with the membrane and to pass through the membrane and affect the interior of the cell. This mechanism takes longer than the simpler one that alters the size of the pores.

One and the same transmitter can have opposite effects, depending on the receptor membrane with which it reacts. Acetylcholine, for instance, can excite the membrane of one neuron and inhibit that of another. Yet some transmitters are always excitatory or always inhibitory. In vertebrates, γ-aminobutyric acid or GABA is always an inhibitory transmitter; glutamate and aspartate are always excitatory.

Transmitters are formed from various chemical substances, the substrate of which is eaten in food. In the chemical reactions that form the transmitters, different substances are made at various stages. In some of these stages, the product formed is itself a transmitter. For instance, from the amino-acid tyrosine, first dopa is formed, then successively dopamine, noradrenaline, and adrenaline; the last three of these are all transmitters.

In some cases it seems to be that certain functions have one main transmitter. Dopamine, for example, is the transmitter of the neurons that wake the sleeping brain; noradrenaline is the hypothalamic transmitter that controls the temperature of the body.

In the case of dopaminergic, noradrenergic and adrenergic nerve fibres, the transmitter is put out at nerve-endings throughout the length of the nerve fibre; this was mentioned above as being typical of the sympathetic system. These nerve-endings along the course of the nerve fibre form little swellings, giving the fibre a beadlike appearance under the miscroscope. Any nerve fibre or blood-vessel being accompanied or surrounded by a sympathetic nerve fibre is effectively in a tube of transmitter; it is bathed in the substance throughout its course.

Transmitters are chemically altered so that they do not act for too long. If they continued to work, rapidly repeated effects on muscles or neurons could not be achieved. As a nerve-ending may deliver many hundred impulses a second, the membrane being affected must be able to respond to each impulse, and so the transmitter must be activated and inactivated at a rate of at least several hundred times a second. There are enzymes at the synapse capable of denaturing the transmitter at this rate. For example there is an enzyme that breaks down acetylcholine into its components, acetic acid and choline; and to all intents and purposes choline has no transmitter properties, being 1/1000th part as active as acetylcholine. In the cases of adrenergic, noradrenergic, and dopaminergic nerve-endings, most of the transmitter is brought back again into the nerve-ending so that it can be used again.

In addition to neurotransmitters, there are neuromodulators. They usually last longer than transmitters. In most cases they have similar action to the transmitter which they accompany. One and the same neuron may put out a modulator and a transmitter. This is like going to get tickets for the opera when there are not many available. The transmitter is the payment for the ticket. The modulator is a present to the box office attendant to soften her up, so that when the payment for the ticket is handed over, she is modulated in your favour and accepts your money for the ticket rather than somebody else's. You can also have modulators working the other way; they tend to reduce the reaction to the transmitter. In this case, the box office attendant is annoyed that you thought of bribing her and she is likely to refuse your money.

Our categories of things and mechanisms are not recognized by the body; and so there may be in some ways no great differences between transmitters and modulators. Often the difference appears to be a matter of duration of effect. GABA can act only for milliseconds, acetylcholine and dopamine can act for $\frac{1}{2}$–1 second, some peptides, such as substance P, can act for a minute or so, and others, such as prolactin, can act for hours. These varying durations are mechanisms for altering the thresholds of post-synaptic neurons so that when excitatory and inhibitory inputs arrive, they have different effects than they otherwise would have had.

Chemically, modulators are peptides. Most of their names are inappropriate as they were named according to the tissue in which they were first found or according to the first function that was investigated. Thus thyrotrophin releasing hormone, luteotrophin, and α -melanocyte stimulating hormone occur not only in the hypothalamus and pituitary gland but also in the eye and in many of the peripheral nerve fibres throughout the body. Vasoactive intestinal peptide acts on blood vessels, dilating them and increasing the local blood supply. In sweating, the transmitter acting on the sweat-glands is acetylcholine; the modulator is vasoactive intestinal peptide. This peptide increases the blood flow so that sweat can be made from the locally passing blood.

Now that the chemical constitution of many transmitters and modulators has been worked out, it has been possible to synthesize them and give them as pills or by injection. That they work when given this way is surprising. But it is less surprising if they act throughout the course of nerve fibres than if they act only in the few minute areas of synapses. Swamping parts of the brain or spinal cord with the transmitter could then be imagined to make up for an absence or deficiency of the substance brought about by some illness. The most successful replacement therapy of this kind has been the treatment of Parkinsonism. In this condition there is atrophy and death of the neurons of the basal ganglia and related regions of the brain that work by secreting dopamine. The patient takes l-dopa, which is changed in the body to dopamine. This reduces the stiffness of Parkinsonism, it often removes the tremor and it can improve the difficulty in starting movements, which is one of the main troubles of this affliction. It is also possible to make other substances to block the action of transmitters. Chemicals that block the action of dopamine are used in the treatment of schizophrenia. One hypothesis is that this disorder is due to lack of noradrenaline in the rewarding system; this system is described on page 138. It is also suggested that in psychotic depression, monoaminergic transmitters are diminished or disturbed in some unknown way. Another hypothesis is that schizophrenia is due to excess of dopamine in some parts of the brain. This idea comes partly from the fact that drugs that help schizophrenia block the dopamine receptors on the post-synaptic membranes. Others think that the dopamine receptors are abnormal in this disease. The present treatment of depression usually consists of giving substances that increase the amount of these transmitters in the brain. Most cases of depression are due to an inherited disturbance of these transmitters, though it is not yet known in what way they are disturbed or if they are secreted in insufficient amounts. Although there is this inherited tendency to become depressed or the opposite, it often needs events in the person's life to bring on each episode.

An indication that mental or psychiatric disorders might be caused by the absence or the wrong working of a neurotransmitter appeared when reserpine was used in the West for the treatment of high blood pressure. In India and Ceylon, a plant called in Europe *Rauwolfia* had been used for centuries by native practioners of medicine. When this plant was investigated by pharmacologists, a substance named reserpine was isolated; it became the first effective drug for lowering the blood pressure. But an unwanted side-effect was depression. If quite normal people became depressed when they were taking this substance, then the state of depression could be induced by a chemical substance, and it might be induced too by a chemical substance made in the body. People in general find it difficult to imagine that their moods and mental behaviour are due to chemistry. Further research on reserpine and related substances showed that it stopped the storage of monoamine transmitters in the central nervous system. These discoveries opened up the era of the treatment of mental disease by drugs.

The cell bodies of neurons are continually making many substances and sending these along their axons. As well as the transmitters, there are solutions of proteins that are sent down the axon and out at the nerve-endings. These substances are supplied to the structure on which the nerve fibre ends; it may be another neuron or a muscle fibre or the skin. This is a two-way traffic. Minute particles of substances also pass the other way, from the tissue supplied, along the axon to the cell body. Some of them do not stop there but pass through the dendrites and the cell-body out through the synaptic gap to the next neuron. In this way, a substance made in a muscle fibre, for instance, might pass into the central nervous system and right up to the brain.

The nerve fibre is not only a telegraph wire; it is also a vacuum transport system. It is like those vacuum tubes they have in some shops which whizz bills and other messages in a little capsule up and down and all over the place. On its outside the nerve fibre is a telegraph wire; inside it is a vacuum communicating system. But it is more cleverly designed than that, for it can send substances in both directions at the same time, and at different speeds.

12 Moving

For God has blessed him in the variety of his movements.
For, tho he cannot fly, he is an excellent clamberer.
For his motions upon the face of the earth are more than any other quadrupede.
For he can tread to all measures upon the musick.
For he can swim for life.
For he can creep.

Plants are merely moved; animals move. Movements are brought about by muscles, and muscles are made to contract by nerves coming from the spinal cord and brain.

In general, small animals move more quickly than large. Small birds move their wings far more rapidly than large birds, and the largest birds prefer to glide and soar on currents of air. One of the smaller humming-birds beats its wings eighty times a second. It is very small, weighing only two grams. There is a very short distance between the wing muscles and the spinal cord, so that the nerve impulses soon reach the muscles. In larger humming-birds, this distance is longer and so the rate of wing-beating can be slower. One weighing twenty grams beats its wings eight to ten times a second. The speed of flight achieved by some birds is amazing. The fastest speed achieved by any animal is the 150–200 miles an hour of the large spine-tailed swift of Asia.

Each nerve impulse arriving at the muscle fibres makes them contract once; this is so for all vertebrates and nearly all insects; but wasps and bees, flies, mosquitoes and some bugs, including the aphids of our gardens, work their wing muscles on a different plan. These muscles contract at a faster rate than their receipt of nerve impulses. This system allows the honey-bee to beat its wings at a rate of 200 to 250 beats a second, the mosquito at a rate of 580 beats a second, and the midge that holds the record at 1046 beats a second.

How the nerves work the muscles

Throughout biology one sees a few mechanisms and a few structures being used in many different ways; there is a general pattern with many variations on it. We have already seen how some of the characteristics of membranes surrounding cells are developed and used in different ways. The passage of ions through the membrane, some passing easily and others with difficulty, governs the mechanism of the nerve impulse; and at synapses this selective permeability to ions is used to excite and to inhibit the post-synaptic membrane. The warmth receptors of the skin which are used for controlling body temperature are used in certain vipers to detect the warmth emitted by their prey.

An example of this variation on a basic theme can be seen in the way nerve impulses are delivered at the neuro-muscular junction. For here, where the motor nerve reaches the muscle, there is a modified synapse, similar to those used within the central nervous system.

When the nerve impulse reaches the nerve-ending in the muscle, it puts out a small amount of acetylcholine. This substance unites with the membrane covering the muscle fibre. This is similar to a synapse in the central nervous system. The region where the nerve fibre joins the muscle fibre is called the motor end-plate. It is an enormously enlarged synapse, thrown into folds. The nerve-endings are similar to those in the central nervous system but they are far larger and are full of vesicles containing acetylcholine. As in the central nervous system, the nerve impulse works by using this chemical transmitter which unites with the post-synaptic membranes. This causes depolarization which spreads along the membrane of the muscle fibre. From the membrane an electrical event passes to the muscle fibre and evokes a biochemical event. That makes the proteins of the muscle fibres contract. At this point, we take leave of the peripheral nervous system and enter the realm of protein molecules; that realm is outside the territory of this book.

The skeletal muscles, those you can see beneath the skin, are all cholinergic, being made to contract by the secretion of acetylcholine. There are many other sorts of muscle in the body; they make up the bladder, the uterus, the gut, the heart and the blood-vessels. The muscle fibres that make up the viscera and the blood-vessels are called smooth or unstriated muscles, the skeletal muscles being known as striated muscles, owing to their microscopic appearances. To make the skeletal muscles contract, nerve impulses have to be brought to every muscle fibre. But the current supplied by the nerve fibres to smooth muscle is passed on by electrotonic spread from muscle fibre to muscle fibre. Neurotransmitters for smooth muscles are noradrenalin, adrenalin, and acetylcholine.

Reflexes for posture and movement

> For thirdly he works it upon stretch with fore-paws extended.

In biology and in engineering there are at least two classes of self-regulating systems—stabilizing and tracking systems. Both of them are used for maintaining posture and for moving. Two examples of stabilizing systems have been discussed so far—the balance of the body and the adjustment of the amount of light to the retina. A typical tracking system is following a moving target with a rifle. In a tracking system, the reference input is continually changing and the output has to follow these changes quickly and accurately. In a stabilizing system the output has to be maintained at the same level as constant, pre-set input. In both systems, the controlling elements have to be continuously informed of what is happening. It would be useless to send out instructions without seeing whether they were being followed or not. The central nervous system has to be kept informed continuously about the rate and the amount of a movement that is occurring, about the position of the limb and of its parts, about the force it is exerting, and about the effectiveness of any correction of error that it is making.

Posture and movement are based on reflexes. The word 'reflex' was introduced in the last century by a neurologist from Nottingham called Marshall Hall to designate the response of a muscle or a group of muscles to a stimulus that excited an afferent nerve. He explained that he chose this word as the muscle reflected the stimulus, just as a wall reflects a ball thrown against it. Since the introduction of the word a hundred and fifty years ago, the meaning has become enlarged and also more rigorous. It is now used to mean an inborn, immediate response of muscles or glands to a particular stimulus affecting the nervous system. Contrary to what people seem to think, reflex responses are not the same on every occasion. The response can diminish or increase, involving fewer or more muscle fibres, lasting a shorter or longer time. The changing pattern of response of reflexes in the lower limbs of human beings with the spinal cord totally divided has been studied by M. R. Dimitrijević and myself. If one keeps on tapping the tendon below the knee-cap to induce the knee-jerk, the amount of response at first increases and then decreases. When it has become very small, it can be brought back to its original size by suddenly increasing the strength of the tap on the tendon or by stimulating the leg in any way.

Neurologists group the muscles of the trunk and limbs into flexors and extensors; in the limbs there are also adductors, abductors and rotators. The movements of vertebrates are mostly based on a pattern of contraction of one set of muscles with simultaneous relaxation of the antagonist muscles; this is called reciprocal innervation. An obvious example is seen in the movements of breathing. As the muscles for inspiration contract, the muscles for expiration relax, and when we breathe out, it is the other way round. To achieve reciprocal innervation, the neurons of one set of muscles have to be excited while those of the antagonist set are inhibited. The afferent nerves from the muscle spindles excite the neurons of the muscle in which they are situated and inhibit the neurons of their antagonists. For certain postures and movements, it is necessary to remove reciprocal innervation; it may be necessary to contract the muscles of antagonist groups together, flexors and extensors, adductors and abductors. This is needed for standing and keeping upright.

Man has been walking about upright for 5 to 10 million years. His way of standing and walking makes use of an arched foot and an erect trunk. His cousin, the ape, walks on flat feet and remains bent at the knee-joints.

Vertebrates which raise their bodies off the ground make use of the very force, gravity, that is pulling them towards the ground, to keep upright. This is done by stretch reflexes; that they maintain posture was discovered by Sherrington early in this century. He showed that stretch reflexes keep the head up and the limbs taut; they hold the abdominal wall and abdominal floor in, so that the viscera do not flop down and forwards. Stretch reflexes adjust the amount of contraction and relaxation of muscles all over the body. A diagram of a spinal stretch reflex is shown in Fig. 12.1.

When a muscle is pulled on or stretched, the stretch stimulates the receptors within the muscle spindles. They discharge impulses to the spinal cord. The impulses end up on the motoneurons of the muscle, excite them, and they send impulses back to the muscle, making it contract. When the weight or the stretch is taken off the muscle, the spindle receptors cease to be stimulated, impulses from the muscle no longer reach the motoneurons, they stop firing off impulses, and the muscle relaxes. Thus pulling the muscle makes it contract, and relaxing it causes it to relax. So that the spindles can be used as the receptors for stretch, they have to be kept taut; this is done by muscle fibres within the spindles. Figure 12.1 shows the main muscle fibre, above it the spindle receptor with the small muscle fibres at its two ends, the afferent fibre from the spindle receptor ending up on the main motoneuron. It also shows a small motoneuron; this is the one controlling the small muscle fibres of the muscle spindle.

This spinal stretch reflex has only one synapse between the afferent nerve fibres and the motoneurons. Monosynaptic reflexes like this one are rare. Most reflexes have several synapses between the afferent nerve fibres and the final motor fibres that adjust posture or bring about a movement. The general tautness or tone of muscles depends on stretch

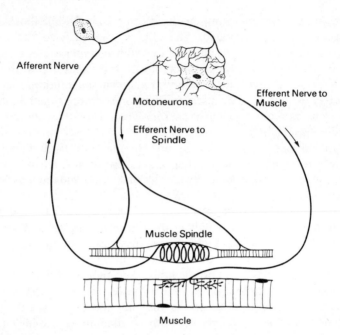

Fig. 12.1. Diagram of spinal stretch reflex.

reflexes having two or three synapses in their path. The contraction of muscles all over the body to adjust for postural changes depends on stretch reflexes with a path up to the cerebral hemispheres and back. The more synapses there are on a pathway, the more modifications can be introduced into the reflex.

Mammals in which the spinal cord has been cut across cannot stand. But chickens which have had their heads cut off can run around the farmyard minus a head; their legs work perfectly, their wings flap in conjunction, and even their balance is adequate. The movements continue until all the blood is pumped out of the carotid arteries, and the loss of blood brings these reflex movements to an end. Snakes continue to perform their serpentine movements after their heads have been cut off and move along the ground. Beheaded eels are capable of all the movements of which eels are capable when possessed of heads. If a frog or toad is decapitated while it is copulating, its headless trunk continues to clasp the female, faithful beyond death.

In man, the spinal cord may be cut through and separated from the brain by wounds, accident or disease. A bullet may be shot right through the spinal cord. This leaves the patient with two separated central nervous systems. He has his brain and a certain length of spinal cord above, and the rest of the spinal cord below; and there is no neural connexion between the two. If this injury occurs in the neck, death comes soon; for breathing ceases.

When the spinal cord gets cut through by some injury or disease process, spastic paralysis develops. In spastic limbs, many muscles are contracting at the same time and so the limb is stiff or spastic. The essential reason is that motoneurons are generally very excitable. They fire off spontaneously and also in response to every sort of stimulation; and they go on firing off impulses for a far longer time than normal. As these motoneurons command the muscles of the limbs and the back and abdomen, the abdominal wall may contract as hard as a board, the back may be arched, and the two legs are held firmly pressed together, either extended straight out or bent up. In the normal undamaged nervous system, there are mechanisms that control this spread of excitement throughout the spinal cord. One of these mechanisms of inhibitory braking is recurrent inhibition. From the nerve fibres going to supply the muscles, a small branch turns round within the spinal cord and goes to a number of motoneurons; it is an inhibitory branch and so it stops the continuous firing of the motoneurons. This mechanism no longer works when the spinal cord is separated from the brain. The lack of inhibition of motoneurons causing spasticity is not the main reason for the paralysis of the divided spinal cord; the main reason is that the spinal motoneurons are no longer connected to the brain, and it is the brain that orders our movements.

In the patients with the spinal cord divided, a condition known as paraplegia, the bladder and bowels work automatically, the patient being unable to control them. They carry on independently, as in a baby. When the central nervous system is intact, this control is organized by many parts of the brain. The front parts of the cerebral hemispheres are the region of most importance for voluntary control. When circumstances prevent us from emptying the bladder and we have to keep it full for an hour or so, it is this part of the brain that stops reflex emptying of the bladder. Like all skilful movements, this control has to be learned and practised. Using this region of the brain, we also make the bladder or rectum empty when we decide it is a convenient moment. Many other animals have acquired these skills. We may observe this in the dog. This animal uses urine to map out his territory; and as we all know he has difficulty in passing a tree or lamp-post without leaving his mark. The quantity of urine secreted is insufficient for this social use; and so we see the male dog cocking a leg and going through all the movements of emptying the bladder, even though there is no urine to pass.

Four-legged vertebrates have three patterns of walking, running, creeping and crawling. In the diagonal pattern they move the limbs in the following order: right forelimb, left hindlimb, left forelimb, right hindlimb. In this pattern, the two limbs on one side are in opposite phases of movement at the same time, the one flexed, the other extended. In the second pattern, the two limbs of one side are coupled together: the animal flexes both the fore- and hind-limb of one side and extends both limbs of the other side. In the third pattern, the animal flexes both forelimbs together and then extends them together, doing the same with the hindlimbs. The first pattern the usual pattern of the human infant crawling and of quadrupeds walking, trotting and swimming. These patterns are built into the spinal cord and they do not require reflexes from the foot touching the ground. You can see this by holding a small dog above a stream or swimming pool. He will make the usual dog-stroke swimming movements as you lower him towards the water. The same movements continue in the water and when the feet touch dry land. The brain sets the pattern of movement going and it then continues as long as the dog needs to move. The pattern in which the two forelimbs flex and extend together with the two hindlimbs working together is the pattern of galloping, leaping and jumping. The pattern in which the two limbs of one side flex and extend together is called pacing. Most quadrupeds do not use it but the camel does; that is what makes its body swing from side to side.

The three patterns can be mixed together. When human beings walk, they use their upper limbs in the trotting pattern, the diagonal pattern of movement. If one uses ones limbs in a pacing pattern, extending the two limbs of one side together and flexing the other limbs, one looks rather odd.

A newborn baby can walk if it is held up. Take a baby and hold him so that his feet are planted on a table. This firm contact causes a reflex contraction of the extensor muscles of the lower limbs; and it is so effective that the baby takes its own weight. Then lean your baby forwards and at the same time extend his head by pushing his chin up. He will then walk beautifully and enjoy it. This reflex walking lasts only about two months. There are other reflex games one can play with babies. For example, hold the baby just by a table; move him so that the front of his leg touches the edge of the table. Lo and behold, the baby reflexly lifts his leg and places the foot on the table. This reflex, occurring in many vertebrates, is called the tactile placing reaction. It also goes off in a few months, as the nervous system matures.

Whereabouts in the brain various reflexes are built in has been learned from the appalling deformed babies born with all the higher parts of the brain absent and replaced by a bag of fluid. Only the spinal cord and the lower levels of the brain are there. These deformed babies breathe, suck swallow and vomit, When the skin around the corner of the baby's mouth is touched, the head is turned round towards the stimulus, the mouth is opened; and if it is touched with a nipple, a finger or a stick, this object will be sucked. A baby like this can yawn, cough, belch and sneeze; it also can perform the reflexes built into the spinal cord. It empties its bladder and bowels, like a normal baby; it sleeps and can be woken up.

Many of the movements organized by the spinal cord and the lower part of the brain are working before the baby is born, as every mother knows. Some mothers-to-be have had a tea-cup kicked out of their hands, the kick coming from within.

Human embryos removed by operation can be kept alive for many minutes; and important researches on these specimens have been carried out in the United States. From these investigations, we now know that movements can be obtained from stimulating human fetuses aged $7\frac{1}{2}$ weeks from conception. The first movement obtainable is a movement of the neck away from the stimulus when the mouth is touched. The $9\frac{1}{2}$ weeks old fetus opens the mouth when stimulated around the mouth; at $10\frac{1}{2}$ weeks, this stimulus makes it carry out swallowing movements as well. At this time it bends its toes and its fingers when the sole or the palm is stimulated. A little later, stimulation around the anus makes the fetus contract the sphincter muscle, closing this orifice.

Reflexes developed when the baby is still in the womb are all ready to be used after birth. The sucking reflex evoked by touch on the baby's lips and the complicated swallowing reflexes evoked when anything touches the back of the throat are ready for immediate use. There are reflex movements evoked by light. During the first few days of life, the baby turns its eyes and head towards a light; but if the light is too bright, it will shut its eyes. Within fifteen days, the baby will follow objects moved horizontally in its field of vision, first with its eyes, and then by turning its head. Within a few moments of birth, the baby turns its eyes, both together, in the direction of a noise made near one of its ears.

But the baby is not just a reflex organism. It arrives ready to explore. It explores the mother's body to find the nipple. Later it starts looking, listening, moving its arms out to touch and feel. It is active, not passive.

Reflexes are not just for standing and walking, for sucking, coughing, swallowing and vomiting. For instance, there are flexion reflexes, having the purpose of removing the limb from something likely to damage it. If something very hot touches you, you find that your hand is pulled away so quickly that it has all happened before you know anything about it. By means of electrical recording it is possible to time the events in this reflex to an accuracy of a thousandth of a second. It can then be calculated that the hand is pulled away before any information reaches the cerebral cortex to tell you what has happened. If you tread on a thorn, it takes about a twentieth of a second for the nerve impulses to get to the spinal cord and back to the muscles pulling your foot away, but it takes a fifth of a second, four times as long, for the impulses to get up to the brain and back to the muscles of the limb. In a giraffe it takes even longer; it would take a third of a second for impulses running in the fastest-conducting fibres to reach the brain from one of its feet.

The organization of the total response to a painful stimulus follows the usual pattern employed among the higher mammals. At first, there is an emergency response, effective, possibly too crude. The event is then reported to the higher parts of the central nervous system, where it can be considered and fitted in with everything else that is going on at that moment. Further action is then taken. This takes longer, but it has the advantage that it fits in better with the total situation of the animal at the time. These higher level contributions are not reflex. They break through reflex responses and substitute something better suited to the whole situation.

Animals with fur or feathers have a scratch reflex, designed to remove insects and other irritants. The pathway of this reflex within the spinal cord is a long one, for something irritating the animal at the back of the head brings the hindlimb forward to scratch this bit of skin. The scratch reflex can easily be evoked in dogs by tickling the skin of the back or sides; you can often get it by tickling them just behind the shoulders. Then the dogs stops whatever he is doing, distributes his weight on three legs, and scratches for as long as you go on tickling him.

Reflexes designed to take care of the body are organized not only for damage arriving from outside. There are reflexes to get rid of irritants already in the body, sneezing to get things out of the nose, coughing to get them out of the trachea, and vomiting to get them out of the stomach.

Changes in reflexes

Reflexes are not inevitable and fixed; but the very first part of a reflex may be difficult to change. They can be controlled, diminished, obliterated, suppressed, amplified and developed. This can be done by all those factors that we call mental, emotional or psychological, including suggestion and hypnosis. The more neurons and synapses there are in a reflex pathway, the more modifications there can be introduced into the reflex. We can do very little to change the knee-jerk and nothing to alter the pupil's reaction to light and dark. But we can train ourselves to suppress the gag reflex, the reflex that makes us retch when something touches the back of the throat. The reflex watering of the mouth, on which Pavlov concentrated, depends largely on training. A convinced vegetarian's mouth would probably not water when he smells steak cooking, whereas most other people's would.

At the lower levels of the central nervous system, the more stereotyped and simple reflexes are organized. They consist of three or four neurons with two or three synapses in between. Above this, further interneuronal pathways are available, the time for the reflex effects taking a little longer and a greater variety of effects becoming available. Above the spinal cord, the different regions of the brain can be brought into the reflex cycle. Further modification of the effects is achieved. And finally the whole brain including the cerebral hemispheres can add their contribution. In this case, we no longer talk of reflexes. But nothing essentially different has occurred. Further and further pathways and synapses have been introduced into the cycle so that more modifications to behaviour can be achieved.

For example, the movements of the legs in running are organized by the lower levels of the spinal cord. This simple and stereotyped movement is then altered so that it becomes the skilled movement of running over uneven ground, jumping over a puddle, and continuing to run while looking back over the shoulder. Swallowing is a simple stereotyped movement organized by the lower level of the brain. It becomes the final part of the more complicated movements of eating, tasting and considering the food.

The more complicated and delicate the movement, the more learning is used, and the greater the part played by the higher levels of the brain. The highest levels of the brain can also control many simple reflex activities. The control of otherwise automatic reflex functions is a speciality of Indian fakirs and those adept in Yoga. Reflexes can also be altered and controlled at spinal level. When the spinal cord is cut across in very young kittens or puppies, a great deal of compensation for this injury to the central nervous system can occur. With care and training, these animals can be taught to walk and stand. The reflexes needed for these skills can be developed in these baby animals far more easily than in adult animals. Kozak and Westerman carried out some important investigations of the changes that can be induced in built-in reflexes of the spinal cord of the kitten. They showed that by rubbing the skin for ten minutes daily or putting a hind-limb in ice-cold or hot water daily, they could alter or suppress the built-in reflexes. This constituted one of the many examples of proof in the laboratory for what has been obvious to clinical observers for a long time: that patients with the spinal cord divided show similar changes in reflexes. Doctors and physiotherapists who treat these patients see many examples of how they can alter, suppress and encourage various reflex postures and movements. They can train the bowels and the bladders of these patients to empty their contents reflexly in response to various forms of stimulation or to do so daily at a certain time.

Standing

Standing depends on balancing, particularly for two-legged creatures like ourselves; and moving requires even better balancing. We only have to move an arm or bend the head backwards, and we have altered the centre of gravity. To deal with this change, some muscles of the trunk and the limbs are contracted and others are relaxed; this happens without us being aware of it. One can do a striking experiment to illustrate this automatic adjustment. We fix electrodes which record the activity of two or three muscles of the legs and then convert this activity into sound, playing it through a loudspeaker. There is silence or almost silence when the person is standing. But if he is given a slight push or if he raises one arm, we hear a thunderstorm of activity in the muscles of his legs. All this reflex activity is constantly going on without us being aware of any of it. It maintains our posture and gives us a firm base on which our movements are built. Like many other more complicated reflexes, these reflexes have to be practised and developed; and the baby and young child spend a lot of time learning to do this.

Standing is based on many reflexes. For one of these, the extensor thrust reflex, impulses coming from the foot go to the spinal cord and make all muscles of the leg contract together, so as to turn the limb into a rigid pillar. When the foot leaves the ground, the muscles of the foot are no longer stretched, the muscles of the leg relax, and the limb becomes loose again.

When we stand, gravity is pulling on our bodies and limbs, tending to make us fall to the ground. But this pull on the muscles evokes their stretch reflexes; the muscles then contract and oppose the pull of gravity.

Thus the very force that tends to make the animal fold up and fall is used to keep it standing upright.

Standing on two legs depends on postural reflexes. They are essential to keep the trunk straight and upright and in line with the head and neck. Postural reflexes also need utricles in the inner ears. Man also uses postural reflexes based on vision; although they are important, they are not essential; we do not fall over when we shut our eyes. When the baby is born, postural reflexes are not yet developed; they start working during the first few months of life. At about the sixth month, the baby reflexly contracts certain muscles to compensate for being tipped when he is sitting. As he becomes better at sitting, these reflexes develop further and they stop him falling over. They become fully developed as he learns to stand.

When we start to walk, we allow the body to lean forwards. This changes the centre of gravity, moving it forwards, downwards and slightly laterally. In order not to fall, one foot has to be moved forwards. When this foot touches the ground, the weight is transferred to it. At the same time the other foot pushes on the ground, giving the propulsive force to move the body forwards. Then this foot leaves the ground and swings forwards. When it reaches the ground in front of the other foot, the heel strikes the ground first. Then the weight of the body is put onto this limb. In normal walking both feet are on the ground together for about a quarter of each step; for the rest of the time we are balancing on one limb. And so walking depends on the good control of balance. The baby cannot walk until he has acquired control of reflexes concerned with balance. The main difference between running and walking is that in running both feet are off the ground at the same time and both feet are never on the ground simultaneously.

The reflexes necessary for standing and stepping are built into the spinal cord. Reciprocal innervation, holding the legs stiff as pillars, the co-ordination of all four limbs in stepping, these are all organized by the spinal cord. In the cat, in which this has been investigated, there are two small regions in the middle of the brain, in the brainstem, in which the total act of walking and running is organized. If this small region is electrically stimulated, the front part of the brain having been removed, the unconscious cat stands up on its legs and begins to walk. As the region is more intensely stimulated, the faster the running becomes. Normally, this brainstem region is controlled by parts of the brain that are further forward. They command the lower regions to walk or run, and these regions merely set the apparatus of the spinal cord in motion.

Once we have mastered the skill of standing, only very few muscles are used. The muscles are contracted just enough to correct the tendency to sway and to keep the centre of gravity in the central line of the body. This economy of the use of muscles is an example of the effect of practice and training. The more used to carrying out a posture or a movement one becomes, the more relaxed one is and the less muscles one uses, the less work is done, the less tired one becomes.

To attain these skills, the child is helped by its mother and others around it. This is not a feature of humans only. Chimpanzees teach their babies to do all the movements of which they are capable. Professor Yerkes, who spent many years studying chimpanzees and gorillas at Yale University, relates that the chimpanzee mother helps her baby 'to stand, first on all fours, then on its feet, and she lures it to walk toward her as she backs away'.

There are some essential differences between a statue of a man made of metal or stone and a man of flesh and blood. The real man can balance, and if he is pushed off balance, he corrects the tendency to fall. All animals which walk on two legs, such as penguins, bears and men, must control the centre of gravity all the time, for it changes with every step and every movement of the trunk and upper limbs. One of the most impressive sights is that of an ostrich or a crane firmly planted on its stilt legs with its head bent right over and its beak touching the ground. But the less beautiful sight of a human being in the same position is really more astounding. For whereas nearly all the weight of the bird remains above its legs and feet and only a very small proportion is bent over in front, with human beings this is not so. If one bends forward with the upper limbs also hanging down, probably a half of one's total weight is hanging well forward of the legs and feet. Many receptors contribute to this achievement. The final co-ordination is organized by the basal ganglia. When the body or any part of it is tilted, or when the ground is uneven, the basal ganglia arrange muscles to compensate for the changing conditions. The basal ganglia are always receiving impulses from the labyrinths. In man, when the labyrinths are destroyed or damaged, the eyes can compensate for the organ of balance. When the labyrinths are destroyed and the basal ganglia have been damaged by some disease, the patient needs his eyes even to keep his head upright; when he closes his eyes, his head falls forward. When the basal ganglia are damaged, the patient is liable to fall if he is pushed, as the compensating adjustments of the muscles are inadequate and late.

The basal ganglia are degenerate in Parkinsonism. Patients with this disorder have difficulty in starting movements, in stopping them, and in changing from one movement to the next. All movements are slow.

Neurons of the basal ganglia that work by putting out the transmitter dopamine are degenerate. This lack can be treated by giving l-dopa, a compound that is changed in the body to dopamine. Neurons working by emitting other transmitters are also degenerate in Parkinsonism; and research is being undertaken to try and make up for the lack of these transmitters.

The contribution of the cerebellum

For he can jump over a stick which is patience upon proof positive.

There is a very large part of the brain filling the back of the skull, looking somewhat like a miniature version of the cerebral hemispheres; it is therefore called the cerebellum. It is shown in Plates 10, 11 and 12. It first developed to organize the information coming from the vestibular apparatus and the lateral line organ in primitive fish. In all animals it remains near the vestibular apparatus; and one of its functions is to co-ordinate movements with the changing centre of gravity and to keep the animal upright and in a correct posture.

The cerebellum underwent much development with the evolution of birds from primitive reptiles; for birds' rapid movements in three dimensions of space demand perfect timing and balance.

When the parts of the cerebral hemispheres that organize movement send impulses to the spinal cord, probably a replica of the instructions is sent to the cerebellum. As the spinal cord carries out the instructions, it reports back to the cerebellum how the movement is being carried out. With these two inputs the cerebellum can function as an error-measuring device, comparing the actual performance with the instructions. It may be, too, that every programme of movement is compared with instructions for this movement stored from previous occasions; and that this allows the cerebellum to correct the movements in relation to previous programmes of the movement.

When the cerebellum is damaged or degenerates, the error between the movement being performed and the original programme of the movement is no longer continuously corrected. The patient walks as if he is drunk. As he stands, he keeps his legs wide apart, giving himself a wide base on which to balance. When he moves, there are jerky tremors of his limbs. The hands overshoot as he tries to reach something. This is because the movement is no longer limited by impulses from the cerebellum. The patient may even be unsteady as he sits; his head jerks continually and his whole trunk may sway. His speech is affected in the same way. The flow of the sentence is broken up into short jerks, for the patient's breathing is poorly co-ordinated with the muscles of the mouth, pharynx and tongue.

The contribution of the cerebral hemispheres

> For he can jump from an eminence into his master's bosom.
> For he can catch the cork and toss it again.

We know from the various animals with which we are familiar that their young are born with every degree of prowess in movement. The newborn goat can stand at birth and in a few hours it jumps around and gambols. It is the same with the deer and the gnu, which immediately after birth get up and follow close to their mothers. Foals too can stand almost immediately and they very soon walk. The new born dolphin can swim, it can remain under water and 'knows' to come up to the surface to breathe. The seal, however, cannot swim and needs to be enticed into the water.

Animals like deer which can jump and run at birth are taught to improve these skills by their mothers; chimpanzees, orang-utans and gorillas teach their babies to climb. Games that human children play are also played by deer and primates. Chimpanzees and deer play 'I'm king of the castle'. Young chimpanzees play 'tag' or 'touch-last'; and when they are brought up with human babies they play the pretence hiding game of 'peekaboo'; and they enjoy making towers of toy bricks and pulling wheeled toys around on string.

Many parts of the brain higher than the cerebellum contribute to organizing movement. 'Higher' does not only mean anatomically higher, that is higher up in the head than the parts of the nervous system just above the spinal cord; it means higher in the sense that these parts have been developed later and are less automatic and more capable of modification in their behaviour. When certain whole sequences of movement are needed, these higher parts of the brain send down orders for these totalities. The higher parts know nothing of flexor and extensor muscles, of the organization of reciprocal innervation, of arranging the muscles and the parts in the right order, of seeing that the centre of gravity is maintained while the trunk is moved forward. The spinal cord can organize the movements of running; the cerebellum and related parts of the brain can arrange these movements so that the animal keeps its balance when running. The totality of running is organized at higher levels of the brain.

Many innate movements of the body need no contribution from the cerebral hemispheres; such movements are crying, sneezing, coughing, swallowing, belching and vomiting. Some other total conjunctions of movement are innate. A young child may throw itself down on its back, and yell with rage; it has never seen anyone else doing this.

If the organisation of a movement is innate, that does not mean that it is present at birth. It means that it manifests itself without needing learning and imitation. In higher vertebrates, many kinds of movements are innate, though they become manifest only at certain times after birth. Walking, running, jumping are innate in man; normally they are learned with encouragement from others, but doubtless infants left to their own devices would acquire these movements on their own. Swimming, curiously enough, is not innate; for although all races develop it, human beings who have not learned it can drown. Man's cousin, the chimpanzee, cannot swim and is frightened of water; he also dislikes rain. The orang-utan cannot swim either. It is not known for certain whether the gorilla swims or not; there are reports that they cross rivers. Professor Yerkes considered that there was no evidence about the gibbon's ability to swim. Certainly a male and female gibbon I knew in Bangkok were not afraid of the rapidly flowing water of a river by which they lived, and they would spend a lot of time fishing floating debris out of the river.

Even complicated sequences of movements may be innate. Squirrels bury the nuts they do not want when they are replete, and press down the earth over their hidden treasure. Every part of this sequence of movements is innate.

When we practise a series of movements, such as those needed for playing the piano, information is repeatedly sent to the spinal cord, to the cerebellum and to various parts of the cerebral hemispheres. Some part of the central nervous system monitors the discharge of nerve impulses that are sent off to perform a sequence of movements. Information about the movement, as it is being performed, is then compared with the pattern of impulses being sent out.

Since all movements are improved by practice, it seems that the pattern of signals sent to the relevant parts of the nervous system must be stored. Otherwise we would be like children trying to do something for the first time whenever we tried to repeat a pattern of movements. There must be a kind of memory for movements. But we do not know how practice improves the efficiency of any skill. It is needed to acquire even those skills we learned so long ago that we have forgotten all about it, the skills of sitting, standing, walking. Practising must be done at the right time. Experiments done in the United States have shown that monkeys brought up with their limbs encased in cardboard cylinders never learn to use them properly, remain abnormally clumsy, and cannot acquire all the deft movements characteristic of their race. In such an experiment, repeated and necessary information has been withheld from many levels of the nervous system at a time when it was essential; if this information comes later, it is too late.

We take for granted all the skills we acquired before we knew what we were doing. For instance, we have to learn to work our two hands together and, perhaps more difficult, to work one without the other, and to do different things with the two hands. The ability to touch with our fingers the things we can see is a skill we learn during the first year of life. This co-ordination of hand and eye is particularly developed in higher primates. It must have been essential for living in trees in an upright posture. Squirrels and parrots seem to have it also. All of this has to be learned. It takes weeks for the child to learn to know the feel of a cube or of a ball in the hand; and this knowledge is not automatically transferred from one hand to the other. All such cognitive skills are normally acquired as the child plays. For children's play is not just a diversion like the golf or tennis of adults. It is an important and essential part of neural learning. All higher mammals play and use this play to train both the sensory and motor parts of their nervous systems. One can see this occurring with otters, dogs, cats and foxes.

So necessary is the stimulation from the environment in some cases that the movements never develop without it. A striking example of this occurred a few years ago in America. For certain work, it was necessary to breed white mice quite free from any bacteria. This meant that immediately after birth the newborn mice had to be taken away from their mothers and placed under bacteriologically sterile conditions. All these mice died. When they were dissected after death, it was found their bladders were full to bursting. Their attendants then realized that none of them had passed urine during their short lives. On observing the behaviour of other mice and their babies, they saw that the mothers licked the babies all over. When the mothers licked their babies' genital organs, the babies emptied their bladders. It was apparent that this external stimulation had to be added to the internal stimulation of a full bladder before the built-in mechanism of bladder emptying could work; without it, the animal could not pass urine and died. Once this was known, they could breed the mice satisfactorily by brushing their genitals with soft paint-brushes. Incidentally, they were surprisingly ignorant about the habits of the animals they kept. Anyone who has kept a bitch which has given birth knows that she noses around and licks the underside of her offspring and that this sets off eliminatory reflexes.

In man, the left cerebral hemisphere is the more important of the two for performing movements; it is the right hemisphere in lefthanded people. The left hemisphere directs the right to carry out movements, to do up buttons, to make signs showing the way, or to stop; but the right hemisphere is bad at directing the left. One would have thought that each hemisphere would have been equally good at organizing the movements of the opposite limbs; but it is not so. The left hemisphere is more important for learned movement; perhaps this is because it is the hemisphere in which speech is organized. The right hemisphere is the more important for movements of the trunk, of the eyes, and for not very skilled movements, such as those of turning round and walking.

From the hemispheres there are two pathways to the parts of the spinal cord that carry out the movements of walking and running. One consists of neurons with very long nerve fibres; they run all the way from the cortex to the motoneurons of the spinal cord. The other consists of linked neurons. In this chain, the last link is from the reticular formation to the motoneurons.

Human beings often make use of speech in learning new sequences of movements. When someone teaches you a new sequence of movements, say a dance or how to swing a golf club, he uses speech to describe and explain it, as well as showing you what to do. And then when you try out the movement, you speak to yourself; you say something like 'I have to move the right foot forward and then bring the left one up to the right one' or 'I must remember to follow through after I have hit the ball.' We use inner speech throughout most of our activities.

Certain kinds of movements develop only under the influence of hormones. Nest-building, sitting on eggs, copulating—these occur only when the correct hormones have their influence on the brain and spinal cord. Under the influence of the hormone prolactin, birds go through all movements needed for constructing nests, though they may never have seen a nest or known what the finished product would be like. In species less developed than primates, the movements of copulation are inborn and do not have to be observed or learned; but they become more efficient with practice. They are inborn but they do not develop till puberty, when certain neurons react to the influences of hormones secreted by the ovaries and testes. No doubt those pretty movements of mother cats as they gently pick up their kittens in their teeth by the loose skin at the back of their necks are not learned but are inborn, though needing the secretion of hormones to come into play. And incidentally the kitten shows an inborn reflex, present at or shortly after birth, when it is picked up in this way; its whole back is flexed, as are its hind-limbs; the fore-limbs remain moderately extended. Thus its hind-limbs are lifted from the ground, it tucks itself into a small space and when it is dropped back into its basket, its fore-limbs are already extended to stop its head hitting the ground.

The effect of hormones on certain sorts of movements can be seen in such an everyday occurrance as a dog passing urine. As we must have all noticed, male puppies do not cock a leg when they pass urine; they crouch a little, round their backs and lower the pelvis. The adult male dog's way of urinating is a secondary sexual characteristic; and it can be induced before the onset of puberty by the injection of testosterone proprionate. Bitches also acquire it if they are given this male hormone. If male puppies are castrated soon after birth, they do not develop the adult male posture for micturition; but they acquire it if they are given this hormone. It does seem curious that the position taken when passing urine should be a secondary sexual characteristic. Doubtless this is associated with the male dog's way of marking out its territory by means of urinary signposts. How the hormone affects certain neurons within the central nervous system to make them work in such a way as to produce a certain posture of the body, we do not know.

Movements organized at lower levels tend to remain intact when disease strikes the nervous system. A common kind of paralysis in man is hemiplegia. The movements controlled by the opposite damaged hemisphere no longer occur, though a few reflex movements organized lower in the brain remain. The patient automatically moves the paralysed arm when he yawns or sneezes though he cannot do so when he wants to pick up a book.

It is no mere figure of speech to say that we are weak with laughing; laughter brings the flexor muscles of our lower limbs into activity. Fear can also bring us to our knees. With these emotions, the body tends to crumple up, bending at the hips and the knees, the trunk flexes, the head and neck bend forward a little. Such movements occurring without our intending to do them show us that the higher levels of the brain, those we use when we intend to do something, are not necessary for all movements.

There is a rare disorder called cataplexy, in which the pathway from parts of the brain particularly concerned with the movements associated with emotion becomes abnormally easily available. Patients with this trouble crumple up and fall to the ground when they experience a strong emotion. Laughing may weaken them so that they fall; you can fell them with a joke. If a patient with cataplexy gets so furious that he wants to hit you, as soon as his emotion gets the better of him, he will fall limp to the ground. I once saw a mother of some young children who had this disorder. When she got so annoyed with them that she wanted to hit them, she just flopped down, unable to move.

13 Pain

Sleep and pain tend to inspire poets and philosophers; micturition and defaecation do not. With psychoanalysts, it is the other way round.

There have always been two different theories of the mechanism of pain, one usually called the quantitative theory and the other nowadays called the stimulus-specific theory. The quantitative theory goes back to Aristotle. The stimulus-specific theory was developed when the scientific investigation of sensation began in the last century.

The quantitative theory considers pain to be result of excessive stimulation: too hot a stimulus, or too cold, too hard a pressure or squeeze, and pain results. The same peripheral nerve fibres are thought to be conducting impulses with the ordinary stimulation as with the painful stimulation; it is just that they are conducting far more impulses per second with the stimulation that causes pain. According to this theory, hot and cold are two extremes of a single temperature-sensing system. A lot of stimulation of the receptors is thought to cause the sensation of hot, little stimulation that of cold, and very intense stimulation causes pain to be added to the other sensations.

The stimulus-specific theory proposes that pain is an independent form of sensation, just as touch is, and warmth and cold are. Each of these sensory systems is thought to be independent of the others, each having its own receptors and each system finally ending in different regions of the cerebral hemispheres.

At present, it seems to be that both theories are right. There are stimulus-specific receptors and nerve fibres, responding to only one kind of stimulus; and there are receptors that respond to more than one kind. Receptors of the muscles report the tension put on the muscle or developed by the muscle itself and nothing else. There are nerve fibres of the skin that are activated only by mechanical events, such as deformation of the skin or pulling or moving it. There are different warm and cold receptors; they are not the two ends of a spectrum, as is required by the quantitative theory. One lot is activated by rising and the others by falling temperature. There are different nerve fibres reporting stimulation that is damaging or threatening to damage the body, and which cause us to feel pain. The stimulus-specific theory of pain and sensation cannot be applied too rigorously. Mechanoreceptors may contribute to pain; nociceptors can cause a sensation of sub-pain.

In the case of the viscera, the quantitative theory fits best. Pain occurs when a large number of impulses are sent to the spinal cord by nerves from the alimentary canal or the bladder. When a moderate number of impulses per second are sent in, one feels the sensation causing the desire to empty the bladder or the rectum.

A sensation is the result of activation of neurons of the cerebral hemispheres. Sensation is not the same thing as the input to lower levels of the nervous system. For this reason one speaks of mechanoreceptors and nociceptors and not of touch fibres or pain fibres, one talks of a noxious or nocuous input and not of pain. Apart from theoretical reasons, this usage is right because some stimulus that is painful to one person may not be so to another or it may be painful on one part of the body and painless on another. One can have pain without damage and damage without pain. Cancer is noxious and can be painless. Phantom limbs that occur after amputations can be painful though innocuous.

Sensations are usually accompanied by emotion. A sudden new sensation in the skin is accompanied by surprise and the emotion of being startled. Sensations can be pleasant or unpleasant. Tickle causes pleasure to young children and it makes babies laugh. Certain rhythms of tactile stimulation or rubbing may be accompanied by pleasure. The right balance of warmth and cold is pleasant, the wrong amount of either is unpleasant. One supposes that the purpose of the accompanying emotion is to teach the animal correct behaviour: correct means tending to aid it in continuing to live and to give birth to the next generation; incorrect is the opposite.

When the operation of leucotomy (discussed in chapter 24) was introduced, it was discovered that the sensation of pain could be separated from its associated unpleasant emotion. When the brain was cut so that the frontal lobes were separated from the thalamus, the patient no longer complained of the pain of cancer and he seemed to be indifferent to it. He could feel pain when he was pricked or when he burned himself, but he no longer suffered from the previous constant pain. Most of the patients said, unemotionally, that pressure on the tumour was still painful but they were obviously not disturbed by the pain. There was a chasm between the affective emotional aspect of pain and the pure sensation of pain.

The kind of pain we feel depends largely on the tissue that is being damaged or irritated and also on what is causing the pain. Blood itself causes pain when it is in the wrong place, that is when it has leaked out of blood-vessels. A lack of vital blood-supply in the right place can cause pain. This happens when a muscle is working and its blood-supply is reduced or cut off. It is the cause of the pain of coronary thrombosis. Suddenly one of the arteries that supplies the heart muscle gets blocked. The heart goes on beating (it may not and then the person dies of a heart attack) with insufficient blood to bring it oxygen. That causes pain. There is similar pain when any muscle goes on working without enough blood supply. It happens in old age when the arteries get furred up, like old pipes. Then the old man has to stop walking to give the muscles of his legs a chance to get more blood while they are resting.

Any kind of stimulation of the pulp and the dentine of the teeth is painful. That is why it hurts when the dentist blows hot or cold air into your teeth. I am hoping that one or two dentists will read this book and blow air on our teeth at the same temperature as our mouths. Damage to bone causes a deep aching gnawing pain. Irritating chemicals injected into muscles cause a similar deep aching pain. The brain can be cut or burned without there being any kind of sensation. But damage to the peripheral nerves is painful; and the pain of cancer is often due to the growth invading these nerves. The kind of pain caused by damage to the skin depends on which layer is being involved: damage to the most superficial layer causes itching and burning pain; damage to the deeper layer causes an ache.

Pain in the viscera feels altogether different from pain in the skin, the muscles or the bones. In general, the activity of the intestines and ureters goes on silently (well, relatively silently) and automatically without giving us any sensation. When this activity becomes more vigorous, we have the sensation that the viscera need to be emptied. When the stomach contains a lot of fluid and is working hard, we may be able to feel as well as hear the gurglings and splashings. When the intestines are contracting hard to push their contents past an obstruction, we get the pain of colic. This is a rhythmical waxing and waning of pain, as the intestines contract and relax. Some viscera tell us that they exist only when they give us pain; these are the ureters, the urethra, the bile and pancreatic ducts. People are amazed to hear that the intestines can be cut through or even burned without this causing any sort of sensation. But this is not really surprising because it is unlikely that they will ever meet these fates and so they have not evolved any defensive mechanisms to deal with such unlikely events. If they are pulled on, that causes pain. For that is something that is likely to occur a few times during a life; when they are working hard to push through an obstacle, then they do pull on the tissues that hold them in place and they are pulled in return.

Some pains make you move; colic of a ureter trying to pass a kidney stone is an example. Others make you lie still; this happens with peritonitis and when there is bleeding in the abdominal cavity.

When a part of the body gets inflamed, substances are made in the tissues that excite nociceptor nerve fibres and cause pain. They not only cause pain but they also make the nociceptors more sensitive to other kinds of stimuli. In an inflamed area, warmth and touch that normally cause only a slight sensation cause pain. One of these substances formed in inflamed tissues is prostaglandin E. Aspirin and related drugs stop this substance being produced; that is how they relieve certain kinds of pain.

When a nerve is damaged or cut through, as occurs when a limb is amputated, nerve fibres grow out of the cut nerves into nowhere. These sprouting fibres are abnormally sensitive to pressure or to being moved, squeezed or stretched; they are also sensitive to noradrenalin which is emitted all around them by the accompanying sympathetic nerve fibres.

When we have pain, we may wish that man were not born to suffer and we are likely to think that pain is all bad. But that is not true. There are a few rare congenital conditions in which the person does not feel pain. In one of these, congenital non-progressive sensory neuropathy, the nerve fibres and their connections in the spinal cord necessary for feeling pain are defective or absent. In another condition wrongly called congenital indifference to pain, it appears there is an excessive amount of endorphin circulating in the body. This is a peptide with actions similar to morphine, which will be discussed below. Or it may be that the neurons of the spinal cord that receive a noxious input are being continually inhibited. Patients having either of these conditions do not reach adult life without scarring large parts of their bodies, without damaging their joints, and without biting their tongues and the insides of their mouths. Pain is protective. It protects against damage from the surrounding world and also against damaging oneself, over-stretching the bladder, biting oneself, swallowing liquids which are too hot.

So far we have been discussing acute pain. Chronic pain is pain that is constant or frequently recurs. This is the pain of arthritis, of backache, of cancer, it is the pain that may follow an attack of shingles in the elderly. Pain going on for a long time can affect the central nervous system for the rest of the person's life. Two examples of a severe and lasting pain affecting neurons permanently are reported in chapter 23. In these cases, certain groups of neurons retain the pattern of firing together as they did when the pain first occurred; when they are excited again, they reproduce the whole pattern of firing; this is a kind of basic memory. Memory implies learning. In some cases, neurons in the brain can be shown to have learned pain. They behave differently, after they have been receiving an input causing pain for a long time. Perhaps one should expect this; for the central nervous system is a learning machine. Learning is necessary for survival. The simplest organisms back in the beginnings of time changed with experience: that is learning. Although it may not be good or necessary to learn pain, it could be that the learning machine cannot decide what to learn and what to leave out. It learns how to change reflexes, how to co-ordinate eye and limb. It seems also to learn unnecessary movements, those unwanted by their performer. This may be what happens when someone develops tics, those involuntary screwings up of the corner of the mouth or movements of the face or head; once learned, almost never forgotten. But learning these movements and learning pain, these are rare. Why this sometimes happens, we do not know.

When some pains have been going on for a long time—and I don't know what length of time a long time is—the behaviour of certain neurons of the thalamus and cerebral cortex becomes changed. This has been found out by operating on the brain under local anaesthetics. We may take an example of a painful fantom upper limb that has come on after amputation. At one time neurosurgeons tried to cure the pain by operating on the opposite cerebral cortex and removing the arm area. The arm area, as will be seen in chapter 18, is a region of the cerebral cortex in the front of the parietal lobe which receives impulses causing sensation of touch and pressure in the opposite arm. Above this region is the same region for the leg and below it the region for the face. In some of the patients with a painful fantom upper limb, the cortical arm area enlarges and spreads out onto the areas of the face and the leg. The constant presence of the painful fantom is also associated with something else abnormal. When the surgeon stimulates this area electrically, the pain from which the patient is suffering is reproduced. Normally stimulation of this part of the brain never causes pain; it causes numbness or tingling, pins and needles, or a need to move the limb. The area has become abnormal in that it now reproduces pain when excited instead of numbness and tingling. The operation of cutting out this area did not work because the pain came back after a few months.

Over the past fifteen years, important advances have been made in the understanding of pain. This subject is more complicated than has been realized for many centuries. Pain and all sensation used to be thought of as being only afferent, as being messages delivered to the cerebral cortex. In 1969, a Canadian psychologist, D. V. Reynolds, reported that he had been operating on rats, burning, cutting or pinching them, and that the rats felt nothing, provided he electrically stimulated a certain part of the midbrain. During this stimulation the animals seemed to feel touch or pressure, but they gave no indication of feeling pain, they had no reflexes suggesting that something painful was going on, there was no change in blood pressure, no change in breathing, no squeaking. Nothing quite like this had been seen before. Usually the electric stimulation of the brain causes something obvious, a movement, a change in breathing, or, if the animal is awake, it shows some sort of behaviour, it looks, it listens, it moves. Although inhibition of neurons of the spinal cord was already known, a complete absence of pain and the manifestations of pain from stimulating parts of the brain was something surprising. Eventually many regions of the brain were found whose stimulation stopped pain being felt. They were all in the central grey matter of the brain: this is the oldest part, already developed in ancestral fish. Stimulation of various neurons in this region excites certain neurons in the medulla oblongata. From these neurons fibres descend to the posterior horns of the spinal cord and to similar regions of the brain that receive an input from the face and neck. These are inhibitory neurons and they act on the nerve fibres from the skin, muscles and viscera where they come into the spinal cord. They are able to obliterate the message before it is delivered at the first synapse within the central nervous system. Thus the inability to feel pain, or analgesia as it is called, from electric stimulation of a region in the midbrain was due to pre-synaptic inhibition of the nerve fibres arriving in the spinal cord with messages of noxious events.

When this electrically induced analgesia had been explained as activating an inhibitory system of nerve fibres, the thought occurred to many research workers that morphine and the related opiates might work by activating this system: could it be that morphine is an effective drug against pain, an analgesic drug, because it excites the neurons that had been stimulated electrically? If this were found to be so, then morphine would be working by inhibiting the incoming impulses caused by noxious stimulation. This could not be the whole explanation of morphine's action against pain because it was known already that it acted at the two levels, on the spinal cord and on the brain. Some research workers then injected morphine in minute amounts into the region of the midbrain from which electric stimulation caused analgesia. The morphine produced the same effects as the electrical stimulation. If the neurons of the medulla oblongata were previously destroyed, then morphine no longer stopped pain; and if this tract of inhibitory fibres had been already cut, then morphine no longer worked. If the tract had been cut on one side of the spinal cord, morphine did not stop pain on that side of the animal; and if the tract had been cut on both sides, then morphine did not work on the lower limbs, below the level of the cut. This evidence showed that morphine, whatever other actions it has, works as an analgesic drug by activating this descending inhibitory system. It also acts directly on the spinal cord. It causes pre-synaptic inhibition of the nerve fibres coming in reporting noxious stimulation, so that their message does not get through to the spinal cord.

It is curious that morphine and other opiate drugs are fixed on to the membrane of neurons of animals, for they are substances formed in plants. If morphine molecules fit into the membranes of certain cells of the body, there may perhaps be some chemical substances in the body that normally fit these sites on cell membranes. Many workers then began searching for what are called endogenous opioids. At present, more than ten substances, all peptides, have been found in the body that have similar actions to opiates. It is probable that only three of these are actually used in the body—to prevent pain and to act on the bladder, alimentary canal and other parts of the nervous system, β-endorphin and leucine–enkephalin and methionine–enkephalin. β-endorphin is made in a group of neurons of the hypothalamus. There is also a peptide made in the pituitary called pro-opiocortin, which is broken down to form other substances with various physiological actions. One of these is β-endorphin; when it is injected into the posterior horns of the spinal cord, it behaves in the same way as morphine. It prevents an input from nerve fibres bringing in reports of noxious events.

At present the way in which β-endorphin is used to diminish pain is unknown. It is perhaps put into the cerebrospinal fluid, the fluid that surrounds the spinal cord and brain and bathes the inside of the brain. It is not rapidly broken down into other chemical substances and so it is likely to go on acting for minutes or even hours.

The two enkephalins were discovered owing to research on endogenous substances with actions similar to morphine: they are general neurotransmitters used in many places within the central nervous system.

The question why there is a pain-preventing and pain-removing system in the body demands an answer. Yet answers to the question 'why' are usually just guesses; the question 'how' is the question that science successfully answers.

It may be that the system is used for sleeping. Sleep is essential; perhaps this system is active during sleep, to allow the animal to sleep in spite of something that would otherwise be painful. Turning off pain may be part of stress behaviour. When you are running away from a tiger, it is better to go on running even if you have sprained your ankle. It is desirable not to feel the pain and not to react to it. The ankle can be attended to afterwards, if there is an afterwards. During stress adrenalin and adrenocorticotrophin are poured into the blood stream. Pro-opiocortin contains two peptides, adrenocorticotrophin and β-endorphin. The presence of adrenocorticotrophin is a hint that during stress a pain-preventing system is being activated.

Another question that comes up is whether we are using this pain-suppressing system all the time; is it that we are constantly inhibiting small inputs that cause some damage and might be giving us continuous pain? The answer appears to be yes. People who have some chronic painful condition such as arthritis or backache, are using this system. If they were not doing so, presumably their pain would be worse.

One wonders too if some people and people under extraordinary conditions are able to bring in this inhibitory system and not feel pain. This may be the explanation of people running swords through their tongues, dancing on red-hot coals or hanging themselves up with hooks through their skins. When these people have been investigated by physiologists, they have been found to be able to induce slow waves in their electroencephalograms. Without training one cannot do this. Not only those going into trance states in order to dance on red hot coal or perform similar acts without being hurt, but Sen Buddhist monks also learn to go into the same state, and they induce the same slow waves in their brains. What is most amazing about those who perform these dangerous dances in religious ecstasy is that they do not burn their feet and they do not get blisters. Those who pierce their skins with nails or swords do not bleed. The only other physiological fact we know about the state needed for these feats is that the sympathetic system is very active at the time. This may cause closing down of the blood-vessels of the skin and prevent the bleeding.

In the last few years everyone has been astounded to watch operations on television being performed on wide-awake Chinese patients, acupuncture analgesia being used instead of a general anaesthetic. Although acupuncture is five thousand years old, its use to stop the pain of surgical operations is new to the Chinese just as it is to us. Like most things in medicine, it was found to work before it was understood how or why. The method consists of electrically stimulating certain regions of the body at a painful or just sub-painful intensity for about twenty minutes before the operation is begun; the stimulation is continued throughout the operation. The needles are put through the skin into the muscles beneath. The intensity of the current is slowly increased so that the local muscles are rapidly contracting and the sensation felt by the patient is pain or just less than pain.

It is probable that acupuncture analgesia—not acupuncture for the treatment of disease—depends on three mechanisms being considered here. There is local presynaptic inhibition, there is inhibition via tracts descending from the medulla oblongata, and there is the production of endorphin. Swedish research workers who investigated acupuncture analgesia found that the nearer the needles being electrically stimulated were to the site of operation, the more effective they were in stopping the pain of theoperation. This acupuncture input was most effective when it was within the territory of the same peripheral nerve as the site of the operation. Within the spinal cord are interactions between two or more inputs. Prolonged excitation of the tactile nerve fibres can reduce the perception of noxious input. The twenty minutes of acupuncture stimulation activates the descending inhibitory tract from the medulla oblongata to the posterior horn neurons. Further, Chinese research workers showed some years ago that twenty minutes of acupuncture stimulation carried out on a rabbit produced some change in the cerebrospinal fluid that could be transferred to another rabbit. Having given the first rabbit the acupuncture, they took the cerebrospinal fluid, and infused it into the cerebrospinal fluid of a second rabbit. This rabbit then had its threshold for pain heightened. This experiment showed that the acupuncture stimulation had caused some substance to appear in the cerebrospinal fluid that acted on the nervous system to raise the animal's threshold for pain. From our knowledge acquired some years later, this substance would be an endorphin. Thus the mechanisms of acupuncture analgesia appear to be inhibition occurring at spinal level, descending inhibition from the medulla oblongata to the spinal cord, and emission of endorphin to act generally.

We are beginning to see the connecting links between acupuncture analgesia used in China for operations, acupuncture done by twiddling or electrically stimulating needles for the treatment of some diseases, the treatment of some chronic pain by electric stimulation with electrodes on the skin, and the treatment of drug addiction, smoking, and alcoholism by electric stimulation of the head. The body reacts differently to slow and fast rates of stimulation, fast being impulses arriving at 80 or more a second and slow being at rates considerably less than this. Fast rates of stimulation activate the neurons in the medulla that send nerve fibres to the spinal cord and inhibit peripheral nerve fibres reporting noxious or painful events. These neurons are connected to enkephalinergic neurons which work by pre-synaptic inhibition. Thus fast rates of stimulation can be effective in stopping pain. Slow rates of stimulation increase the amount of β-endorphin in the cerebrospinal fluid in patients who have constant pain. These are the rates used in acupuncture and in electric stimulation for chronic pain. For the treatment of morphine and heroin addiction, high rates of electric stimulation are used, the current being passed through the head or ears. It thus seems that this stimulation brings enkephalinergic neurons into activity and the naturally produced enkephalin replaces the morphine or heroin at the synapses where the drug was previously acting. The patient no longer has a craving for the drug as his naturally occurring transmitter is being mobilized to replace the drug.

14 Awake and exploring: relaxed and sleeping

Selection and paying attention

For from this proceeds the passing quickness of his attention.

If one were to design a nervous system, one would probably have had the receptors signalling all events to the central nervous system and have left the brain to sort out this mass of incoming messages. The ear might report every sound, the eye everything to be seen, and the nose all smells floating in the air. A million impulses would reach the nervous system every second. If this input were not reduced, there would be an overloading of the lines and the whole system would get clogged up. If much of it did get through, we would be too pre-occupied to act and incapable of responding.

Selection is necessary as so much is always going on. The sun is shining, there are long shadows on the far side of the wood, there are pine-needles on the ground, and a robin is threatening just inside his territory. But none of this matters to the deer, sniffing the wind and pricking up its ears. It selects the unexpected, the new smell arriving on the wind and it listens for the sounds that may come with it. The animal is alert, seeking information. It is also neglecting the great bulk of stimuli that arrive. Only some aspects of the environment interest us. If we are thirsty, we have to be looking out for water; when hungry, we must be searching for food. Our attention and our interest are arranged by our needs; and the need that is predominant at any time will make us attend to those aspects of the environment likely to satisfy it.

By using a tape-recorder, we can easily observe how well the nervous system selects what it wants to know. When we play back what we have just been recording, we will be astounded to hear a clock strike in the middle of it. We would have sworn that at the time we were recording, no clock struck; yet there it is, on the tape. The tape-recorder does not select; it records everything indiscriminately.

What the brain needs to have is news; and news, as it says, is something new. The input has to be reduced so as to allow important news to come in. This means selection. The nervous system needs to control its own input, to play up one input and to play down another.

The first problem is how to reject the vast number of impulses arriving at the central nervous system so as to attend to those that could be important. In terms of radio engineering, the animal has to discriminate the signal from the noise. The nervous system has various ways of increasing one input and decreasing others.

Selection starts at the receptors. Controlling nerves supply the cochlea, the receptors of the vestibule, the olfactory receptors and the muscle spindles. The input from the skin is controlled as it enters the spinal cord. We are all familiar with the first control of the visual sense organs, our eyelids. They are the first element of selection in the visual input. We can cut off this input merely by shutting our eyes. Marsupials can do the same with their ears; they have a muscle which closes their outer ears when they go to sleep. Hippopotami can also close their ears like this and they use these muscles when they go underwater. Apart from shutting the eyes, we can adjust the amount of light that reaches the retina by altering the size of the pupil.

Inhibition is used also to highlight an important input. It can reduce the number of impulses coming in so effectively that it can block out the message altogether. Inhibition can be used to bring out contrasts. We discussed this occurring in the retina. This mechanism of surround inhibition is used throughout the central nervous system.

In the centre of the brain there are a great number of neurons that appear to alert the higher levels of the brain and prepare them to take note of an arriving input. They are in the core of the older parts of the brain (Fig. 18.1); they are called the reticular activating system. It is a two-way system; for it sends impulses to all parts of the cerebral hemispheres to alert them, and it receives impulses from the cerebral hemispheres to activate it.

When something catches your eye, impulses pass from the optic nerves to the reticular system and then they are relayed to the cerebral hemispheres to tell you what is happening. It is probably the reticular formation that alerts you. You must be vigilant, ready for rapid flight or to turn on the aggressor.

A pain will wake you and demand attention. The different sensations are usually accompanied by feelings—surprise, familiarity, pleasure or aesthetic appreciation. Touch and hearing are liable to alert you. If one is lying dozing out of doors, the smallest of flies has merely to alight on ones forearm and one suddenly wakes up and pulls ones arm away before one knows what is happening; and how much more alarming it is when the fly crawls up ones nose or into ones ear. If we tread on a nail, one level of our central nervous system causes us to feel pain, to make us have an unpleasant emotion, and to localize the pain to the lower surface of the foot. Other levels receive the message and deal with it according to their needs, interpreting the information as demanding action, such as raising the blood pressure, constricting the blood vessels of the upper limbs, stabilizing the body on the unpricked limb and withdrawing the pricked limb from the ground. At a higher level in the central nervous system, the input arising from treading on the nail has more complicated effects. It not only is sent on to parts of the cerebral cortex for further analysis, so that the animal feels pain in the foot and can try and work out what has caused that pain. It is also sent to sensory areas for other inputs, hearing, vision, vestibular sensation. It may inhibit these other inputs, so that attention is focused on the foot; or it may heighten these inputs, so that all afferent channels become more important, so that attention is focused on every sort of sensation.

The distribution of the input within the central nervous system needs to be a changing one, continually capable of being re-distributed. For instance, the passage of food along the alimentary canal does not usually need to occupy our consciousness. Our consciousness—what we call 'we'—must be left free to enjoy music. But if something goes wrong, if there is a traffic block in the alimentary canal, an obstruction, then the usual afferent impulses coming in from the canal are increased and finally the neural substratum of consciousness is made aware of what is happening. If we then get colicky pains, we can use the tools of consciousness—knowledge, reasoning, planning—to take steps to get rid of the obstruction.

Important work on the selection of the input was carried out by Hernández-Peón in Mexico and California. He found that if an animal's attention is distracted from one kind of stimulation and is turned to another, the size of the electrical response being recorded is decreased. One of the first experiments he published was done in this way. He recorded the nerve impulses coming along the visual pathway while a light was repeatedly flashed in front of a cat's eyes. Then he brought a tin of sardines up to the cat's nose or else he whispered something in its ear. When he did this, he found that the nerve impulses coming in from the flashing light ceased to arrive at the visual region of the cerebral cortex. When the smell of sardines was removed or the whispering was stopped, the nerve impulses due to the flashing light returned to their original number. These experiments could also be done the other way round, the visual, odorous, or painful stimuli obliterating the auditory input. When Hernández-Peón showed the cat the sardiness or a live mouse in a glass, the auditory input from repeated clicks was suppressed. It was also suppressed by the smell of the sardines or by a painful stimulation of one of the paws. From these experiments it was concluded that when a cat's attention is focused on one sort of stimulus, a regularly repeated and unimportant stimulus into another afferent channel is not permitted to reach the primary receptive area.

Hernández-Péon later carried out some of these experiments in man. He found that the nerve impulses coming in from the eyes were greatly reduced when the person was engaged in conversation, when he was solving an arithmetical problem or when he was asked to remember something. And what is more interesting, he found that when he suggested to the person that the brightness of the flashing light was being altered, the action potential he was recording from the brain was correspondingly altered. If he said the light was being made brighter, the action potentials got far bigger and when he suggested that the intensity of the light was being reduced, the response became less. All this was done without actually changing the intensity of the light. Similarly it was found that the volleys of impulses arriving at the primary tactile area or primary auditory area could be reduced by giving the person problems or just by engaging him in conversation. Also the number of impulses arriving at the higher centres of the brain diminishes when the stimulus is continued regularly and becomes monotonous, as had previously been observed in the cat.

When an event stops being new, it becomes less important and loses priority; the lines must be cleared for new events. For the nervous system, an event is new if it is changed in any way. If a click is repeated, the nerve impulses caused by each click gradually fade away. But if the pitch of the sound of the click is raised or lowered, if the click is suddenly made softer or louder, then the response in the cochlear nucleus is immediately brought back to its original size, for this is different from the previous input. It may be important; and so it constitutes the kind of information the brain wants. When this occurs at the higher levels of the central nervous system, it is familar to us all. A monotonously repeated sound may not keep us awake and it may even help us to sleep; we soon cease to hear it. But if it changes in any way—by dropping a beat, or by changing its pitch—our attention is involuntarily turned to it again.

With practice one can learn to neglect one sensory input. Everyone who uses a microscope learns to pay no attention to the input coming in from the eye that is not looking down it; one does not close that eye. I have already mentioned how one does not hear extraneous noises when recording something with interest. Similarly one can learn with practice to neglect a lot of nearby noise and to attend to what one is doing. It could be that the brain inhibits the particular input when we are concentrating on something else. If this is so, it is not that we take no notice of the neglected input; it actually would not come into the brain or spinal cord. Ballet dancers learn to suppress the input coming in from the vestibular apparatus when they keep turning rapidly. They use their eyes instead and avoid a conflict between the inputs from the vestibule and from the eyes and in this way they cease to feel giddy or to have nausea.

We have talked of descending control of afferent pathways to the higher levels of the brain without saying what parts of the brain exercise this control. Each primary receptive area of the cerebral cortex is able to control its own input, its own afferent pathway. For instance, the visual area of the cortex can control the retina and the relays on the visual pathway, and the auditory area of the cortex can control the inner ear and the relays on the auditory pathway. The sensory area of the cerebral cortex controls the input to the spinal cord arriving via the nerves from the skin, muscles and viscera. Descending control of this input also comes from a central region of the midbrain and from part of the medulla oblongata.

In the centre of the brainstem, as was mentioned above, is a specialized mass of cells called the reticular formation. It goes up into the midbrain and down into the spinal cord. This mass of short, intertwining neurons forms a part of the brain from the earliest vertebrates onwards; in fact, in the lower vertebrates, the central nervous system has little else than this structure. In the reticular formation, the neurons are short with short axons, and the dendrites overlap and intertwine. There are enormous numbers of these neurons, so that this neural formation is like a net, and so is called reticular. It is a very slowly conducting system. Faster conducting systems evolved later.

The reticular formation is concerned with the basic functions of living, with breathing, with controlling the heart and the blood pressure, with sleep and waking, with being vigilant and resting. To keep the animal alive in a world full of creatures eager to eat it and at the same time to keep it eating and drinking, is the function of the reticular formation. It stops messages reaching consciousness when the animal has to sleep, it allows them to wake the animal, and then gives priority to what is most important at the moment. In order to sort out what comes in from the world, it is connected to all afferent tracts of nerve fibres.

The sensory input is distributed to the reticular formation in two ways. In one way, each sensory input goes to general neurons so that one neuron receives impulses coming from, say, auditory, tactile, and visual channels. In the other way, private lines predominate; a group of neurons receives only visual or only auditory input. It may be that the neurons receiving many different sensory inputs are a part of the mechanism for making the animal attend to everything happening or about to happen and that neurons receiving single sensory inputs form a part of the mechanism for focusing attention on one kind of sensation. The reticular formation of the brainstem and hypothalamus and thalamus excites the cerebral hemispheres and keeps the cerebral cortex active and alert. It also brings about relaxation and repose and prepares the animal for sleep. These two regions work reciprocally. When there is an increased input to the brain, the alerting system is activated, and as the input diminishes, the reposing system comes to the fore. The reticular formation also receives masses of nerve fibres from above, from the cerebral hemispheres. Presumably this is how thoughts, ideas and emotions take control of both parts, either arousing our interest or letting us relax.

When the alerting system of the reticular formation is active, impulses are rushed down to the spinal cord. They go to the motoneurons of the muscle spindles, making all the spindles tense. This is like tuning the strings of a violin. They are then ready to be played upon.

This action of the reticular formation on the muscles of the body is present throughout waking life and also to a certain extent during sleep. People who are psychologically tense unconsciously keep their muscles active and tense; and those who are relaxed allow their muscles to relax. The activity of muscles in people about to be executed has been investigated in the United States. As would be expected, these people have most of their muscles actively contracting. Many anxious people are in the same state all the time. They feel that most conditions of living threaten them; and they react like those facing death, being frightened and apprehensive.

Sleeping and waking

For there is nothing sweeter than his peace when at rest.

Nearly all animals sleep; and no one knows why. Fish have periods of inactivity akin to sleep. The sea-mammal, called the porpoise in England and the bottle-nosed dolphin in America, submerges when it sleeps but it comes up twice a minute for air, waking at each breath. When asleep, it keeps one eye open, scanning its environment. Snakes and lizards sleep with their eyes open, having no movable eyelids. Bats and flying foxes sleep when they are hanging with their heads down. Man spends about a third of his life asleep.

Sleeping habits differ greatly between the various species of vertebrates. Deer sleep for only very short periods, but when they are asleep they are deeply unconscious and can be touched without being woken. Sheep and domestic cattle sleep very little. It is usually thought that they sleep so little because they have a stomach designed to digest cellulose. For this purpose, they have a special stomach called a reticulo-rumen, which is the first of their stomachs. For this to work properly and to empty, it must be kept in an upright position; and to keep it upright the animal has to keep its thorax upright; it must not lie down. If it went into deep sleep, the thorax and head would fall onto the ground, the rumen would not empty properly and the gas formed during digestion would not pass up the oesophagus and be belched out of the mouth. As domestic cattle spend so much of their time eating and the rest of their time ruminating, there is almost no time left for lying down and sleeping. Calves and lambs still at the breast do sleep, and so do very old cattle and sheep. It appears to me that Brahminy cattle do sleep, for I have seen them in Northern Queensland and in India lying down apparently asleep, their heads turned to one side, resting on or just by their hindlimbs.

Hediger, from his great experience of animals in the wild, in zoos and menageries, concludes that animals which eat vegetation and which are the prey of the carnivores sleep very deeply but for a short time; they also copulate quickly, and their young can stand and walk at birth. Antelopes copulate merely for seconds, their offspring can run within half an hour of birth. Bears, which have no natural enemies, except for that universal enemy of all living creatures, man, copulate for hours, and their cubs are born in an immature state. The punishment for killing animals, one hopes, is that we will be reincarnated as antelopes and not as bears.

Even when asleep, an animal must be alive to danger; and so animals choose places to sleep where danger is least. And when asleep, they must be prepared to wake suddenly. The cry of her baby in the night must waken the mother, while the radio blaring across the street should not waken her, otherwise she will be tired and tense in the morning. Even the real lord of the jungle, the elephant, is very sensitive to anything moving at night. Hediger spent a lot of time studying elephants asleep in Africa, in zoos and circuses in Europe. He found he could never creep about quietly enough not to waken them. When elephants sleep, they put their heads on the bodies of their comrades and even rub their hindquarters hard against each other without waking each other up; but they would always wake immediately a human being made the slightest noise. Herbivores are woken so easily by noise that that is why, Hediger says, there are no photographs of antelopes sleeping; no one has been able to get close enough.

Horses normally sleep about 7 hours of the 24. They lie down flat for deep sleep but they can dose off while they are standing. The European swift can sleep while flying. Apparently soldiers can sleep while marching. This means that the neurons working innumerable muscles are active, as well as neurons of the labyrinths, and those co-ordinating these activities.

Sleep is not just passive relaxation of wakefulness. There are neural structures in the brain that actively cause sleep. When certain neurons are electrically stimulated the animal goes to sleep; when others are stimulated, it wakes up. The sleep-inducing and awakening neurons are scattered in many regions of the brain. They are in the most primitive parts of the cerebral hemispheres, that is in the front parts of the temporal lobes, in many parts of the hypothalamus, in the thalamus and in the reticular formation throughout the central core of the brain. When the neurons concerned with sleep in the front part of the hypothalamus are destroyed, the animal no longer sleeps. In the epidemic of encephalitis lethargica that occurred after the First World War this part of the brain was damaged. These patients had strange sleep disturbances. If these neurons are experimentally stimulated in an animal, the animal becomes sleepy. It looks around for somewhere cosy, becomes quiet and relaxed, curls up and goes to sleep. It remains asleep for hours without these neurons being stimulated again. When the waking centre is active, it activates the cerebral cortex. The animal becomes lively and ready to face the world.

A Russian surgeon reported a case of a soldier on whom he operated during the war against the Germans. A metal fragment had entered the patient's skull and had lodged in the hypothalamus. When the surgeon, operating under local anaesthesia, tried to pull the piece of metal out, the patient immediately fell asleep. The surgeon then stopped as he thought the patient had gone into a state of shock. After a few minutes the patient woke up, and when questioned said he had had an irresistible desire to sleep. The surgeon finally removed the metal fragment on the third attempt; on each occasion when his forceps moved the piece of metal in the hypothalamus, the patient went to sleep.

Waking and sleeping still occur after the entire cerebral hemispheres have been removed or are not working; and they occur too in babies born without hemispheres and in patients in whom the hemispheres have been destroyed.

In the nineteen-fifties, a great step forward was made in our knowledge about sleep when Kleitman and Dement in the United States recorded the electroencephalogram throughout a whole night's sleep. It then became clear that only parts of the brain are inactive during sleep. Some parts are inactive during some stages of sleep, others at other stages. There are two kinds of sleep, rapid-eye-movement or r.e.m. sleep and slow-wave sleep. The name r.e.m. sleep comes from the fact that at this stage of sleep there are rapid irregular movements of the eyes behind closed eyelids. In this phase, heart-rate and breathing are fast and not very regular, and the brain and the penis get more blood than during waking life. During slow-wave sleep, the heart beats slowly and regularly and breathing is slower than during waking life. When we go to sleep, we start off with slow-wave sleep. The deepest phase is reached after about half to one hour. After we have spent about one to one and a half hours in this phase, the first phase of r.e.m. sleep arrives. During a night there are four to six periods of r.e.m. sleep, each lasting between ten and thirty minutes. Young adults spend up to a quarter of their sleep in the r.e.m. phase; babies spend far longer and old people far less. Old people also spend less time in the phase of slow sleep.

An interesting experiment was carried out in the United States showing that the r.e.m. phase is related to higher cerebral activity. A group of people wore inverting spectacles all day long. Inverting spectacles make the whole world appear upside down. This extraordinary change in the experiencing of the environment demands constant adaptation and learning. During this time of learning, These people spent a longer part of their nights in r.e.m. sleep.

If people are woken during the r.e.m. stage of sleep—this is recognised by continuous recording of the electroencephalograph—they nearly always say that they were in the middle of dreaming. But if they are woken at other stages of sleep, only rarely do they say they are dreaming. It is not known whether this means that dreaming occurs mainly during r.e.m. sleep or if it means that dreams are remembered during this stage and forgotten during deeper sleep. In either case, it is obvious that we remember only the merest fragments of our dreams, the parts occurring just before we wake up.

Nightmares occur during r.e.m. sleep, as so do most of our dreams. But walking in ones sleep takes place in slow-wave sleep, during the deeper phases. Lady Macbeth was not alone in seeming to be looking for something nor in talking when she walked in her sleep; both are common in sleep-walkers. If the sleep-walker is woken, he is not dreaming at the time and he can recall nothing.

Visual dreaming is not equivalent to r.e.m sleep. R.e.m. sleep is important at birth; at this time there is no visual imagery. Newborn kittens have r.e.m. sleep before their eyes are open. Also men who have had their entire cerebral hemispheres damaged by head injury or disease have r.e.m. sleep.

It is almost certain that other mammals than man dream. They show the same r.e.m. sleep. Before the electroencephalograph was used to investigate sleep, many experiments had been done on animals' dreaming. For example, sausages were put in front of the noses of sleeping dogs, in Germany, of course; the dogs would then make chewing movements and wrinkle the skin around their mouths. Records have been kept of the movements sleeping puppies make from the moment of birth. At the end of the first week, they make lip-smacking and sucking noises; later they snarl and utter minimal barks; later still they make running movements.

Sleep is upset in many diseases, but there is one disease that is really a disorder of sleep. This is narcolepsy; it occurs with cataplexy, which was mentioned at the end of chapter 12. Patients with this complaint have to go to sleep during the day; this may happen for periods of 5 to 15 minutes six or seven times a day. From each little nap they wake up quite restored. These patients fall off to sleep very quickly and their sleep is restless and disturbed. They walk in their sleep. And some of them have short periods of waking during the night just as they have periods of sleeping during the day.

There is another rare disorder of sleep called sleep paralysis. Nurses on night duty occasionally have this. When the person with this disorder is tired, tending to fall asleep, or if they suddenly wake up, they go to move and find they are quite unable to move even a finger. This total paralysis lasts from a few seconds to a few minutes. During the time, they may be very frightened and can have visual or auditory hallucinations, like dreams.

One of the tortures used by governments of all civilized countries is to deprive their victims of sleep. If one is prevented from sleeping for three days and nights, one tends to get a temporary psychosis, hallucinations and paranoid delusions. This state is induced on purpose by brain-washers.

Most people wake every morning at about the same time. At this time sleep is light, and it may be that the daily visual and auditory stimuli wake us. But this is not the whole matter; for these stimuli have all the insignificance of familiarity. In winter it may be dark, in summer light. More remarkable is our ability to wake ourselves automatically at some unusual early hour, say five o'clock. This is not a perfect mechanism; for usually we wake before this set time and keep waking ourselves up several times before five; and then the final waking may occur after five. It is likely that the parts of our brains concerned in the waking are the cerebral cortex and part of the reticular formation concerned with alerting the brain. But how one sets this mechanism going, no one knows.

Sleeping and waking alternately over the 24 hours are examples of circadian rhythms (circa, about; dies, a day.). Other activities that rhythmically recur are the activity of the bowels and changes in body temperature. Much research work has been done to learn whether these rhythms are intrinsic, being organized by some kind of internal clock, or extrinsic, being ordered by some recurring event in the world around us, such as the length of daylight or changes in environmental temperature, or whether they are due to a combination of both factors. This is often difficult to find out as the internal clock tends to have the same cycle as repeated external events. The cockroach, for instance, is fairly inactive in daylight and busy at night. If cockroaches are kept in continuous daylight, they still run around at the time when night should have fallen. Thus their activity depends on their internal clocks and not on the dark.

What is curious is that many circadian rhythms of human beings have a 25 hour cycle. This has been learned by putting people in underground rooms or caves where daylight does not penetrate and where factors such as humidity, temperature and atmospheric pressure can be kept constant. This 25 hours varies a little from person to person but it is almost always more than 24 hours. If a person in such an experiment usually got up at 8 in the morning, by twelve days he would be getting up at 8 in the evening, thinking he was getting up at his usual time in the morning. This independence of the usual 24 hour cycle shows us that we have an intrinsic oscillator, independent of the earth's rotation. Yet in normal living, this intrinsic rhythm is changed to a 24 hour rhythm. Aschoff and Wever in Germany have done extensive and very long-lasting experiments to find out what changes the intrinsic 25 hour rhythm to the usual 24 hour rhythm. Although the periodicity of light and dark is important for certain species, this plays no role in man: keeping man under varying periods of light and dark does not alter his circadian rhythms. The factor that does govern the 24 hour periodicity is the earth's magnetic field. This field changes in a 24-hour cycle as the world turns on its axis. When in experiments people are isolated from the magnetic field of the earth, they have the circadian rhythm of 25 hours. When they are returned to the earth's magnetic field, they have the usual 24 hour cycle. In these experiments the subjects are totally unaware of being influenced by any outside agency; they do not know that their internal clocks have changed from 25 to 24 hours; and they do not know when they are living within this field or when it is excluded. We have no idea what part of the body senses the magnetic field, nor whether it is all the cells of the body or some particular sensory receptors.

The earth's magnetic field is influenced by the sun. The possible effects of solar activity on ourselves and other living organisms could be observed better if cyclical events were noted in relation to the 27 day period of revolution of the sun around its axis instead of in relation to lunar months or to the arbitrary calendar.

The intrinsic rhythm generator has been studied in *Aplysia*, a large snail. In this animal there are neurons in the central nervous system that fire off volleys of impulses at the end of every 12 hours. If these neurons are dissected out and put in a dish surrounded by necessary nutrients, they continue to fire off with their 12 hour rhythm. Thus this rhythm of firing is a property of the cells; it seems to depend on their biochemical characteristics. This is an example of neurons behaving as time-keepers.

15 Needs, desires, and emotions

For he will not do destruction, if he is well-fed, neither will he spit
without provocation.

During the last quarter of a century, a new science has been evolved:
ethology, the study of animal behaviour. This is mainly the child of
Konrad Lorenz. It is related to the anatomy and physiology of the
nervous system, as any science of psychology has to be.

Just as fifty years before, Freud had uncovered his ears and listened to
his patients, so Lorenz opened his eyes and looked at the animals around
him. What he saw was animals imbued with energy, inquisitive, active,
always busy, and each one preoccupied with the others of its group. That
is all obvious to anyone who looks at animals without having had any
training in a psychological laboratory. But at the time Lorenz began
observing the animals among whom he lived, psychologists regarded
animal behaviour as consisting of chains of reflexes or as being responses
to stimulation. In reality, motivation comes from within. The brain
leads the animal to seek from its environment the things that are
necessary for its survival. The brain gives the animal its appetites and
makes it carry out acts of behaviour designed to satisfy them. It
translates needs into desires. People think of the brain as the organ of the
mind, as the source of the intellect, of thinking, of ideas. It is all that, and
it is much else besides. It is mainly the organ of motivation, the part of
ourselves that makes us do everything we do.

Lorenz thinks of animal motivation in the following way. There are
certain basic instincts, each with energy at its disposal. The energy
mounts up until it is discharged; after it has been discharged in the
consummatory act, it gradually builds up again. And this cycle of
damming and discharging of instinctive energy makes animals spend
their time seeking the stimulation that will discharge the energy. The
necessity for discharging instinctive energy is what makes animals active
and inquisitive, so that they move around the world exposing themselves
to danger. There are cues that serve to make them discharge this
instinctive energy in an act, named 'releasers'. As the fulfilment of
desires is pleasant and the inability to fulfil them is unpleasant, animals
learn by a natural system of rewards and punishments.

The animal's desire or need to perform certain acts of behaviour differs at various times. One factor causing the difference is the amount of hormones circulating in its body and affecting its tissues, including its brain. Depending on the presence of hormones, features of the environment may stimulate the animal or they may evoke no interest. From the animal's point of view, the stimulus is not the same on every occasion; it depends on the animal's internal state. If we present a male trap-door spider to the female, we might imagine that this stimulus is always the same, being the male of the species. However, the response of the female spider to this constant stimulus varies a great deal. She may live contentedly with him for several months, she may live with him for only a day or two, or she may eat him straight away, rather than await the inevitable tedium of married life. The male never knows what sort of reception he is going to get; he may be invited to the marriage bed or he may be invited to a supper, not to eat but to be eaten. The same stimulus—male trap-door spider—releases different behaviour in the female, depending on factors within, such as whether she is ready to mate or whether she has recently mated.

The more important the stimulus from the world without, the less motivation there need be from within, and vice versa. When there is much motivation, an otherwise inadequate stimulus from the environment will suffice. Or if any kind of releasing mechanism fails to be found in the outside world, the total innate reaction can be manifested spontaneously without being triggered off by stimulation. This behaviour, reaction to a stimulus which is absent, is called vacuum activity or reaction to deprivation. Such vacuum activities have often been observed in birds and other animals reared apart from their fellows, and so there is no question of them having been learned. The existence of vacuum activities shows us that such acts of behaviour are innate and inherited.

Lorenz has reported instances of whole episodes of behaviour being manifested in the absence of the essential stimulus. He had a starling brought up in captivity and accustomed to receiving its food from a dish. This bird would fly up and carry out the complete motions of catching a non-existent fly; it would focus on it, swoop on it, apparently catch it, and swallow it. It had never seen another bird catch an insect. Waxwings have been seen catching non-existent insects during frosty weather, when no insects are around. Similar *in vacuo* behaviour has been seen in humming-birds. They fasten non-existent materials for nest-building to non-existent twigs. Whether the birds are actually experiencing hallucinations of the missing objects, we do not know. We do know, however, that humans under conditions of maximal deprivation often do have hallucinations; these are a sort of mirage, supplied by the imagination, driven by the need. It may be that dreams should be considered as such hallucinations. Hallucinations satisfy to some extent, and that perhaps is their purpose and the reason for their existence.

When a drive has recently been adequately satisfied, the stimulus must be ideal in every respect to serve as a releaser of behaviour. Even then, only a token reaction may be produced. A correct stimulus no longer works when the need for it is absent. Once the need has been satisfied, the animal will not respond to the very stimulus that previously evoked the response. For instance, a stimulus that gives rise to certain behaviour during the breeding season is meaningless and causes no response when it occurs at other times. This is common observation. When we have just finished eating a meal, another excellent meal placed in front of us evokes different behaviour from what it had previously done when we were hungry. Sexual stimulation that would evoke copulation in the male when he has not copulated for a long time does not do so when it occurs shortly after several copulations. Thus satiety reduces or stops the drive and the desire; but only for a time.

Among human beings, consciousness is used in the continuous seeking to satisfy needs. How far it is used in other animals, we do not know. Obviously it is used by the animals we know best, dogs and cats, tigers, lions and elephants. Because we use consciousness, we tend to overvalue conscious awareness, thought and planning; and we find it difficult to imagine how an animal acts effectively without this conscious thinking.

Professor Richter at Johns Hopkins University in Baltimore devoted many years to the study of animals choosing a correct diet. He deprived rats of an essential ingredient, for example, vitamin B1 or calcium. The animals were put in a kind of self-service shop. He and his colleagues would then observe what foods and how much of them the rats chose. From these investigations we have learned that animals choose those foods that supply the elements which they need. If a rat is deprived of a certain vitamin, it would choose foods rich in that vitamin. Female rats would take a lot more fat when they were lactating; the amount reverted to average when the litter was weaned. When rats were provided with pure protein, starch, sugar, fats and vitamins, all substances previously unknown to them, they chose a well-balanced diet. Richter also did experiments in which he upset the animal's metabolism by removing some endocrine glands. When the parathyroid glands are cut out, the body loses its calcium and retains too much phosphorus. Richter has shown that rats in which the gland has been cut out have a craving for calcium and a diminished appetite for phosphorus. He has also shown that pregnant rats choose a particular diet; they take an increased amount of calcium, phosphorus, protein and fat, all of which they need to build the fetus and to produce milk.

In these examples, we are observing how the animal's needs induce its desires. We do not know how this comes about; but we know that it does so through its taste receptors. If the nerves coming to the brain from these receptors are divided, the rat no longer makes these life-saving choices in its diet. In the case of salt-depletion, brought about by removal of the adrenal glands, Richter found that the rats deprived of salt had a lower threshold for the taste of salt; they were able to taste salt dissolved in water when the concentration was 15 times less than that which normal rats could taste.

If a rat gets nausea from any taste, it will always avoid that taste in the future; one trial is enough to put if off. It can even be put off tastes that it usually likes, such as sugar. It is therefore difficult to kill rats by poisoning them. Richter found that rats could be poisoned only when the poison was so well mixed with the food that its taste was masked or when the poison was insoluble in saliva so as to be tasteless.

Similar mechanisms, whatever they are, operate in human beings; or rather, they tend to until they are altered by implanted social influences. That untrammelled human infants act like this is known from a few cases reported in the medical literature. A particularly striking case was reported by Richter and Wilkins from Baltimore. A little boy, aged three and a half, had been born with a great deficiency of the adrenal glands. This had the effect of upsetting the body's control of its salts so that the child was constantly deficient in sodium, the most important element of all. The boy had a natural craving for sodium chloride, common salt. From the age of one, he had always taken large amounts of salt. At this age, the little boy started licking the salt off pretzels. He would chew salt biscuits and bacon; after he had got the salt out of them, he would spit the rest out. He eventually discovered the salt in the salt shaker, and then showed a great appetite for it. His mother reported to the doctor what had happened when the child was eighteen months old. 'When I would feed him his dinner at noon, he would keep crying for something that wasn't on the table and always pointed to the cupboard. I didn't think of the salt, so I held him up in front of the cupboard to see what he wanted. He picked out the salt at once; and in order to see what he would do with it, I let him have it. He poured some out and ate it by dipping his finger in it. After this he wouldn't eat any food without having the salt too. I would purposely let it off the table and even hide it from him until I could ask the doctor about it. For it seemed to us like he ate a terrible lot of plain salt. . . . After we gave it to him all the time he usually didn't ask for it with his dinner; but he wouldn't eat his breakfast or supper without it. He really cried for it and acted like he had to have it.' All the foods the boy liked were salty ones. And, interestingly enough, the first word he learned to say was salt. He took a lot of water too, which he also needed. The sad end to this tale is that when the little boy was taken into hospital, he was given an ordinary diet, with no extra salt; and he died.

The behaviour of this little boy, not only so sensible but so necessary, comes as a surprise. We think of the brain as being able to plan the future, making use of its experience of the past. But that the brain should possess this kind of intuitive or instinctive knowledge comes to us as a surprise. We always overestimate consciousness. It is unnecessary for animals to know the purpose of their activities; all that is needed is that they should behave in the right way.

How the animal's needs come to cause its appetite is a large subject which still being investigated. They physiological mechanisms differ for different needs and among different species. In higher mammals both hunger and the sensation of feeling full depend on receptors in the stomach and on the concentration of glucose in the blood. If blood from satiated rats is transfused into hungry rats, these rats will stop eating. Another substance, glucagon, secreted by the pancreas, also plays a role in providing the sensation of satiety. Another and different mechanism is that of osmoreceptors in the hypothalamus. They are sensitive to the osmotic pressure of the plasma of the blood, and they can make the animal eat or stop eating.

Hormones, to be discussed in the next chapter, also play a role. Before an animal goes into hibernation or migrates, it needs to eat more; and so it needs to have a bigger appetite. More of what it eats at that time is converted into fat, for that is a better fuel than carbohydrates. A hormone secreted by the pituitary does both these things; it increases the appetite and it converts carbohydrate and protein of the food into fat depots. In birds, it is probable that the hormone prolactin makes the animal have the need to move off on its long journey of migration.

An animal's needs are not only the obvious ones, eating, drinking, and avoiding enemies who prey upon it. Depending on the species, the baby animal may need to cling to its mother, to push its behind up against the side of the nest, as does the baby cuckoo, it may need to skip and jump, to strengthen its legs and learn to use them. In species akin to ourselves, such as the anthropoid apes, we can see the distress of the young animal if it is prevented from satisfying its basic needs.

As the young animal gets older, the needs and the consequent desires become more complicated. Again, depending on the species, it has general social needs. It may need companionship; without it, the animal cannot develop normally and will never function as a proper member of its social group. Yerkes, who knew chimpanzees better than anyone did at that time, has written of them:

The need for social stimulation, such as is provided by companions, becomes so strong during late infancy and early childhood that isolation causes varied symptoms of deprivation. In addition to overt behavioral expressions of distress, there is general physiological dysfunction. Taken forcibly from companion or group and left alone, the ape cries, screams, rages, struggles desperately to escape and return to its fellows. Such behaviour may last for hours. All the bodily functions may be more or less upset. Food may be persistently refused, and depression may follow the emotional orgy.

Monkeys have been brought up in complete isolation in order to find out what effect this has on their psychological health. These monkeys became psychotic; they had the kind of psychosis called catatonia, in which there is no emotional expression and probably no feeling of emotion. In their brains there were abnormalities in the activity of neurons of the sensory part of the thalamus and of the septal region, a part of the brain concerned with experiencing pleasure.

Chimpanzees are very ready to accept other animals as companions, human beings, orang-utans, gorillas, dogs or cats. It is the same with the young gorilla. Hediger has related how a child gorilla in a zoo succeeded in tricking its young lady keeper into its cage one evening; the latch of the lock clicked shut; and so she had to spend the whole night being hugged and loved by the poor lonely young gorilla. The social needs of animals in zoos are not considered; and in the arguments for and against having zoos, this inevitable deprivation is one of the reasons against imprisoning animals.

After puberty, reproduction demands that the animal should mate and found a family. After mating, the animal experiences the needs and emotions associated with preparing a home for the young. This brings about nest-building in birds, rodents, and sticklebacks. After birth of the babies, there follow the emotions associated with the succouring and protection of the young, retrieving them and bringing them back to the nest in the case of rodents, teaching the fledgelings to fly in the case of birds, and for man all those thousand things from changing the nappies to earning enough money to send them to school. For the species needs to be firmly established and in higher animals this means being taught the knowledge acquired by its forbears.

Some emotions aid the satisfaction of desires. They add to the energy provided by each basic need and drive. All emotion can be totally removed by cutting out certain parts of the brain. When this state is induced, the animal is inactive. A man will just sit or lie wherever he happens to be and he does not bother to feed himself or get up to get himself something to drink.

Emotion increases the energy of drives; or it may be that emotion provides the energy of our drives. The emotion of aggression is needed to make the animal establish its territory, to provide enough food for itself, its mate and its young brood-to-be. The painful emotion of fear is needed to make animals flee from their enemies. Painful emotions result from being unadapted to the environments; their purpose is to make the animal adjust better.

If the environment provides no stimulation, most animals experience boredom. This is a negative emotional state, though its unpleasantness is different from that associated with an inability to satisfy a strong internal need, such as hunger or thirst. Boredom is commonly seen in animals kept captive in zoos and in animals under domestication. In the zoo, it is observed in members of the cat family, showing itself in their compulsive pacing up and down and ritualized turning movements, to a psychiatrist so reminiscent of the behaviour of some human compulsion neurotics. If boredom occurs in animals under natural conditions, it may act as a spur in the search for necessary stimulation. In man, we know from introspection that it can lead to satisfaction in imagination, to the wish-fulfilments of dreams and daydreams, and to many kinds of substitute gratifications.

Many emotions are not for ourselves alone; they are produced for their effect on others; and they are a basic way of communicating with others. Subtle emotions are understood by other members of the same species. More basic emotions such as fear, readiness to fight, and emotions accompanying pain or pleasure are understood by other mammals or perhaps by all other vertebrates. We can tell when a dog or cat is in pain or is about to fight us; dogs can tell when the stag is frightened and about to flee and when it is about to attack them.

It may well be that some other mammals recognize the emotions we are experiencing and expressing better than we do. Possibly they detect our fear or our intended aggression towards them. I do not mean the obvious threatening behaviour, when we pick up a stone or a stick, or obvious fleeing, as we turn our backs and start running away. One has the impression that they understand the meaning of our scarcely expressed intentions before we would know those of another man. It may be that we give off smells which our poor olfactory systems cannot detect but which the sniffing dog and deer understand and which warn them of our attitudes.

Reactions to emotions are not the same in everyone; people have different constitutions. Some react to difficult situations by increasing the activity of the parasympathetic nerves to their stomachs and bowels; others cause changes in the blood vessels of the coverings of their brains and get migraine; others induce spasms in muscles and get headaches, backache, pains in their chests. Others do not express states of emotion or stressful psychological conditions physically, their bodies are not used to play out the dramas of their lives. They deal with them in the outside world. They create emotional situations, they quarrel with all their friends, they become involved in traffic accidents; or they get depressed or neurotic in many ways.

Sometimes shocks of a psychological kind can affect the endocrine balance of the body. Horror and continual fear can cause overactivity of the thyroid gland. Some disorders result from the continual use, perhaps in an unbalanced or pathological way, of the parts of the autonomic nervous system. Nervous children frequently empty their bladders; so do elephants. Bats and monkeys pass their urine on to their assailants, using their bladders as offensive weapons. Perhaps this frequency of passing urine in children and some adults is a relic of this manner of showing aggression. Some adults, when nervous, get diarrhoea, others get constipation. Elephants and camels too are very prone to diarrhoea when they are anxious or upset. Many kinds of monkeys use defaecation as an offensive weapon. Travellers in South America have reported how irritated troops of monkeys will defaecate on them from above, their ability to hit the target being excellent. In chimpanzees and gorillas, micturition and defaecation occur with strong emotional states. It is the same with ourselves. There is no doubt that certain chronic disorders of the lower bowel, such as ulcerative colitis, are caused by psychological and emotional events. They have been produced experimentally by prolonged stimulation of the hypothalamus. Also when a certain region of the hypothalamus is stimulated several times a day in monkeys, the animals develop ulcers of the stomach and duodenum. In man, psychological factors can cause gastric and duodenal ulcers and they can equally cause them to heal or not to heal. It is commonly found that an ulcer suddenly becomes worse or it starts to bleed when an upsetting psychological event occurs. There are several mechanisms known which could bring this to pass. One of the effects of adrenocorticotrophic hormone is to make the stomach secrete acid. When electrodes implanted in the hypothalami of animals are constantly stimulated, too much of this hormone is secreted, and the animals eventually develop gastric or duodenal ulcers or ulcers in the colon.

There have been one or two famous patients who have had openings made between their stomachs and the belly-wall and who have been observed by doctors aware of the importance of psychological influences on the body. Instruments could be passed through this hole, the inside of the stomach could be looked at and samples of the gastric juices could be taken. Every American and British doctor remembers hearing about such a case when he was a student. For this was a patient whose case was published by his doctor, Dr Beaumont in 1833 and who rejoiced in the name of Alexis St Martin.

In our own time two doctors at the New York Hospital, H. G. Wolff and S. Wolf, studied another patient with a gastric fistula. They had the advantage of having the modern psychological and sociological outlook as well as quantitative methods of investigation and colour photography at their disposal. In order to study human gastric function, they employed their subject, Tom, as a laboratory worker; they also got to know him so well, that they knew how any of the stresses, upsets or pleasures of day-to-day life would affect him psychologically. Knowing how Tom would be feeling in various circumstances, they could correlate this knowledge with the state of his stomach.

Fear had the following effects on his stomach.

Sudden fright occurred one morning when an irate doctor, a member of the staff, suddenly entered the room, began hastily opening drawers, looking on shelves, and swearing to himself. He was looking for protocols to which he attached great importance. Our subject, who tidies up the laboratory, had mislaid them the previous afternoon, and he was fearful of detection and of losing his precious job. He remained silent and motionless and his face became pallid.

At the same time the mucous membrane of his stomach became pale and it secreted less than the normal amount of acid. These effects lasted for five minutes after the doctor had found what he was looking for and had left the room. The mucous membrane of the stomach also remained pale with diminished secretion of acid, when Tom was sad, discouraged or was reproaching himself about anything. This effect resulting from his mood or other psychological factors would override the physiological effects due to food. For instance, beef-broth would cause an increase in the bloodflow in the stomach and the secretion of acid. But these would not appear if Tom was feeling depressed. If he was feeling resentful, there would be an increased secretion of acid with dilatation of the blood vessels, and a great increase in the movements of the stomach. Quite different reactions were shown by the stomach when Tom was feeling hostile and agressive. On these occasions, the stomach was in the same state as it would be at the start of a big meal: the amount of acid secreted was three times the normal and the mucous membrane was 'turgid, engorged and much redder than usual'. On another occasion, the investigators found that when Tom's face was red with anger and resentment, so was his stomach. Anxiety also caused an increased secretion of acid, abnormal redness and increased blood supply of the stomach; and when the anxiety persisted for weeks, so did these changes in his stomach. In Tom's case, this readiness of the stomach to receive a meal was unassociated with his feeling hungry or having a good appetite; on the contrary, he had no appetite. But in some patients, anxiety and resentment cause hunger, and these patients may eat a lot at the times when they have these emotions.

A doctor living in Chicago has recorded his own case. He had the interesting habit of examining his own gastric juices by sucking them up by means of a stomach tube every morning. One day thieves entered his house and killed his landlady. On that day, his gastric hydrochloric acid was double its normal strength. For the following ten days, he expected to be shot by the gangsters in revenge for helping the police track them down; during this time the concentration of his gastric acid remained very high. After he had moved to what he considered a safe place, his acidity returned to normal.

The actual feeling of emotion is a mixed mental and physical experience. Fear and anxiety are felt in the pit of the stomach. When certain parts of the cerebral hemispheres are stimulated in conscious patients, the patients experience this feeling, and they cannot say if the sensation they feel is a physical one in the centre of the abdomen or if it is a mental or psychological one. When the same parts of the cerebral hemispheres spontaneously discharge, as they do in epilepsy, patients experience before the actual fit this sensation of fear or anxiety in the pit of the stomach.

Emotion will suddenly send up the blood pressure and this may cause a cerebral haemorrhage and death. Aubrey has recorded that when the Earl of Dorset was Lord Treasurer, he was giving evidence at a trial.

The Lord Treasurer had in his bosome some writings, and which as he was pulling-out to give in evidence, sayed 'Here is that will strike you dead!' and as soon as he had spoken these words, fell downe starke dead in the place.

Aubrey comments:

An extraordinary perturbation of mind will bring an apoplexie: I know several instances of it.

16 The centre of the brain: the hypothalamus

The hypothalamus is in the centre of the brain; this is shown in the drawing of Fig. 16.1. It is immediately above the pituitary gland and below the thalamus, as its name indicates; and it is surrounded by the massive cerebral hemispheres.

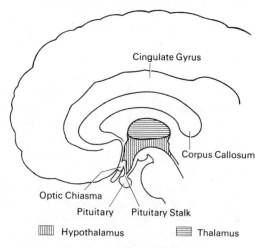

Fig. 16.1. The brain has been cut through, from front to back to show the position of the hypothalamus and thalamus.

The first physiologist who conceived of the idea of investigating the anatomical basis of animal behaviour was W. R. Hess of Zurich, and he spent most of his life doing this. Hess brought an altogether fresh way of thinking about physiology and anatomy; he has provided all research workers too with one of their most useful ways of investigating the nervous system. This technique consists of introducing very fine electrodes into the brain, the leads of which come out through the skull; they are left in place for ever. After the operation, the animal recovers rapidly and goes on living its normal life, unaware of the electrodes in its brain. We know this, as the identical procedure has been carried out in human patients. When the animal is living its usual life, the electrodes can be stimulated; this excites the neurons among which the electrodes are placed. The effect on behaviour of stimulation of these neurons can then be observed; and thus one can learn about their function. Stimulation may be repeated whenever observations need to be made.

Nowadays the stimulation is done by remote control; no wires are fixed to the electrodes. When enough data have been collected, a destructive current is passed through the electrodes, which destroys the little block of brain tissue lying between the two electrodes. This is painless too; the animal feels nothing. Then the effect on the animal's behaviour of life without these neurons can be observed. When the animal is finally killed, microscopic examination of the brain is carried out to find out exactly which neurons were destroyed. In these, as in all experiments on animals, the way of killing is absolutely painless. The animal is given a large dose of a barbiturate drug, which sends it to sleep, and it never wakes again.

The more fundamental a function is, the more completely it is organized at lower neural levels. The hypothalamus organizes whole entities which we see as acts of behaviour. Lower neural levels control various components of an act of behaviour; each higher level then adds its contribution, in accordance with what it has received from all the neurons connected to it. For example, the rhythmical movements of breathing are arranged at the level of the spinal cord and of the basal part of the brain. The hypothalamus alters the basic rhythm, the rate and depth of breathing, when it is organizing acts of behaviour, such as running away, fighting, sleeping or waking up. Breathing has to be altered in accordance with various states of emotion; and when bosoms heaved, as they did in Victorian novels, it was presumably the hypothalamus that did it.

Hess conceived the hypothalamus as organising two opposite kinds of behaviour: relating oneself to the external world and attending to the needs of the body. The first uses mainly the sympathetic nervous system and the second the parasympathetic system. The second aspect of living is restorative; it includes digestion, elimination from both ends of the alimentary canal, elimination of urine, and sleep; and also hibernation for those who hibernate and aestivation for those who aestivate. The hypothalamus is the organizer of circadian rhythms. The hypothalamus controls the production of heat by the metabolism of the body, including the body temperature. If the part of the hypothalamus controlling body temperature is destroyed, the animal is at the mercy of the environmental temperature. It cannot shiver; it cannot close down nor dilate the blood vessels of the skin. The control of temperature is achieved by the hypothalamic control of the sympathetic nerves. The nerves of this system call still work when the hypothalamus has been destroyed, but having lost their central control they work in response to local conditions and not to serve the total requirements of the body.

Other instances of the general neural pattern of organization are the acts of micturition and defaecation. When these acts are ordered by the hypothalamus, it is not merely a matter of emptying the bladder and rectum. The animal performs these acts according to the way of its species, the whole skeleton and musculature being organized, the adult male dog micturating on three legs while cocking the fourth. Although these acts are performed in a normal manner, they are not fitted into the programme and circumstances of the animal's life unless the cerebral hemispheres are in control; for these highest levels of the brain are necessary to take stock of a total situation and to organize behaviour accordingly.

One can observe the hierarchical organization of the brain by comparing the behaviour of an anencephalic baby with a normal baby. Whereas the deformed baby with only a medulla oblongata is able to suck and swallow when something touches its lips, a baby with a hypothalamus can demand food from its parent. By opening and shutting its mouth and making sucking sounds and movements, it makes its needs clear to the parent.

Reward and punishment

For he purrs in thankfulness, when God tells him he's a good Cat.

We know that in art and science discoveries are often made by mistake. The worker may be investigating one problem and he finds something different of greater importance. In 1954 in Montreal, Olds and Milner were studying the physiology of the reticular formation by means of electrodes implanted in the brain. One day the electrodes were put in the wrong part of the brain of a rat, in a region in front of the hypothalamus. Milner and Olds noticed that after this animal's brain had been electrically stimulated, the rat would always return to the place where the stimulation had occurred. The rat seemed to be seeking the stimulation, just as a hungry animal looks for food in the place where it had previously been fed. In fact, the stimulation in the brain acted like a reward in the kinds of experiments that laboratory psychologists do. The electrical stimulation was in fact a reward and it could be used in teaching animals to run mazes and to solve problems. The conclusion was that this stimulation was giving the animal pleasure. Since their observation, this work has been confirmed in cats, dogs, pigeons, monkeys, dolphins, goats, goldfish, and man.

The regions of the brain that give the animal pleasure when they are electrically or chemically stimulated are now called pleasure or reward centres. Olds spent the rest of his life doing experiments related to this discovery. He connected the implanted electrodes to a circuit incorporating a lever that the rat could press with its forepaws; when it pushed the lever, it stimulated its own reward centre. Rats got such pleasure from doing this that they would keep on pressing until they fell asleep or dropped from exhaustion. In some other experiments, he put very hungry rats in cages with stacks of food; these hungry rats preferred pressing the lever to eating. Rats would run mazes and solve puzzles or even put up with a painful electric shock to a paw, all for the pleasure of pressing the lever and stimulating the pleasure centre. Unlike coventional rewards given in training the animal, this reward never reached satiation level and never ceased through habituation. In normal life, rewards lose their potency: enough is enough. But animals with electrodes implanted in reward sites in their brains tend to go on stimulating themselves. Destruction of the reward centre at operation makes animals indifferent to whatever happens and incapable of showing any emotion.

One of the reward centres is the septal area situated just below a thin membrane called the septum pellucidum. It is around the anterior commissure shown in Plate 12. It is connected with the temporal lobes above it and with the hypothalamus below. There are also reward centres in the hypothalamus and temporal lobes connected to the septal area, in the thalamus and in the midbrain.

Olds went on to find other parts of the rat's brain that the animal obviously disliked having stimulated; he called these aversive centres. However, the idea of aversive centres is less definite than reward centres; for a region electrically stimulated might have caused the animal to have pain or anxiety, fear or any unpleasant emotion. In man parts of the brain can be electrically excited that cause pain, fear, or anxiety; but one would not conceive of the regions as being aversive centres.

We do not know, then, if connections to aversive centres give the animal punishment when it does the biologically wrong thing, but we think that the animal learns correct behaviour by being rewarded with pleasure. Once an animal has some experience of living, it will remember from previous occasions that the discharge of energy in the instinctive act is associated with relief and pleasure; or it will remember that a certain conjunction of circumstances was accompanied by unhappiness or pain. In the nature of things, the animal is forced to avoid pain and discomfort; and so it is taught to avoid the state associated with these emotions and feelings and to seek the opposite state.

It seems probable that it is the same pleasure centre that rewards hunger as rewards sexual stimulation. Eating enough food excites the pleasure centre. How eating too much excites the aversive centre or inhibits the pleasure centre, we do not yet understand.

Professor Robert Heath of Tulane University in New Orleans had the idea that as schizophrenics show and seem to experience no pleasure, stimulating the region of the pleasure centre in these patients might be a good form of treatment. He put electrodes into the septal region, stimulated it, and then instructed the patients to carry on stimulating themselves. The manifestations of pleasure were not striking. But some neurosurgeons have implanted electrodes in the septum in patients with severe pain in cancer and allowed the patient to stimulate the area. During stimulation and for a long time afterwards, the patients no longer feel pain; instead, they get a contented or a happier feeling than mere contentedness. Heath continued his work on schizophrenia by introducing transmitter substances to the septum down a fine tube. This did have good effects, and brought about a remission of the illness for many months in several patients.

Fighting and fleeing

> For when he takes his prey he plays with it to give it a chance.
> For one mouse in seven escapes by his dallying.

Hess found that when he stimulated certain regions of the hypothalamus of the cat, the animal would become agressive and attack or else it would be submissive and would run away. Hess called these two patterns of behaviour, fighting and fleeing, the defence reaction. The reasons for putting them together was that the neurons producing both kinds of behaviour were next door to each other and both ways of behaving are used for saving the animal's life.

Physiological experiments led Hess to conclude that these two reactions must be closely linked. Many years later ethologists concluded from the observation of animals behaving in the wild, that agression and fear are two aspects of one kind of behaviour. Both aspects of defence are manifested by animals as far apart as fish, birds, and mammals; and they occur in social animals living in groups. If an animal is seeking a territory and it happens to enter a territory already occupied, it may let itself be chased off. When it is the proud owner of a territory, it favours the law that says 'Trespassers will be prosecuted' and it will do the prosecuting itself. Which aspect of the defence reaction the animal manifests depends chiefly on the location of the trespasser. If the trespasser has intruded well into the property, its intrusion will be met by aggression. If the intruder is only on the boundary, aggression will take the form of threat. In either case, the intruder is likely to flee. When neighbours meet at their common boundary, both animals show mixed pictures of flight and fight.

Animals living in packs like wolves also show both manifestations of the defence reaction. When a wolf threatens another one, it will either go on threatening or else it will submit, depending on the behaviour of the animal being threatened. Similarly household hens show both aspects of the defence reaction in the establishment of pecking order.

Which aspect of the defence reaction is shown depends, according to Hediger, on the critical distance between the animal and its enemy. When this distance is considerable, the animal will go off, either by walking away or by fleeing; when the distance is small, the animal will attack. The actual distance differs from species to species, and in the same animal from time to time. Hediger's concept covers the general observation that an animal when cornered will fight; and naturalists know that this applies also to timid animals, such as small antelopes, rabbits and mice. Before attacking, all or nearly all vertebrates threaten; they prefer to scare an enemy rather than fight.

The kind of behaviour induced by stimulating electrodes in the hypothalamus differs from similar behaviour arising naturally. Under normal living conditions, the defence reaction is integrated into the animal's total activity. Aggression or flight is preceded by preparatory behaviour and is followed by a slow cooling off. Before attacking, the cat threatens. When it attacks, it directs its attack well, aiming at the face or the eyes of its enemy. The agressive behaviour of a cat being stimulated artificially by means of electrodes in the hypothalamus is directed at any living creature near it. The behaviour is carried on somewhat like that of an automaton.

In experiments of this type, when no human being or other animal is in the laboratory, the stimulated animal behaves as if it sees another animal; as far as one can judge, it behaves as if it has an hallucination. When these experiments are done on pigeons the pigeon circles round a non-existent animal, preparing either to attack or flee.

If the neurons of the flight reaction region of the hypothalamus are destroyed in a rat, the animal no longer runs away from a place where it has been hurt. One can put a rat in a cage in which part of the floor is electrified; if the rat steps on that part it gets a shock. A normal rat immediately gets off this bit of floor. But if a rat in which these neurons have been destroyed is put in the cage, it will remain on this very spot.

From experiments such as these one learns that a certain region of the brain can organize totalities of behaviour. One then has to find out how this region plays a role in the behaviour of the intact and living animal.

When a person feels the emotion of fear, there is neural activity in certain parts of the cerebral hemispheres and in the hypothalamus; these two regions are connected together. The parts of the cerebral hemispheres concerned are some large masses of grey matter in the front part of the temporal lobes: they are called the amygdala, as earlier Greek-speaking anatomists thought they looked like almonds. The neurons of this region can excite and inhibit neurons of the hypothalamus; they can cause fear or stop fear; they can induce rage or prevent it.

Hess found that when he stimulated certain neurons with a minimal electric current, the animal would show a state of vigilance. As the current was increased, the reaction would become more intense, finally becoming an actual attack with all the manifestations of fury. The usual bodily changes which are a part of fight or flight occurred. The cat would look for someone on whom to vent its rage; it usually found the experimenter, one is pleased to note. Its fur would stand on end, its ears would be laid back on its head, it would arch its back or crouch ready to spring and then jump at the experimenter, biting and scratching him. If another cat were placed in the cage, the stimulated cat would attack it, even though it was normally friendly or perhaps even afraid of the other cat. When the current was switched off, the animal quickly calmed down and went on doing what it had been doing before. When other nearby regions of the hypothalamus were stimulated, the cat showed typical signs of fear and tried to run away.

Probably, in real life, the display of the rage reaction is organized by the hypothalamus. It may be that the amygdala brings subtlety into the reaction, modifying it according to the rapidly changing circumstances resulting from aggression. The highest levels of the brain provide the animal with consciousness and memory, enabling it to organize these acts of behaviour in accordance with its previous experience.

Hess's work was extended in Munich by von Holst and his colleagues. They implanted permanent electrodes in various regions of the brain of domestic chickens and stimulated them by wireless transmission while the birds lived their normal lives in the farmyard of the Institute for Physiological Behaviour. Depending on which region was stimulated, the bird could be made to exhibit various elements of the defence reaction. It showed various kinds of attack and of flight. It behaved as if it was confronted by a comrade higher in the pecking order when no other hen was there; or an animal low in the pecking order puffed itself up and lorded it over its superiors when it was among them in the yard. It suddenly made the mating call, it picked non-existent seeds off the ground, drank non-existent water when other parts of the brain were stimulated. When the stimulating current is only slight and is then slowly increased, successive parts of a total act or behaviour appear. At first the hen becomes alert, then she gets up, walks about, and finally jumps off the platform on which she is placed, at this stage showing the complete flight reaction. A whole territory of investigation of the brain and behaviour is being opened up by using a combination of two or more electric stimulations, by altering their timing, and by combining electric stimulation with natural stimulation and relating these to the needs the animal has at the time of the experiment.

Aggression increases at puberty and at times of breeding. This is undoubtedly the effect of androgens; but it is not yet known which neurons are affected by the hormones responsible for this change in behaviour.

Mating

> For having consider'd God and himself he will consider his neighbour.
> For if he meets another cat he will kiss her in kindness.

The total act of copulation is organized in a part of the hypothalamus and the neighbouring septal region. Cats with the cerebral hemispheres removed can still preform sexual intercourse if they are placed in the right position. The parts of the hypothalamus concerned are not the same as those organizing the defence reaction. In fact, these two functions are opposed. For a sexual act to take place, fight and flight have to be prevented. Females have to cease to be aggressive and become receptive. The neurons of the hypothalamus concerned with sexuality perform their function only when they receive gonadal hormones in their blood supply. The hormones change these neurons in some way, though in what way we do not yet know.

Patients with lesions here sometimes get an increased libido and strong sexual appetite. This is about the same region of the brain as causes a strong feeling of pleasure when it is stimulated. One patient had this part of the brain disturbed by a clot of blood. When she was in hospital waiting for an operation to remove the clot, she would ask any man who was visiting to come to bed with her, then and there, in the ward. After the operation to remove the clot had been performed and the lady was again behaving normally, she was most embarrassed when questioned about her unusual conduct.

This part of the brain can be ruined in less skilful boxers, as it is particularly vulnerable to the trauma of repeated head injuries. Some of these men become placid and indifferent, they lose all interest in sex and they may become impotent.

Also in epilepsy originating in the deeper parts of the temporal lobes, the sex drive may be abnormal. The commonest defect is much diminished libido than in healthy people; these patients have diminished sexual responsiveness and they do not experience orgasm. If their kind of epilepsy is treated by the surgical removal of the damaged temporal lobe, the sexual drive becomes normal or even excessive. It is apparent that when these parts of the brain are removed, sexual activity becomes more intense and more frequent.

One sees that many epileptic saints and holy psychopaths may well have had an abnormally low sex drive and no interest in sex; hence their antagonism to sexuality and their failure to understand the behaviour of normal human beings.

When electrodes are implanted in the hypothalamus of the rabbit and the activity of the neurons is recorded, it has been seen that sexual intercourse creates a great deal of activity among the neurons concerned with sexual behaviour. When these neurons are excited into activity, they stimulate the pituitary gland to secrete the luteotrophic hormone that causes ovulation. Once the amount of this hormone in the circulation reaches a certain level, chemoreceptors in the hypothalamus stop the hypothalamic neurons stimulating the pituitary gland. In this example of the sexual activity of the female rabbit, we can see how one act follows another. A certain activity, in this case copulation, is caused by the actions of hormones on neurons in the hypothalamus. This activity in turn excites related neurons in the hypothalamus, and they act upon the pituitary to cause ovulation. Once this has been achieved, the balance of hormone secretion is again altered, so that no more ova are discharged, and the next stage in reproduction can be prepared with the implantation of the ovum in the uterus.

Although grooming and care of the fur are not sexual activities, they may be mentioned here. When cats were stimulated by Hess in the front part of the hypothalamus and in the septal region, they stopped doing

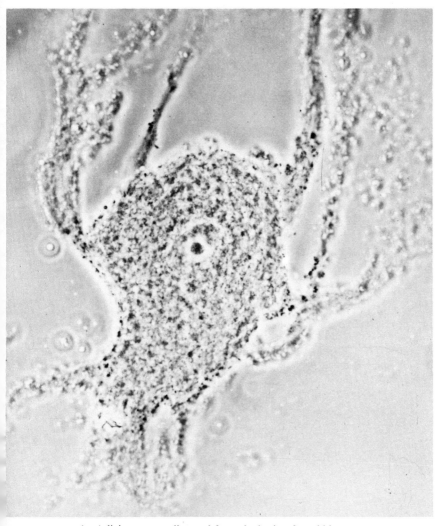

1   A living neuron dissected from the brain of a rabbit

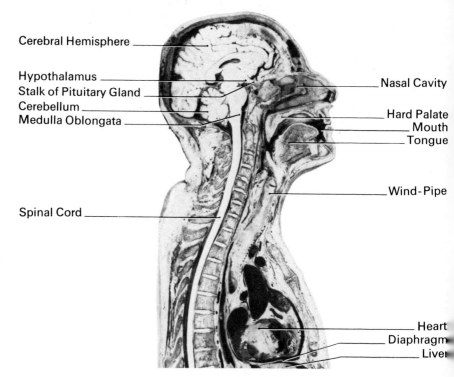

Cerebral Hemisphere

Hypothalamus
Stalk of Pituitary Gland
Cerebellum
Medulla Oblongata

Spinal Cord

Nasal Cavity

Hard Palate
Mouth
Tongue

Wind-Pipe

Heart
Diaphragm
Liver

2   Mid-line section through a man

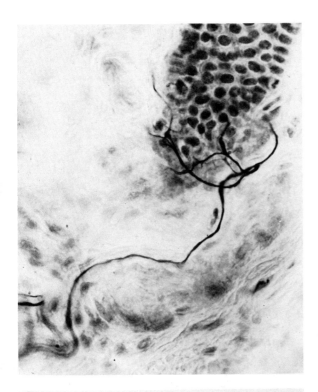

3 A nerve fibre in the skin of a man's finger

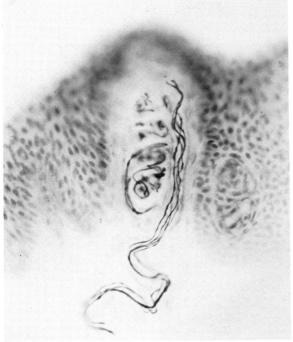

4 Several nerve fibres ending in a sensory receptor in the skin of a man's finger

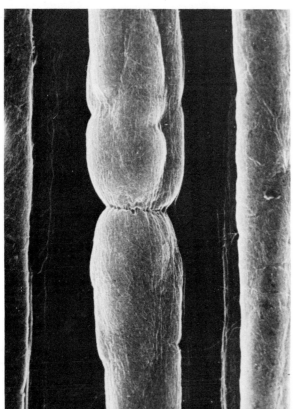

5 Scanning electron microscope study showing a node on a myelinated nerve fibre

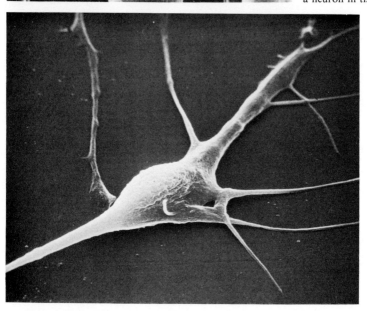

6 Scanning electron microscope study showing a neuron in tissue culture

Nerve
endings

Cell body
of neuron

Membrane surrounding
cell body of neuron

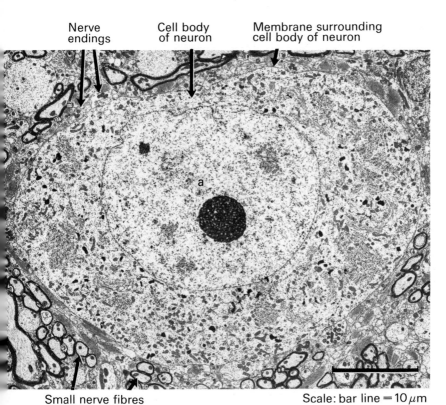

a

Small nerve fibres

Scale: bar line = 10 μm

7   Electron microscope study of a cat's motoneuron

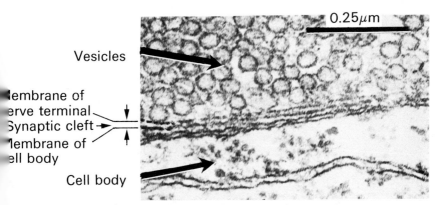

0.25 μm

Vesicles

Membrane of
nerve terminal
Synaptic cleft
Membrane of
cell body

Cell body

8   Synapses between nerve-endings and a motoneuron in a cat

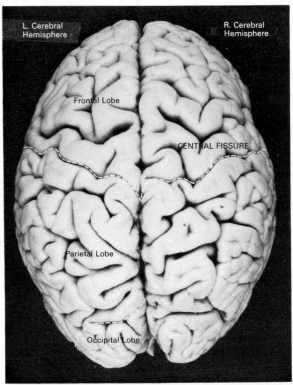

9 The brain of a fifty-year-old man from above

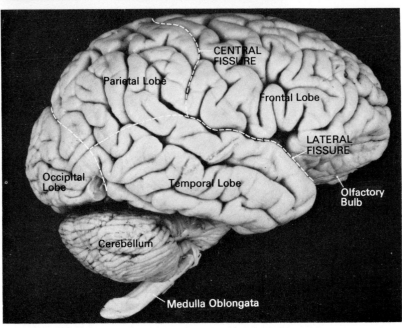

10 The same brain from the right side

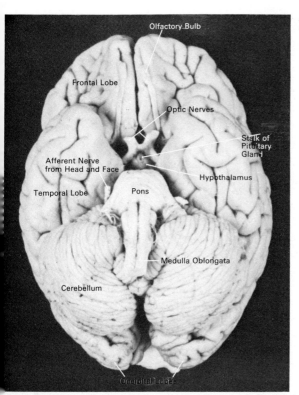

Olfactory Bulb

Frontal Lobe

Optic Nerves

Stalk of Pituitary Gland

Afferent Nerve from Head and Face

Hypothalamus

Temporal Lobe

Pons

Medulla Oblongata

Cerebellum

Occipital Lobe

11 The same brain from below

12 The same brain from the left side

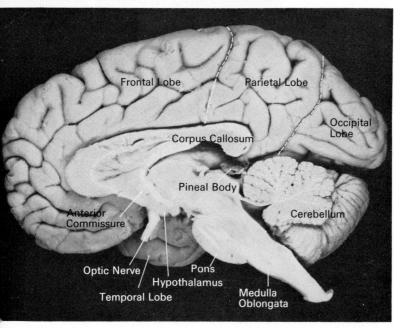

Frontal Lobe

Parietal Lobe

Occipital Lobe

Corpus Callosum

Pineal Body

Cerebellum

Anterior Commissure

Optic Nerve

Hypothalamus

Pons

Temporal Lobe

Medulla Oblongata

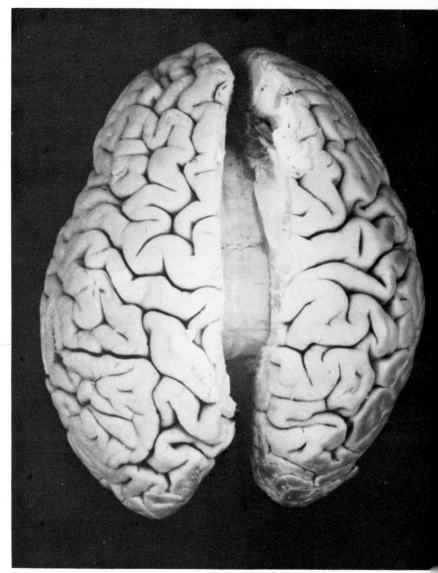

13 An adult man's brain dissected to show the corpus callosum

whatever they happened to be doing, and groomed themselves in that thorough manner typical of cats. They would usually go on till they had finished, although the stimulation had ceased.

Eating and drinking

For tenthly he goes in quest of food.

All parts of the central nervous system make a contribution to such important activities as eating and drinking; yet the hypothalamus is apparently the main centre organizing these acts. It controls the intake and output of water and the metabolism of fat and carbohydrates. It makes the animal aware of the need to eat and drink and it is essential in making it feel replete when it has had enough. What an animal chooses to eat is the concern of the cerebral hemispheres. They retain the knowledge of what is edible, they remember where it is to be found, and they direct their possessor's steps in search of it. When they are experimentally cut out, the animal will chew and swallow anything put into its mouth.

There are certain groups of neurons in the hypothalamus that when stimulated make the animal go round sniffing everything to find out if it is edible or not. The animal eats voraciously. When a strong current is used, the animal will eat anything, even chewing wooden sticks. In certain experiments, male rats with electrodes implanted in this region were put in cages containing both a lot of food and some females on heat. The males immediately showed interest in the females. When the current was turned on to stimulate the neurons organizing eating, the rats all left the females alone and started eating. When the current was turned off, they would stop eating and again take an interest in the females. Thus the desire to eat could be induced and made pre-eminent by stimulating these neurons. If the electrodes are left in permanently and are frequently stimulated, the animal goes on eating and eating, eventually becoming exceedingly fat. If it is allowed to stimulate these neurons itself, the animal will go on rewarding itself with food continually for 24 hours or more. Two research workers in Warsaw have proved that the animal actually feels hunger. They trained a goat by means of the conditioned reflex technique to raise its foot whenever it felt hungry and wanted to eat. They then implanted electrodes into this animal's hypothalamus. Whenever they stimulated these neurons, the animal raised its foot.

There are some other neurons nearby which, when stimulated, stop the animal eating. Destruction of these neurons makes the animal eat far too much. Thus destruction of the eating-excitatory neurons or stimulation of the eating-inhibitory neurons stop the animal eating and drinking. It will die of starvation in the midst of plenty.

Hunger depends on many things. There are glucose receptors in the hypothalamus that sense the amount of glucose in the passing blood; when it goes down, the animal feels hungry. But it is not only a question of glucose; fatty acids and amino acids in the blood also play a role.

There are other neurons in the hypothalamus which control drinking. If they are destroyed, the animal loses the urge to drink; it will still go on eating normally. Various parts of the brain are connected to these neurons and play a role in organizing the amount of fluid the animal will take. An important region is the amygdala of the temporal lobe (see Fig. 16.2). In the hypothalamus are neurons sensitive to the shrinking and swelling of cells; these are osmoreceptors. They play an important part in making the animal feel thirsty or that it has drunk enough. Feeling that one has had enough to drink also depends on receptors in the stomach wall which report that the stomach is full. The glucose receptors and osmoreceptors of the hypothalamus also react to the temperature of the passing blood. When the temperature starts to rise, one feels thirsty but not hungry; cooling the blood makes one hungry. The neurons of the brain that organize eating are adrenergic and those organizing drinking are cholinergic.

However, choosing a correct diet is more complicated than that. For animals not only come to eat a right amount of food, they eat a proper variety. Nearly all animals have to take a varied diet; and they do so by stopping eating a certain food even when there is a lot of it available and by eating something else, even when there is less of that food around. One factor is the availability of the food; but another and important one is whether they want that food or not. And this is determined somehow by internal needs.

There are other neurons in the brain of the rat that on being stimulated make the rat hoard food. Perhaps there are similar neurons in the brain of man. Hoarding is one of the actions that is not stopped by a consummatory act. Other actions of this kind are playing and exploring.

There are also needs to eat and drink unrelated to hunger and thirst. Babies need to carry out a certain amount of sucking however much fluid they get; indeed experiments have shown that the amount of sucking is more important than the amount of milk. This is an inborn drive, a need to carry out the sucking act.

The autonomic nervous system

When one is running for one's life, one is using every part of the nervous system, balancing, increasing the force and the rate of the heart, looking with ones pupils wide open, quietening the bladder and the alimentary canal. This means using the sympathetic nervous system. When one is relaxing in safety, digesting, eating, secreting saliva and juices throughout the alimentary canal, one is using the parasympathetic system.

The final transmitter acting on cells that respond to parasympathetic nerve fibres is acetylcholine and on those responding to sympathetic fibres is noradrenalin. The sympathetic system also has at its disposal a large store of adrenalin in the adrenal glands; this gland pours out adrenalin and some noradrenalin into the passing blood. Most nerve fibres below a certain size put out their transmitters throughout their course. This includes the sympathetic fibres. There are minute swellings on the fibres at which the transmitter substance is put out; in fact on sympathetic fibres there are about 330 000 of these swellings per cu. mm of nerve fibre. These nerve fibres have their effects in a different way from larger myelinated fibres which release their transmitter only at a few final nerve terminals.

Most muscle fibres are cholinergic; the transmitter used is acetylcholine. But there are non-skeletal muscles, as was mentioned in chapter 11, which make up the alimentary canal, the uterus and the blood vessels which are noradrenergic. They are contracted by noradrenalin from the sympathetic nerves and by adrenalin arriving in the bloodstream.

The sympathetic system wakes up when we wake up. It is stimulated far more when our emotions are aroused, particularly the emotions of aggression, fear, and sex. A mere token of such activity brings in the sympathetic system. Even talking activates it. A sudden shout or merely driving a car speeds up the heart rate. In motor racing, heart rates of 200 a minute have been recorded. If a stimulus is startling enough, the pupils dilate, eyelids retract, the hair stands on end and the bronchi dilate. Everything is organized for action. Glucose is poured out of the liver and rushed to the muscles. The blood-vessels of the muscles are opened up and those of the intestines closed down. Blood is sent to the skin and sweating is started, to evaporate the water of the sweat and keep the animal cool.

In fish and reptiles the colour of the skin is controlled by the sympathetic nervous system. It can be made darker or lighter by spreading out or contracting cells called melanocytes. These cells contain a dark pigment, melanin. Changing the colour of the skin is protective behaviour. It is a part of the defence reaction, and is used both for camouflage and for striking terror into an enemy. Mammals have lost the ability to control skin colour, for it would no longer work once you have got fur. But when you lose your fur, as man has, you can't get it back. This is the usual principle in evolution. Sometimes a species can achieve a similar mechanism or a similar weapon via some other evolutionary path; but once one has lost a part or a mechanism during evolution, that identical part or mechanism is not developed again.

The salivary glands are supplied by parasympathetic and sympathetic nerves, the main supply being parasympathetic. The parasympathetic system is quietened during anger and excitement; the mouth is dry owing to less activity of the salivary glands. It may be difficult to swallow as the chewed up food is insufficiently lubricated. Weeping is also a parasympathetic activity; and so are defaecation and urination. Most of copulation is also parasympathetic. Erection and ejaculation depend on parasympathetic nerves. Sympathetic nerves play a small part; they close off the bladder at the start of ejaculation to stop the semen going into the bladder.

Most acts of behaviour are not just sympathetic or parasympathetic. It is more complicated and subtle than that. Although the skin has to have a good blood supply to evaporate sweat, the immediate and first action of sympathetic activity is to constrict the blood-vessels of the skin. Anxiety and anger both make one pale. But facial pallor can also be due to a fall in blood pressure due to fear. Behaviour is very different according to whether an animal is bravely attacking or slinking away. In most cases it tends not to run away as that provokes pursuit. But there are no general principles here. A small antelope surprised by a lion runs for its life, because the lion is a poor runner, and so it will probably escape. The lion kills by hiding in the bushes and then leaping on the antelope, which it kills with luck, before the antelope knows what has happened. The pattern of an animal's behaviour is different for enemies swooping from the skies and those approaching on land, for enemies of one's own species and those of other species. A good picture of sympathetic activity associated with aggression and fleeing is given by Professor Yerkes, who spent many years of his life with chimpanzees.

When a cow approached, the apes would retreat in alarm; but when the potential threat to safety chanced to walk away it was boldly chased and threatened. There were corresponding sudden changes of bodily attitude and appearance in the apes and indications of secretory and excretory processes. When it is aggressive the chimpanzee is likely to march or run forward erect, swinging its arms and seeming to swell in size, partly because its hair rises. It stamps or beats the ground and bangs anything near that will resound. Often it screams, barks, or shouts, with its mouth wide open and the lips drawn back to expose the teeth. A chimpanzee retreating is an entirely different creature. Its hair lies flat, its body seems to shrink as if to escape attention, and it runs away quietly. Unless, indeed, every hair stands on end with terror and the challenger becomes a capering ball of fur. In all these cases and apparently correlated with the strength of the stimulus, frequent defaecation may occur, or, less commonly, urination and vomiting.

All sorts of sudden events and chronic stresses alter the balance of the two parts of the autonomic system. Both parts are continuously played upon by the emotions. In man, anger causes the secretion of noradrenalin, anxiety causes the secretion of adrenalin. And adrenalin itself causes a feeling of anxiety.

The hypothalamus has four principal ways of using these two parts of the autonomic nervous system; it can diminish or increase the activity of the sympathetic system and diminish or increase the activity of the parasympathetic system. Only in extreme circumstances does it both decrease the one system and increase the other. Normally both systems are active all the time, their activities being harmoniously balanced according to the needs of the moment.

In addition to the general activation of the sympathetic system, there are local sympathetic reflexes. Every harmful and painful stimulus brings out two sympathetic reflex responses: a local spinal response; and a longer supraspinal response in which impulses are sent up to the medulla oblongata and others return to the spinal cord. This second response is more general and brings in sympathetic activity over the general region of the body that has been stimulated.

The alimentary canal is controlled by sympathetic and parasympathetic nerves. The sympathetic quietens it, for general activity demands peaceful internal action. The parasympathetic activates it for you can digest at your leisure when you are relaxed. Throughout the alimentary canal, parasympathetic nerves excite all the glands into activity so that they secrete their enzymes and lubricants to digest the food. In many carnivores, the smell of blood activates the parasympathetic nervous system so that their mouths water and enzymes are secreted throughout the alimentary canal.

The parts of the brain in which the parasympathetic centres are located are the same parts that contain the rewarding or pleasure centres; these are the regions that the animal will endlessly stimulate in itself by pressing the lever. The parts where the sympathetic centres are located are parts that the animals do not stimulate if the permanent electrodes are implanted in them. It appears then that the parasympathetic centres give a feeling of contentment and pleasure whereas the excitement or agitation of sympathetic activity is not welcomed.

The transmitters of the sympathetic and parasympathetic systems, adrenalin, noradrenalin, and acetylcholine, are not the only chemical substances used in the alimentary canal. There are also local hormones, produced by cells of the alimentary canal called paracrine cells. Many of these local hormones are produced by the food as it passes along. For instance, fat in the food passing through the duodenum induces the secretion of cholecystokinin. This hormone acts on the gall-bladder, making it contact and pour out bile; the bile is needed for the digestion of fat. Paracrine cells of the pancreas also produce this hormone; here it makes the pancrease secrete insulin, and insulin is needed to digest carbohydrate.

Over and above the hypothalamus

The hypothalamus does not initiate behaviour. That is the function of the cerebral hemispheres. The hemispheres collect information from all input channels, make a total and meaningful picture from it, supply the picture with suitable emotions and memories, and then organize a programme of behaviour.

There are certain parts of the cerebral hemispheres that are closely related to the hypothalamus. For example, the orbital cortex, which is the part of the cerebral hemispheres lying above our eyes, connects to the front part of the hypothalamus that commands the parasympathetic system and the back part that commands the sympathetic system. Many parts of the temporal lobes are connected to the region of the hypothalamus which controls the pituitary gland and the secretion of hormones.

The earliest parts of the cerebral hemispheres to develop during evolution are called the limbic lobe. This lobe is made up of various parts, which are shown in Fig. 16.2; they are the cingulate gyrus, the hippocampal gyrus, the uncus and the amygdala. They are related most directly to the hypothalamus.

One notices incidentally from the names that these nomenclators lived around the Mediterranean; they were in fact Romans. A part of the brain was called the olive; here we have the amygdala, an almond and the hippocampus, a sea-horse. The amygdala was developed in fish to

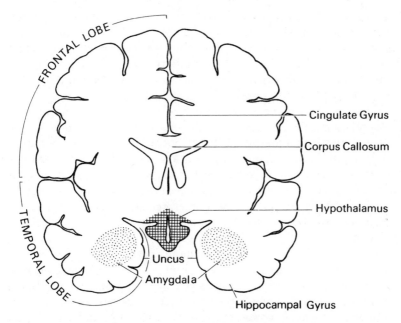

Fig. 16.2. The human brain cut from side to side to show the position of the hypothalamus and the parts of the limbic lobe, amygdala, and uncus.

interpret the inputs of taste and smell. In higher animals, all sensory inputs are relayed to this grey matter.

As we have seen already, within the hypothalamus are groups of neurons capable of organizing sexual activity, eating and drinking, and the defence reaction with its two aspects, flight and aggression. The first two, sex and eating, could be seen as being opposed to the third, the defence reaction. Probably the neurons organizing the defence reaction inhibit those concerned with eating and sex, and vice versa.

When the amygdala and hippocampus are removed experimentally, there is an increase in sex and eating and a decrease in defence. It appears that a system of braking has been removed from the activities of sex and eating and that a brake has been put on the defence reaction. As these activities may work reciprocally, merely one mechanism may have been removed when these parts of the temporal lobes are cut out, for the removal of one brake might suffice to obtain the whole result. Eventually, however, these animals do show rage, but the provocation had to be very high. Evidently what had changed was the threshold for aggressive reactions; as would have been expected, the animal was still capable of manifesting them.

Further experiments have shown that if these operations are carried out on animals in which the gonads had previously been removed, or if they are removed after the operation, then the sexual components of the behaviour did not appear. This supports other evidence that the hypothalamic nuclei organizing sexual behaviour function only when supplied by hormones secreted by the gonads.

What the hypothalamus receives has already passed through the cerebral hemispheres. The animal behaves by responding to the situation in which it finds itself. Before it can respond to this situation, all the inputs have been integrated and assessed. This is the function of the cerebral hemispheres. What is occurring is related to past experience and in the higher vertebrates it may also be related to a probable future. Only when the situation has been interpreted and judged is a line of behaviour ordered and the hypothalamus called upon to organize this behaviour.

It works similarly with regard to more simple aspects of behaviour too, such as defaecating, eating, and drinking. It appears that when we imagine a delicious meal or see, smell or start tasting food, we are activating the insula, and, as we have seen, this part of the cerebral hemisphere is closely connected with the hypothalamus. And so, the smell or taste or just the thought of food activates the hypothalamus and the parasympathetic system. This makes our mouths water; and farther along the alimentary canal, other digestive juices are similarly secreted, and the movements of the stomach and duodenum are increased, all ready to receive the meal.

It is possible that the cerebral hemisphere-hypothalamus circuit can be short-circuited at every level. For instance, the foot is pulled off the thorn of the cactus before the cerebral cortex knows what is happening. Something sudden and potentially dangerous alarms the animal before it knows what it is. The alarm reaction is set off by certain regions of the mid-brain. The whole nervous system is alerted, and the cortex is made vigilant to find out what has happened. The cortex does not need to find out and then spread the alarm throughout the central nervous system; though things can also happen in this order.

There is one other situation in which it may be that hypothalamic behaviour is in control, the cerebral hemispheres being short-circuited: fleeing in panic before an unknown horror. Many people in a panic-stricken crowd have no idea why they are fleeing. They are wholly taken up in terror and the urge to flee, and that organizes their behaviour. The contributions of the cerebral hemispheres, reasoning, memories of past experience, planning play no role.

It is likely that the same occurs in boxing or other fighting when one loses one's temper; and the skilful boxer may try to make his opponent do so if he can. For the man who has lost his temper may be wilder but he has lost his cunning. All that he has learned and remembers, all his strategy and his planning has gone. These are the contributions of the cerebral hemispheres. It may be that when one loses one's temper, one short-circuits the cerebral hemispheres and acts with the hypothalamus alone.

The relationship between the cerebral hemispheres and the hypo-thalamus is not merely one of inhibition. In normal life, it could be that the hemispheres call upon the hypothalamus to produce the patterns of behaviour organized in this structure when the total situation of the animal demands them. Now that the patterns of behaviour obtainable from experimental stimulation of the hypothalamus have been observed, it appears that such acts of violent behaviour are almost never seen in pure form in natural conditions. For what was seen in these experiments was somewhat different from what is seen in normal life. When the cerebral hemispheres are in control, the animal is capable at all times of reviewing the situation. It is not merely a wildly fighting object or a wildly fleeing animal. Its behaviour is related to the total situation. A bird will be aggressive when it is attacked within its own territory; it will be far less aggressive when it is on the border of its territory; it will flee when it is attacked in someone else's territory.

Hypothalamic behaviour is adjusted and graded by the hemispheres. Using its cerebral hemispheres, the animal can appreciate the whole situation and is able to choose. The cerebral hemispheres provide a means of delaying direct responses. Above all, they integrate the basic ways of behaving into the whole situation. When the animal is hungry the cerebral hemispheres organize the finding of food. When it is thirsty, they are needed for finding water. They keep the record of previous experience, they know the landmarks in the country, the paths to the water pools, they remember the smell of approaching rain; they are the end-stations of all sensory inflows, so that they know the sight, the smell, the sound, the combined sensations of water.

17 Broadcasting information: hormones

Nerves are not the only messengers; there are also chemical messengers. These are the hormones. They are of two kinds. Those secreted by endocrine glands, acting generally; and those secreted by paracrine cells, acting locally. If the obvious analogy for nerve fibres is the telephone or telegraphy, then the analogy for hormones is radio. There are then two broadcasting systems, a local radio station serving just a few houses, and a general station for the whole country. The control of the general broadcasting stations belongs to the central authority of the brain. Just as there are many broadcasting stations, so there are many different hormones. The programme is broadcast far and wide, but it can be picked up only by those with sets tuned to receive it. So it is with hormones. They are poured into the bloodstream and sent all round the body; but they bring meaningful messages only to those cells tuned in to receive them.

Hormones might be thought of as drugs manufactured in the body. Nowadays the chemical constitution of most of them has been worked out, and they are also manufactured by the pharmaceutical industry. The practical result of this is that if our own bodies give up making them, we can take them artificially, by swallowing them or having them injected.

Endocrine and paracrine glands are factories producing chemical substances which they make out of the various products brought to them in the bloodstream. Endocrine or ductless glands pass their products directly into the bloodstream; other glands, such as tear glands or salivary glands, have little pipes or ducts through which they pour their products into the special place designed to receive them.

Hormones have obvious effects on behaviour. They give the animal desires in order to make it perform those functions that are needed by his species. The environment in which he lives also stimulates his desires and satisfies them. Potential sexual objects generate desire. It is found in rats that maternal behaviour can be kept going for far longer than normal by the presence of the young. If, as fast as the rat's babies are being weaned, they are replaced by a new litter brought to the mother, the mother rat will continue to show maternal behaviour for several months instead of the normal period of a few weeks. She builds nests and retrieves the wandering young; and without being fanciful, one may presume she feels the emotions related to these maternal acts. It is the same for most kinds of mammals and birds. It has often been observed that a childless woman soon after adopting a child conceives and starts to produce children of her own. Whether this is really so or not has not been examined statistically, as far as I know. It may well be true. The presence of the baby acts as a constant stimulus to parts of the brain, altering the balance of secretion of hormones, and this may allow fertilization to take place.

Changes in the tissues of the animal and changes in its behaviour brought about by the secretion of hormones are obvious to bird-watchers and owners of cats. (Does one *own* a cat or is one owned or merely tolerated?) The cock bird's change in plumage together with its change in behaviour appear in spring with the hormones causing mating, nest-building, and bringing up the young. The bower bird of Australia and New Guinea collects its favoured coloured objects, arranges them in its bower, and then dances before this back-cloth. The weaver-bird of Africa, obeying its inner compulsions, makes its hanging nest. In our own islands at the end of winter, birds such as the peewit and the bunting, which had lived contentedly together in flocks; go off on their own. Every male acquires a territory; and as he does so, he acquires a new personality and a new kind of behaviour towards his former friends. He becomes aggressive and eager to fight anyone entering his new domain. In the few species in which this subject has been investigated, it is the increasing length of daylight that starts off the new behaviour.

Hormones are not the only instigators of total behaviour. Thoughts and imagination can bring about the secretion of hormones. Thoughts are the activity of cortical and hypothalamic neurons, and these neurons connect to others controlling the pituitary. Thus imagination can call forth the hormones that can then re-stimulate the very same neurons in the brain. This is a positive feed-back mechanism; it can cause an ever-increasing demand made by the animal on its fellows and its surroundings till this cycle is broken by the factors that satisfy the desires and bring the relief of satiety. Similarly, the secretion of hormones can be stopped by thought. Grief suppresses lust far more effectively than religion.

To such questions as do hormones form behaviour, or does behaviour produce the hormones, the answer is that both are true. Hormones produce needs and desires which do not occur until the hormone reaches the brain. In its turn, behaviour influences the brain, and this affects the secretion of hormones.

One of the surprising general facts learned from many thousands of experiments on rats is that the pattern of behaviour of each sex is built into both sexes; and yet under the normal circumstances of their lives each one manifests only its own sexual pattern. That each sex has in its brain neurons capable of organizing the sexual activities of the opposite sex is shown by the results of the injection of male hormones into females and female hormones into males. In rats each sex then shows the behaviour of the opposite sex so successfully that it is treated by other rats as if it were of the sex belonging to the hormone injected; for instance, castrated males injected with female hormones are treated by other males as females. These injected males build nests, an activity normally carried out only by females after puberty; they retrieve the young and bring them back to the nest, behaviour normally shown only by females after the birth of their young. It is remarkable enough that a female rat, raised in isolation knows how to build a nest. It is extraordinary that male rats, who are never normally called upon to do such a thing, also know how to do it, once they have been injected with the female sex hormone, progesterone.

Bird watchers also have seen evidence that the behaviour of each sex may be built into the nervous system of both sexes. Sometimes among those birds in which the male normally feeds the female in courtship, the opposite has been witnessed: the female will feed a male or other females. Aristotle recorded in his book on the generation of animals that two female doves will form a pair if there is no male available; this has frequently been corroborated for many other birds.

The sex of a person, like the moment of death, may be uncertain. There is sex according to the chromosomes, sex according to the kind of gonads possessed by the person, testes or ovaries, sex according to the internal organs that are not seen, such as the uterus or the seminal vescicles, or sex according to the obvious external sexual organs; and the whole body can be influenced towards a feminine or masculine form and behaviour in accordance with the secretion of hormones.

There are certain times in the life of an animal when its nervous system is particularly sensitive to sex hormones. One period is very early on in life. In rats, this is before birth and for a few days after birth. This period is certainly later in monkeys and man but it is not known when it is. In the rat, experiments have been done to learn about the effects of hormones given before or at the time of birth on subsequent sexual behaviour, manifesting itself at puberty. If at this early period, the baby rat's nervous system is receiving a lot of the male hormone, testosterone, then this rat will probably behave as a male when it reaches puberty, regardless of whether it is a male or female. Under normal conditions, this might happen. Hormones pass from the bloodstream of the mother across the placenta into the bloodstream of the baby. If an abnormal amount of testosterone were getting into the baby female rat, then at puberty this rat would not have the cyclical events characteristic of the female reproductive system. This female will then choose female sexual partners and will behave as a male throughout its life. It is the same with male rats injected before birth with female hormone: they will always behave as females and at puberty will present themselves to male rats for copulation. Also if the baby male rat is castrated during its first day of life, it will behave as a female for the rest of its life. All of these effects are due to the hormones affecting the nuclei of certain cells in the brain.

This is not the same for the monkey. Female baby monkeys given injections of testosterone show certain masculine qualities but when they reach puberty they behave as females. Humans resemble the monkey; social factors seem to be the most important determinants of sexual behaviour. Studies of human hermaphrodites show that the sexual role assigned to the child and in which it is brought up determines its behaviour. If the child is brought up as a boy, it will prefer girls when it reaches puberty and if brought up as a girl it will prefer boys. Ritual circumcision, practised by the adherents of certain religions, sometimes cuts off the penis along with the foreskin. These children are usually brought up as girls, and they behave as girls in all respects. Incidentally, human homosexuals of both sexes have normal amounts of pituitary and sex hormones.

There are always two factors interacting, the intrinsic data of the body and the environment in which the body lives. The effect of length of day-light on behaviour is brought about by the pineal gland. Those animals which have third eyes have optic nerves connecting this eye with the pineal gland; the third eye of the lamprey is immediately above the pineal, in the middle of its head. Animals with two eyes have nerve fibres going from the retina to the hypothalamus. There, it is likely that they contribute to the centres organizing circadian rhythms. From here the sympathetic nervous system is involved, sympathetic nerves controlling the pineal gland. The pineal itself acts on the hypothalamus and the hypothalamus controls the pituitary gland. It does so by preventing the pituitary from secreting its hormones that stimulate the gonads. At puberty, this control is relaxed and the action of these hormones on the testicles and ovaries brings about the appropriate physical and psychological characteristics. In some animals, it is the duration of daylight that affects the pineal; and so it is the length of day and night that rules sexual life. In many birds, this relationship between daylight and reproduction seems to have been developed so that the parent birds have enough time during the long days to collect insects to satisfy the voracious appetites of their young. In their case, the rhythm of life, the onset of puberty, the times of mating and producing young, as well as the time of migration, are all set by the length of daylight, reported to the pineal gland.

The pineal is just near the fluid-filled passage in the centre of the brain. It pours its hormones into the cerebrospinal fluid whether this is the route by which they reach the hypothalamus and pituitary is not known for sure. These hormones are melatonin, some polypeptides, and a derivative of serotonin. In all species, including man, as far as we know, these hormones are built up only at night. Thus the seasonal length of night and day rules reproduction. As the days draw out, less pineal hormones are made, the pituitary is allowed to secrete its hormones, the gonads enlarge and become active. By the summer, sexual activity is at its height. As days draw in, the opposite occurs; more hormones are secreted by the pineal, the pituitary is inhibited and sexual organs atrophy.

Young Syrian hamsters have to be born in the spring. This animal hibernates during the winter, and while it hibernates, its testicles are atrophic and no spermatozoa are produced. As the duration of daylight starts to be more than half the twenty-four hours, the secretion of pineal hormones decreases, and the gonads respond to the hormones of the pituitary. Things happen rapidly then; the young are born sixteen days after hibernation stops.

Although it would be presumptuous to extrapolate from hamsters to humans, it has been claimed that human sexual activity increases during prolonged sunlight, even though the nights are short. A travel agent told me that what people want on holidays is sun and sex.

Melatonin also has another role. It contracts pigment-containing cells, their pigment being melanin. Contraction of these cells makes the animal's skin light and relaxation makes it dark. Thus in the sun animals may become darker and those that live in caves have the unearthly pallor of troglodytes.

The effect of the pineal gland on the pituitary is shown up when a tumour of the pineal gland develops. The hormones produced by the tumour can stop the pituitary secreting its own hormones and the patient comes to the doctor with all the manifestations of lack of pituitary function. If the tumour stops the pineal gland forming the hormones that inhibit the pituitary, then puberty comes on abnormally early. Girls of three years old may develop breasts and start menstruating. In boys the changes that occur produce such well-developed muscles that the condition has been called Infant Hercules, where boys of four years old have big muscles, and their voices break; their genital organs enlarge and they can successfully perform sexual intercourse.

The brain is not to be thought of as loftily surveying all that is going on. It is itself a part of the body and subjected to all the influences coming from the body. It receives the same blood that circulates through the whole body and has passed through the liver, heart, and lungs. The blood comes to it full of food, digested and broken down, from the intestines, full of oxygen from the lungs. The blood coming from the endocrine glands contains their products, the various hormones. All these products, oxygen, food, drink, and hormones affect the working of the brain. The brain arranges for hormones to be circulated; and it receives these hormones in the blood that continually bathes it. It can sample the concentration of hormones in the blood, and according to what it finds it adjusts the further secretion of hormones.

The whole brain is connected to the hypothalamus, the hypothalamus controls the pituitary, thus the brain controls behaviour, growth of the animal, and the phases of growth, puberty and the stopping of sexual activity. The organization of hormones by the hypothalamus and the pituitary is a self-adjusting system. The amount of hormone put into the blood-stream to circulate everywhere throughout the body is adjusted in relation to the amount already there. To sense this concentration, there are chemoreceptors in the brain and in the pituitary itself. The pituitary also sends its hormones directly back to the neighbouring region of the hypothalamus. This is a hormonal feed-back system, typical of control systems of the body.

The passage of these various substances between the hypothalamus and pituitary and back again is made easy by large blood-vessels, filling the pituitary stalk. Cells that are affected by a hormone are called its target cells or receptor cells; they are within the central nervous system and all over the body. The target cells of the pituitary are affected by hormones or transmitter substances of the hypothalamus. These substances are usually called hormones but they might be equally called transmitter substances; for they are emitted by short neurons of the hypothalamus. They are named in relation to their effects on the secretion of pituitary hormones. Some make the pituitary release hormones, others act to stop it emitting them. Thus there is thyroid releasing hormone that makes the pituitary put out thyroid-stimulating hormone; and there is somatostatin, which stops it putting out growth hormone, also called somatotrophin.

It is amazing how quickly hormonal effects on behaviour are produced. One example of rapid action comes from the world of insects. The singing of the male grasshopper attracts the female who, hearing it, arrives post-haste and ready for copulation. But when the act is finished, the very same song no longer attracts her. It has been found that the reason for the female's changing her mind is that during copulation the male has injected a hormone with its sperm; and this hormone suppresses the activity of certain neurons in her brain. When these particular neurons are active, the female longs to hear the music of the serenade; but when they are inactive, either this music is not heard or noticed or it means nothing to her.

The pituitary consists of an anterior and a posterior lobe; in many species there is also an intermediate lobe. Human beings do not have an intermediate lobe, except when the female is pregnant; after the birth of the baby, it regresses. The anterior lobe secretes somatotrophin or growth hormone, thyrotrophin, prolactin, pro-opiocortin and two gonadotrophic hormones, follicle-stimulating hormone or follitrophin and luteinizing hormone or lutrophin or interstitial cell-stimulating hormone. The posterior lobe does not produce any hormones but it stores two that it receives from the hypothalamus, vasopressin or antidiuretic hormone and oxytocin.

Hormones are either steroids or peptides. Peptide hormones can usually be broken down into other hormones, peptides with shorter chains of amino acids. They react with the membrane of their target cells, under the influence of local enzymes. Steroid hormones pass through the cell's membrane and alter the character of the cell nucleus. This finally has the effect of altering the entire tissue.

Neurotransmitters affect their target cells in the same ways. They can unite with the cell membrane, they can pass through the membrane into the cell, or they can pass through the cell into its nucleus. In some cases, there is no difference between a transmitter and a hormone. The same substance can be circulated around the body as a hormone or put out locally as a transmitter. Examples of hormones and transmitters that act by staying united with the membrane of the target cell are the peptide hormones and the adrenergic transmitters; hormones that pass through the membrane and affect the interior of cells are steroid hormones and thyroid hormones.

Follicle-stimulating hormone and luteinizing hormone act on the testes and the ovaries. Pro-opiocortin is a long chain of amino acids, which is broken down to β-endorphin, corticotrophin, and melanotrophin. β-endorphin affects the secretion of insulin by the pancreas. How it prevents a noxious input causing pain has been discussed in chapter 13. Corticotrophin is also known as adrenocorticotrophic hormone or ACTH. Melanotrophin is particularly important in reptiles, fish, and amphibia, enabling them to change their spots and thus to imitate the lighting and colour of the environment.

Growth is dependent on neurons of the hypothalamus; they induce the pituitary to secrete somatotrophin. Heredity is an important factor determining the size of a person; no doubt it acts through affecting the amount of somatotrophin. If the neurons controlling growth are destroyed in experiments in animals, the secretion of somatotrophin ceases and the animal stops growing. If the neurons are artificially stimulated, too much somatotrophin is formed and the animal gets very big. Small children usually have normal amounts of somatotrophin; but some people with gigantism (the opposite of dwarfism) are found to be forming excessive amounts of the hormone.

Giants are formed before puberty, when the skeleton can still grow; after puberty, the ends of the bones become permanently fixed to the shafts, and no further growth in length can occur. Tumours of the pituitary gland may secrete excessive amounts of hormones. When a great deal of somatotrophin is secreted after puberty, there is a condition known as acromegaly. The bones become thick and deformed, particularly the bones of the hands and feet and face. The sinuses of the face get larger; that makes the voice deeper. This condition is associated with diminished secretion of gonadal hormones. In females menstruation stops; in both sexes there is decreased libido and infertility.

In some rare cases of excessive secretion of somatotrophin in men, the breasts have secreted milk. At the same time there are emotional changes, the men manifesting maternal instincts and longing to have children. The two gonadotrophins, follitrophin and lutrophin, act on the testes and ovaries. Follitrophin affects the follicles of the ovary, making them produce the female hormone, oestradiol. In the male, it acts on the tubules of the testicles which produce the spermatozoa. Lutrophin acts on the interstitial cells of the gonads. In the female it causes the expulsion of the ovum from the ovary; in the male its effect is to cause the production of androgen. In both sexes, lutrophin makes the gonads grow at puberty.

The secretion of gonadotrophins, no doubt like that of all hormones, is influenced by psychological factors. In those animals in which smell is a guiding sensation, the presence of the smell of the opposite sex influences the amount of these hormones. Female mice do not produce gonadot-rophins when they live among a lot of other females; they need the smell of male mice. It has been found in experiments that the presence of one male is enough to negate the effect of the smell of thirty females.

What is more surprising is that infant female mice, exposed in infancy to the smell of the adult male mouse, come to choose adult male mice as sexual partners when they reach sexual maturity. But if infant females are reared only with other females or with males daily sprayed with perfume, then they have no preference for males on reaching maturity. The period during which the presence or absence of male odour has this effect is very short. This is an example of imprinting. In this case, it is olfactory imprinting; in most other cases investigated so far, imprinting has been visual.

To come back to the case of man, there are some tumours that prevent the pituitary from developing normally. Gonadotrophins are not made and puberty never comes. In these patients the growth of the skeleton continues for longer than usual and so these people have abnormally long limbs. The voice does not break; the man has fine, soft hair and does not need to shave. With the enormous population nowadays, there must be quite a number of such eunuchs around. It would be a good idea to train some of them as alto singers. Instead of castrating infants for the Pope's choir as used to be done for the greater glory of God, we could obtain singers in a normal way. The female counterpart of a eunuch does not seem to have been studied or have aroused as much interest as the male.

The male hormone secreted by the testicles is testosterone and the two female hormones made by the ovaries are oestradiol and progesterone. These hormones, acting at puberty, enlarge the genital organs and cause a growth of hair on certain parts of the body. There is enlargement of the larynx and sinuses in both sexes; this is more marked in the boy and accounts for his voice breaking. In the male, these hormones enlarge the muscles. There are important psychological changes in both sexes, due to the action of the hormones on the central nervous system. In those cultures that frown on sexual activity before marriage, the adolescent's adaptation to his society is made more difficult.

Oestradiol makes female rats ready for coitus; they come up to other rats and present their rear ends in a posture inviting sexual intercourse. Testosterone makes male birds sing, take possession of a territory and get ready to fight other males.

Prolactin makes females maternal. The baby sucks the nipples; this stimulus sends impulses to the spinal cord; they are relayed and go on to excite the hypothalamus. The hypothalamus makes the pituitary secrete prolactin, which fills the breasts with milk. This is another control system: the baby stimulates milk secretion by sucking; when he ceases to suck, the milk supply dries up. Prolactin is unable alone to supply good enough milk. Adrenocorticotrophic hormone is needed and also oxytocin to eject the milk. Prolactin injected into virgin female rats or castrated male rats makes them behave like mother rats. They retrieve baby rats and bring them back to the nest. Without this injection, both are indifferent or even antagonistic to the young. When prolactin is injected into cocks, it makes them behave towards chicks as hens do, instead of showing the usual superior male indifference. In virgin hens, it causes broodiness; in certain virgin fish, it produces nest-building. In the human male, it seems to have no function. In some birds it acts in both sexes, preparing them for migration by putting on fat before the long journey.

Melanotrophin makes the skin pigmented. Adrenocorticotrophic hormone also does so, but it is less strong. Oxytocin is another hormone essential for reproduction. It is produced by both physical and psychological factors. The stimulation of the genital organs of the female makes the hypothalamus pass the hormone down into the posterior pituitary, from where it is sent off in the blood stream. When it reaches the uterus, it causes the muscle of the organ to make rhythmical contractions; these movements help the spermatozoa reach the ovum. The violent movements of the uterus during labour also make the hypothalamus secrete large amounts of the hormone; this again helps the uterus make rhythmical contractions, thus helping the expulsion of the baby. After the baby is born, sucking the breast stimulates the same neurons of the hypothalamus and more of the hormone is produced. In this phase, it aids the expulsion of the milk. Thus it is seen that each subsequent step in reproduction is induced by the previous step. Oxytocin is also made in the male, but it is not yet known what function it has.

The right osmotic pressure of tissues and the blood has to be maintained all the time. This is done by vasopressin, also called the anti-diuretic hormone. Diuresis is the formation of much urine and so anti-diuresis prevents this. Fluid is retained or excreted to maintain a constant osmotic pressure. Vasopressin controls the amount of water taken up from the alimentary canal and the amount of urine put out by the kidneys. Various kinds of stress increase the amount of vasopressin secreted. If some disease process stops the hypothalamus sending down vasopressin into the pituitary and thence into the bloodstream, then there is a condition called diabetes insipidus. What is usually called diabetes is diabetes mellitus, in which the urine contains glucose and so is sweet, hence mellitus. Diabetes insipidus, with insipid as opposed to sweet urine, is also characterized by the patient drinking a great deal of fluid and passing large amounts of urine. In this case, it is due to the kidney being unable to re-absorb sufficient amounts of water when it is not supplied with the antidiuretic hormone.

The adrenal or suprarenal gland caps the kidney, hence the name. They are really two quite separate glands, medulla and cortex. The cortex produces three different steroid hormones, glucocorticoids, androgens, and mineralocorticoid. The medulla forms two hormones, adrenalin and noradrenalin. These hormones have the same effects on most tissues of the body. They are needed for activity and so they put glucose into the blood to be burned for energy. It is probable that aggression makes the glands secrete more noradrenaline. Taking examinations and parachute jumping put out more adrenaline. Tense, anxious, and passive people appear to secrete more adrenaline than others. A further action of these hormones is to act on the pituitary to make it secrete adrenocorticotrophin. This hormone also affects the reticular formation of the brain. The effect of this is probably to make the animal more vigilant, more aware of what is happening in the outside environment. Other ways of coping with stress are organized by the whole brain, the higher levels of which assess the situation. They excite the relevant neurons of the hypothalamus and the hypothalamus makes the pituitary secrete β-lipotrophin, which is then broken down into corticotrophin and β-endorphin.

The pituitary controls the thyroid, which secretes a hormone, thyroxin. The amount of thyroxin put out depends on the animal's activity and vigilance and the surrounding temperature. A cold environment demands more thyroxin to keep the animal warm. The thermostat is a part of the hypothalamus. This acts on the pituitary which then secretes thyroid-stimulating hormones. Stress, rather surprisingly, tends to stop the thyroid putting out thyroxin.

The nervous system itself needs the secretion of the thyroid gland; without this hormone it neither develops nor works properly. Children born without thyroid glands are cretins; they are mentally defective, for their brains do not grow adequately. When the amount of thyroid secretion is insufficient later in life, the tendon reflexes become slow; and this is used as a test for diminished thyroid secretion.

We still know very little about melanotrophin and its relation to the melatonin secreted by the pineal gland. When man has an excessive amount of melanotrophin, the skin and the mouth become pigmented. This happens in Addison's disease, a disease in which the suprarenal glands are destroyed by disease.

The effect of hormones secreted by the testes and ovaries on the nervous system of animals and thus on their behaviour is something man has known about for several thousand years. For he has understood that the removal of the testes alters the behaviour of male animals. More than two thousand years ago Aristotle reported that when the ovaries of sows are removed, their sexual desires are also removed. How man discovered the effects of these operations and how this knowledge became so general, we do not know.

Hormones secreted by the testes in males and the ovaries in females have the expected influence on the animal's behaviour: nearly all animals deprived of their gonads have no sexual interests and show no sexual behaviour. Among human beings, however, women may continue to have sexual desire after their ovaries have been removed at operation or after they have atrophied at the menopause. Cats, as we can all observe, are different. Female cats who have had their ovaries removed respond to the propositions made to them by tom-cats with hate and not with love. But if a minute pellet of oestrogen is injected into the correct part of the hypothalamus, their behaviour changes and they accept the proposals. In many species of mammals this reversal of behaviour occurs naturally. The presence and absence of sexual hormones in the bloodstream occurs in alternating cycles; it is not necessary to remove the ovaries to observe their effects on behaviour. Those hormones that have mainly sexual effects have effects on the aggression-submission aspects of behaviour in some animals. Whether they act on the parts of the hypothalamus that organize attack and flight behaviour is not yet known. The female of the American marten normally lives contentedly with the male, but when she is on heat she turns on him and fights him. On the other hand, the female short-tailed shrew chases the male away unless she is on heat, and can be so aggressive that she may kill and eat him.

When the ovaries of a female animal such as a rat or a mouse are transferred to a male and the testicles of a male to a female, the animal's behaviour changes in the expected direction: the male behaves like a female and the female like a male. Although in the act of copulation, different postures and different patterns of movement are needed from the two sexes, yet the muscles are used correctly and in the correct order by the animals injected with the hormone of the opposite sex. When injections of hormones are carried out in the correct sex before the onset of puberty, the changes in structure and behaviour normally occurring at puberty take place within a few days. Testosterone propionate injected into immature or castrated males induces male copulatory behaviour. When it is injected into male chicks, they start, fifteen days after being hatched, to crow like cocks and to make propositions to females. As has been related, virgin female rats can be made both to build nests and retrieve the young when they receive prolactin. The neurons organizing these aspects of female behaviour do not do this unless they are acted upon by ovarian hormones. If the ovaries are removed before puberty, these females do not manifest the appropriate behaviour towards the male for copulation to take place. But after being injected with female hormone, they will crouch in the appropriate position. However, such experiments do not always lead to the expected result. It has been found that testosterone injected into the hypothalamus of male rats induces strong maternal behaviour.

Among the anthropoids, sex hormones have different effects in the different species; the higher species are less under the control of hormones than lower species. Interestingly enough, the male macaque monkey is more sensitive to the hormones of the female macaque than she is herself. Although the female macaque with ovaries removed may still present herself for sexual intercourse, the male will not touch her. Moreover, male macaques do not groom females without ovaries, grooming being partly a sexual activity in monkeys. The amount of grooming the male gives the female macaque is related to the amount of oestradiol injected into the female spayed macaque. We do not know what features of the female make her attractive to the male. Certainly the male's frequency of copulation is related to the female's menstrual cycle; but her behaviour is less influenced by this cycle than his is, for she will present herself for copulation at any time.

The effect of androgens on aggressive behaviour has been studied in many varieties of vertebrates. When testosterone is injected into farmyard hens, they become aggressive and move up in the pecking order. Androgens injected into both sexes of the following animals increase aggression: American lizards, turtles, valley quails, rats, cocks, hens, fish. The domestic hen calls other hens to food just as the cock usually does. Presumably these hormones act on certain neighbouring neurons in the hypothalamus.

The removal of the testes tends to remove aggressive behaviour. Male rats castrated in the first few weeks of life are as aggressive as female rats and much less aggressive than the males. Normal male aggression can be restored by giving them testosterone.

Castration has less effect on man than on other mammals. One of the results of castration is, as Shakespeare tells us in *Antony and Cleopatra*, that the subject may still have the desire but lack the performance. A eunuch may have erections, may feel orgasms but will not have seminal emissions. It is said that this state may continue for years after castration. Such eunuchs were much prized in Arab and Turkish harems. The kind of eunuchs who owing to some disease or abnormality have never arrived at puberty can have erections; they may be capable of insertion but not of ejaculation. In all of these cases, giving androgens gives the capability of emission.

Young women who have had their ovaries removed or destroyed by disease continue to feel a need for sexual intercourse. In human beings the higher levels of the brain make up for deficiencies of sex hormones governing sexual desire and behaviour.

The effect of male hormones on those nuclei of the hypothalamus that organize aggressive behaviour is more complicated in primates than in species lower in the evolutionary scale. Among chimpanzees, the male is usually dominant; but when the female is on heat, she becomes the dominant one and the male accepts this dominance without question.

In the case of man, apart from direct physiological factors, behaviour is affected by all he has learned and experienced, including the immense influence of other people in the present and, more important, in the past. In man, the organization of behaviour in accordance with cultural factors has become overweeningly important. This means in anatomical and physiological terms that the fore-brain is very important and that the influence of hormones is correspondingly less important. This is why man is more intellectual and less emotional than other animals.

Boys with hypogonadism treated by androgens become more aggressive. They sometimes feel more self-confident; and this occurs before the development of secondary sexual characteristics.

18 General plan of the human brain

Western medicine was born on the island of Cos four hundred years before Christ. Hippocrates, its great originator, first understood the functions of the brain. The following lesson has come down to us.

Some people think that the heart is the organ with which we think and that it feels pain and anxiety. But it is not so . . . From the brain and the brain alone arise our pleasures, joys, laughter and jests, as well as our sorrow, pains and griefs. Through it, in a special manner, we acquire wisdom and knowledge, we see and hear, we distinguish the ugly from the beautiful, the bad from the good, the pleasant from the unpleasant . . . By the same organ we become mad or delirious, we are inspired by dread or fear. It brings dreams, inopportune mistakes, groundless anxieties, blunders . . . The brain is the messenger for the intelligence.

This view became established owing to the support given it by Galen in the second century A.D. But it was lost to Europe when the Roman Empire was overrun by savages from the east. When Christianity took over, human behaviour ceased to be based on a real thing, the brain, and was considered to arise from a wisp of nothingness, the soul. It is difficult for us to conceive of the ignorance of our ancestors in these matters. At one time in Europe, it was believed that the brain was nothing but a bag of mucus; and people thought that when one had a cold and ones nose became filled with mucus, then a part of the brain was coming down the nose through little holes in the base of the skull.

The philosopher is the first cousin of the priest. And most philosophers have continued to speculate on what they call mind–brain relationship without knowing how to do experiments to find the answers to their questions. Meanwhile scientists have gone ahead with their painstaking investigations, based on the belief that the nervous system and its manifestations are subject to the usual laws of physics and chemistry. This approach, and no other one, has obtained results, so that we already know a lot about how the brain works. And the mysterious world of the unknowable, known only to the priests of all religions, shrinks year by year.

The brain, like the rest of the nervous system, consists essentially of neurons. All of them are present when the baby is born, though they are not then all functioning. They are irreplaceable; if we lose any on the journey to the grave, they are lost for ever. In this respect, neurons differ from other cells of the body; for other cells divide, increasing their number to make up for losses to repair the damage done by accident and disease, and to increase the tissues for growth. By the time we come to die, owing to general wear and tear, injuries and pathological processes, and the narrowing of blood vessels, we will inevitably have lost many of the neurons we were born with.

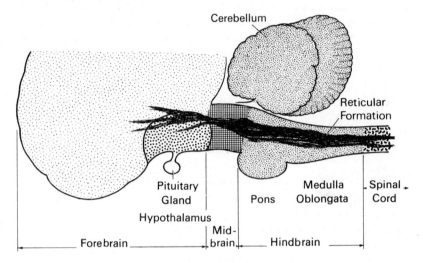

Fig. 18.1. Diagram showing how anatomists usually sub-divide the brain.

Anatomists have various ways of subdividing the brain; the usual way is shown in Fig. 18.1. The upper end of the spinal cord enlarges and opens out to become the medulla oblongata. The cerebellum originally developed out of the floor of the hindbrain; the pons, or bridge, developed in the floor of the hindbrain to take nerve fibres round the floor to the cerebellum. The three structures, medulla oblongata, pons, and cerebellum make up the hindbrain. Coming further forwards is the midbrain, which consists to a large extent of passing nerve fibres, those going up to the forebrain and those coming down to the spinal cord. Above the midbrain there is the forebrain. It consists of the two cerebral hemispheres with all the masses of grey matter within them, the limbic lobe with the septal area, and the hypothalamus. Throughout the centre of the brain is the reticular formation.

Within the members of a species, size of brain is not related to intelligence. Very intelligent men and women have had smaller and lighter brains than half-wits. Brain size among human beings is dependent on height. Women have smaller brains than men because they are shorter. Dwarfs too have small brains, because they are short. It seems to be that among all mammals, the difference in brain size is related to the animal's ability to learn. Man's brain is not the largest of any animal's; the porpoise's, the whale's and the elephant's are bigger. But in relation to the animal's total size, the whale has a small brain, one of the smallest of any mammal's. The larger the brain, the less closely packed are its neurons. This may allow them to have more synapses. Man's cortical neurons are less densely packed than those of other primates; and one must admit that he is more intelligent. Thick layers of cortex may imply neurons with more and larger dendrites, and that too means more interconnexions; and they may be necessary for learning. One must remember that the bee and the ant lead astonishingly successful lives and they have minute brains. But they are almost incapable of learning. Dealing with everything that turns up in the world by learning is a way of evolution that seems to be no longer available to them.

Although the rest of this book will be about the cerebral hemispheres, these parts of the brain are not essential for life. They are an added feature, appearing late in evolution and provided only for the later models. All essential functions had been built into the previous models for some millions of years.

Mammals have made a great advance, nevertheless, in developing this part of the brain. Even the most primitive mammals have many layers of neurons in their cerebral hemispheres, whereas most animals lower in the evolutionary scale have only one layer. In most of the cortex of primates, there are six layers. These layers provide the animal with a hundred thousand neurons per sq.mm. of cortex, and a hundred thousand million neurons in the whole cortex. Any of these neurons could be connected to twenty-five thousand other neurons.

Brains of different animals differ according to which aspects of the world particularly concern them. Smell is a sense that we despise; there is no Royal Society of Olfactory Arts. Yet the cerebral hemispheres first developed to cope with this sense. They started in the ancestors of present-day fish. The whole existence of fish depends on this input. Smell was always related to the alimentary canal, and so the chemoreceptors of taste and smell developed in the mouth part of this canal. These senses are essential for the fish to find good food and to regurgitate bad and for it to find a sexual partner, and in some cases to avoid predators and to keep with its kith and kin.

As the vertebrates continued to develop and as their brains evolved, other sensory inputs developed, and they also acquired end-stations in the forebrain. But the first sensory system to develop remains immediately connected with the parts of the forebrain that organize emotion. By the time the South American mud-fish evolved, more than half the sensory input was devoted to smell. The next group, the reptiles, relies less on smell, and this sensory input occupies less of the forebrain. In their brains, there develops the hippocampus, the part of the cerebral hemispheres related to the hypothalamus, as was seen in chapter 16. Reptiles used their tongues as tactile organs to examine the world, and so they evolved a large sensory tactile region in the forebrain. When birds developed as an offshoot from reptiles, smell lost its pre-eminence; the sensibility of the beak and the tongue became more important. But most important was vision. Birds developed large visual areas of the brain to receive impulses from their all-seeing eyes with their large visual fields. But birds are not the main trunk of evolutionary development; they are out on a limb. The main trunk continued with the first mammals, and they used smelling rather than seeing. Smell remains the most important sense for most mammals today. It was the few mammals who took to living in trees that developed sight and neglected smell; for life among the branches of trees demands good eyesight. And so man, returning to the earth from the trees, has good sight and a poor sense of smell. From examining the brain of an animal we can thus tell whether the animal was orientated towards hearing or smelling, whether it had big eyes or a well-developed nose. For within the phylum of vertebrates, among the various classes and species, the same parts of the brain subserve essentially the same functions. As the development of the skull is necessarily related to the size and development of the brain within, we can deduce from examining the skull of extinct animals what sort of life the owner of that skull once had. One can know whether it lived mainly visually or relied mainly on smell; just as from an examination of its teeth, we know whether it lived on meat or vegetables and fruit.

The cerebral hemispheres do so many things that one can hardly say in a few words what their functions are. From a distant viewpoint, we should consider them as the last intermediate neurons between the afferent and the efferent neurons. They add necessary complications to the never-ending task of adaptation to the environment. They add vast numbers of intermediate neurons between the input from the environment and the response of the animal to this input. They store the animal's own experience of life, all that the individual has learned. From earlier experience, from the pain of previous deprivation and the pleasure of previous satiety, the animal has learnt when to produce the copulating, sleeping, fighting, fleeing, eating, drinking, micturating, and defaecating organized by the hypothalamus. These patterns of behaviour are integrated into the animal's life by the cerebral hemispheres. They choose the moment, the occasion and the place, for the right behaviour.

It was known to Greek medicine that an injury to one side of the brain causes paralysis of the limbs of the opposite side of the body; and from this it was deduced that movements of one side are organized by the opposite cerebral hemisphere. The rest of our knowledge of the forebrain was acquired during the last century from the study of patients with neurological disorders during life and the careful investigation of their brains after death.

The easiest way to get an idea of the general shape and construction of the brain is to go to the butcher's and buy one. It is unlikely that he has a human one, but a sheep's or a bullock's is sufficiently like the human one to make no difference.

Four photographs of a human brain are shown as Plates 9, 10, 11, and 12. The brain is shown from above, below, and from the right side, and the left side of the right hemisphere is shown after it has been divided from the left hemisphere.

The hemispheres are divided for convenience into lobes. The front half is the frontal lobe; it is separated by a fissure, called the central fissure, from the parietal lobe behind it. The part at the back of the skull is the occipital lobe. They are shown in Plate 9.

In Plate 10 all four lobes can be seen. The cerebellum is below the occipital lobe and the medulla oblongata is below that. Beneath the frontal lobe, the slight projection is the olfactory bulb, which receives the olfactory nerves coming through the skull from inside the nose.

Plate 11 shows the brain from below; this surface sits on the floor of the skull. The frontal, occipital and temporal lobes are seen; the parietal lobe does not reach the undersurface of the brain, and so it cannot be seen in this view. A great deal of the temporal lobe is seen in this photograph. Within this part of the temporal lobe is the hippocampus and amygdala. Behind the hemispheres is the cerebellum with its folds and furrows, narrower than those of the cerebral hemispheres. It is at the back of the brain, situated just above the neck. Between the two cerebellar hemispheres is the medulla oblongata, which continues below into the spinal cord and above into the pons. In front of the pons, in shadow, is the floor of the hypothalamus, and in its centre is the stalk of the pituitary gland cut through. Bordering the hypothalamus are the two optic nerves joined together. In front of them are the two olfactory stalks ending in front in the olfactory bulbs, which receive the olfactory nerves. On each side of the pons are the two afferent nerves from the face and head through which all sensation reaches the brain.

All four lobes of the right hemisphere can be seen in Plate 12. The cerebellum is also cut across and so its cut surface is seen. The medulla oblongata and the pons are cut through. In front of the cerebellum the pineal body can be seen. Here Descartes placed the seat of the soul. The large curved bridge of the corpus callosum has been cut through; this is the main structure connecting the two cerebral hemispheres. Another and more ancient bridge can be seen above the opitic nerve; this is the anterior commissure. The hypothalamus is behind the optic nerve. A large mass of white nerve fibres can be seen descending into it; these fibres come from the temporal lobe of the other side.

Our bodies are bilaterally symmetrical, most structures being in pairs. We have two arms, two legs, two eyes, two kidneys. The whole body is not built on this plan of course, for we have one heart, one liver, one pancreas. If we have two eyes, two ears, two limbs, the brain has to be built on the same bilateral plan. We must have two optic nerves from the eyes, two auditory nerves from the ears, and parts of the brain related to the opposite side of the body. A brain built on this double plan runs the danger of behaving as two incoordinated organs. This is overcome by building bridges between the two halves; in anatomy these bridges are called commissures. They are present throughout the spinal cord, the hindbrain and midbrain. In the later-developed parts of the brain they are more obvious, as this part of the brain is more obviously constructed in two halves.

The cerebral hemispheres, when cut, are seen to be made up of white matter and grey matter. The grey matter is along the outside of the hemispheres and so it is called the cortex (Latin: rind or bark; French: *écorce*, which also gives us cork, the rind or bark of the cork oak). The white matter consists mainly of nerve fibres, and the grey matter of nerve cells. The surface of the cerebral hemispheres is thrown into ridges and furrows, so as to get a large sheet of cortex into the restricted space of the skull. On account of this folding, about two-thirds of the cortex is hidden from view, being folded into the depths of the furrows.

The general plan of the working of the hemispheres will now be considered.

The main afferent pathways end up in the thalamus (shown in Fig. 18.2). This is the highest part of the older brain; it is from the thalamus that the cerebral hemispheres developed. How the inputs to the cortex of

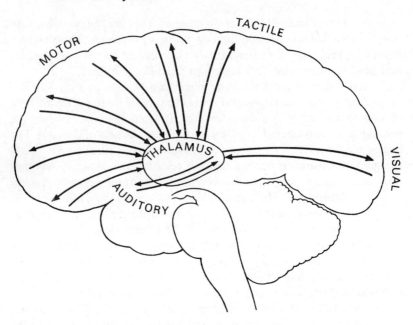

Fig. 18.2. Some connexions between the thalamus and the cerebral cortex.

the hemispheres from the thalamus are arranged can be seen in Fig. 18.2. The main sensory pathways cross the mid-line and go to the opposite thalamus and cerebral hemisphere. Each kind of sensation has its own territory in the thalamus; though there is also some mixing, two or three kinds of sensation having their inputs going to the same region of the thalamus.

In the nineteenth century, neurologists divided the cerebral cortex into primary sensory, parasensory or secondary, and association areas, and motor areas. Each primary sensory area sends its connecting nerve fibres to the surrounding area, which is its parasensory or secondary area; it sends no fibres to any other area. Each secondary area is connected with its corresponding area of the opposite hemisphere and to every other secondary area of the same hemisphere. After the secondary areas come the association areas. These are concerned with elaborating sensory information, with joining together the input from the various sensory channels to make a whole. It looks like fish, it smells like fish, it tastes like fish, so it must be fish. The association areas are interconnected; and finally they are connected to motor areas. The higher the animal in the vertebrate scale, the larger proportion there is of association areas.

The primary receptor area for the sense of smell is in the olfactory bulb, shown in Plates 10 and 11; this is a prolongation of the brain, situated above the nose. From the olfactory bulb, bands of nerve fibres run to the secondary olfactory area in the under-surface of the temporal lobe. As was said before, the nerve fibres of this system do not go to the thalamus. The fibres of the optic nerve go to several regions of the brain, the two most important being to two separate regions in the midbrain. They form relays there, fibres going on to the occipital lobes and to the borders between the occipital and the temporal lobes.

In man, the nerve fibres originating in the left half of both eyes go to the left occipital lobe and those from the right halves go to the right lobe. Thus everything we see on the right is relayed to the left lobe and everything on the left to the right lobe. As we would expect in an animal as visual as man, visual areas of the hemispheres are large. They occupy the entire occipital lobes and spread forward onto the boundary regions of the parietal and temporal lobes. Above the ear and deep in the upper part of the temporal lobe is the primary receptive area for hearing. It receives from both ears but mainly from the opposite one. Between this region and the secondary region for smelling is the primary region for taste. There is a long and wide strip of cortex along the front of the parietal lobe, running from the vertex of the head to above the ear, which is the primary receptive area for all the varieties of touch, pressure and kinaesthetic sense; this is called the somaesthetic area. Below this region and in front of the visual area is the receptive area for vestibular sensations, the sense that one's body is where it is in space, with the feet on the ground and one's head upright.

The inflow from the world is at first selected and controlled at the level of the receptors. It is then distributed to various parts of the spinal cord and the lower levels of the brain. It finally reaches the higher levels of the brain. When this inflow reaches the forebrain we become conscious of sensation. It is probable that at the level of the thalamus in the centre of the cerebral hemisphere, we are conscious of pain and of a crude sort of tactile sensation, of pressure, of being touched. It seems probable that affect is added to sensation in the thalamus. When this part of the brain is damaged by injuries or disease, every sort of sensation acquires an unpleasant quality. Severe pain can occur spontaneously. All sensation is felt excessively. Pleasant smells such as lavender become repulsive. Even a draught causes the patient pain. It is fortunate that this lesion occurs only rarely, since disease attacks the just and the unjust indiscriminately.

The neurons of the cerebral cortex are arranged in layers and columns. One might think of this by imagining a modern building with sixty floors or so and a forest of stanchions; then reduce this to a millionth part of its size, and squash it up a little, both vertically and horizontally. The neurons communicate with each other in both directions: up and down along individual stanchions or columns, and sideways along the floors or layers. The columns are arranged at right angles to the surface and the layers are parallel to it.

19 Exploring man's living brain

It is about a hundred years since we began to learn about the functions of the different parts of the cerebral hemispheres. Before this higher level of neurology could be studied it was necessary to conceive the idea that various parts of the hemispheres might carry out various functions. It was taken for granted over a hundred years ago that each hemisphere works as a whole, the one reduplicating the functions of the other. The first investigator who denied this was Franz Josef Gall, an anatomist and neurologist working at the end of the eighteenth and beginning of the nineteenth century. Gall is known mainly as the founder of phrenology, a subject that is usually thought to be nonsense. In fact, phrenology was not only an original conception of how the brain is organized; in many ways it was the right one. In the first place, Gall took it for granted that the physical organ of the brain engenders the mind. For this heresy in the so-called enlightened eighteenth century he was expelled from Roman Catholic Austria. Secondly, Gall put forward his belief that higher neural functions are localized to certain regions of the cerebral hemispheres. The orthodox view at that time was that the brain worked as a whole and that there are no separate parts having different functions. Again, Gall's view is the correct one. The mistake the phrenologists made was in their choice of functions to localize in the cerebral hemispheres. This however is no easy problem. We still cannot answer satisfactorily questions about what are the basic brain functions that can be localized in the cerebral cortex. For instance, the ability to draw well is not a single function, organized by just one part of the cerebral hemispheres. It needs the skilful use of the fingers, vision and visual recognition, the various cerebral functions that make up the representation of three-dimensional space on a two-dimensional surface, the ability to form the concept of space, and many more functions of different regions of the cerebral hemispheres. But the recognition of colours is carried out by certain neurons in parts of the back of the hemispheres. The phrenologists thought they could localize within the cerebral hemispheres such functions as language, calculation, hope and philoprogenitiveness. They were right about language. They were wrong about calculation; but until a few years ago most neurologists regarded an ability to calculate as a basic cerebral function. They were wrong about hope; perhaps they should have sought it in the human breast. As for philoprogenitiveness, they were not very far wrong, for there are certain parts of the brain that organize sexual function.

The nineteenth century thinker and physiologist, G. H. Lewes, nowadays known mainly as the husband of the novelist George Eliot, wrote in 1871: 'Gall rescued mental function from metaphysics, and made it one of biology . . . In his vision of psychology as a branch of biology, subject to all biological laws and to be pursued on biological methods, he may be said to have given the science its basis.'

The most serious mistake the phrenologists made was to think that the indentations, bumbs and dips on the surface of the skull resulted from the underlying parts of the cerebral hemisphere. Another mistake was to imagine that if a faculty is particularly developed in someone, then the part of the cerebral hemisphere in which that faculty is located will also be large and well-developed. Gall's method of locating faculties within the brain was absurd. For instance, looking back at his schooldays, he remembered that two of his schoolmates had had good verbal memories and large eyes, and so he connected verbal memory with protuberant eyes; he concluded that the faculty of verbal memory is in the frontal lobes just behind the eyes.

During the second quarter of the nineteenth century, most large towns in Britain had their phrenological societies. Phrenology provided people with an interest in psychology, just as has psychoanalysis in our own time. And, again like psychoanalysis, it was accepted far more readily by imaginative writers and untrained intellectuals than by biologists and medical men, who were in a better position to judge it. Serious thinkers about the brain soon came to regard the subject as quackery and phrenologists as charlatans, which indeed they became; and so the contributions of phrenology to neurology have been neglected. Yet they actually had an influence on French and British neurology by way of some scentists who may not have fully realized how their thinking had been influenced. In France Bouillaud was sympathetic to phrenology as a young man; he later played an important part in getting French anatomists and neurologists to accept the idea that speech was carried out by a certain local region of the left cerebral hemisphere. Broca put forward the arguments in support of this idea; he had also been influenced by phrenology as a young man. In England the thinker Herbert Spencer was most interested in phrenology as a boy and a young man. He had a great influence on Hughlings Jackson, a most important thinker in neurology of the last century.

Knowledge of the function of the parts of the cerebral hemispheres has been acquired in three main ways. One is the electrical stimulation of the brain in living animals, including man; this is the subject of this chapter. Another has been by the removal of parts of the cerebral hemispheres or the division of connections between parts; this again has been done in animals and man. The third way has been the correlation of naturally occurring disorders studied during life with the lesions found in the brain after death. We first learn how things go wrong, and then deduce how they work when they go right. We learn from the abnormal; we deduce physiology from pathology.

Lesions within the cerebral hemispheres can destroy the end-stations or the connecting links or both. Destruction of the end-station is just like destroying a railway terminus. Both sorts of termini, railway and cerebral, have afferent and efferent functions. One receives and sends off trains; the other receives and sends off nerve impulses. Destruction of the links between stations disconnects the two stations; it is the same whether the connections are railway lines or nerve fibres.

The most important neural disorder that has contributed to our knowledge of the brain is epilepsy; and the first worker to make use of this material was the founder of British neurology Hughlings Jackson. He was in a good position to study the disease as he could observe it in his wife, who had the variety now known as Jacksonian epilepsy. And so, like Father William, he could argue each case with his wife. Jackson concluded that epilepsy is due to the spontaneous firing of groups of neurons. When fits start with visual, auditory, olfactory, or gustatory hallucinations they do so because the neurons normally occupied with vision, hearing, smelling, and tasting are spontaneously active. If, after the patient's death, the lesion causing the fits is found, it will show which parts of the brain are normally concerned with those functions. When, for instance, a fit starts with a tingling numb sensation in the right foot, and a lesion is found in a certain region of the left hemisphere of the brain, it may be concluded that this region is where sensation of the right foot is organized. If neurons of the receptive area for smelling spontaneously discharge in a fit, the patient will be aware of a strange smell.

The preliminary features of the fit which the patient experiences are called the aura. An aura may be a sensation of vertigo, tingling spreading up a limb, butterflies in the stomach, an overpowering fear, or the vision of a scene from the past. When the features of the aura are correlated with post mortem evidence of the location of the lesion causing the fit, we learn where in the cortex the neurons subserving that function are located.

Using this method, Hughlings Jackson showed that certain parts of the hemispheres are mainly concerned with movements and neighbouring parts are concerned with the sensations associated with movement. He also showed that when a part of the front of the temporal lobe is stimulated by the epileptic discharge, hallucinatory states appear, with strange disturbances of the awareness of reality and of oneself as a part of reality. He described this state by saying that the patients show 'dreams mixing up with present thoughts', and he called it 'double consciousness'. Now that we know more about psychopathology and about normal psychological mechanisms, we realize that sometimes repressed psychological material accompanied by strong emotion comes to the patient's consciousness during this early part of a fit.

It is interesting to find that Dostoyevsky in describing his own fits described the kinds of epilepsy starting in the temporal lobe twenty years before Jackson did. As his kind of fits were not recognized as being a part of epilepsy at that time, both Dostoyevsky and his doctors believed his attacks were partly or entirely hysterical. Dostoyevsky's accounts of his fits, given in his letters, his dairies and his novels, are so well described that one can say without doubt that they began in the left temporal lobe of his brain.

The method that has been most useful in investigating the function of the brain, electrical stimulation, was first used in 1804. A physiologist called Aldini stimulated the brains of animals in the slaughter-house immediately after they had been killed; he observed that the muscles of the opposite side of the body showed movements. He then took his investigations a step farther by stimulating the brain of a freshly decapitated man; and he observed movements of the opposite side of the face (it is unknown whether the head felt this or not). The cerebral hemispheres of living human beings were first stimulated electrically in 1874 by Roberts Bartholow, professor of medicine in Cincinnati. He was able to pass the electrodes through the skulls of two patients as the bone had become softened and rotted away by abscesses. As he expected, he produced movements of the limbs of the opposite side.

A great step forward in the study of the brain was made in 1870 by Fritsch and Hitzig. As no facilities were provided by the Physiological Institute of Berlin for this work, they started their investigations in Hitzig's wife's bedroom. They explored the surface of the hemispheres of lightly-anaesthetized dogs. From such stimulation they worked out in detail what parts of the cerebral cortex control what movements. They showed, among other facts, that Gall's main idea was right—that the brain does not work as one single organ, but that different parts of it perform different functions. Stimulation of certain parts of the cerebral hemispheres caused movements, whereas stimulation elsewhere caused nothing observable. Obviously, parts of the brain concerned with sensation, with thought, emotion or remembering, could not show up in dogs with this stimulation technique.

The next step forward was made by Foerster in Germany and Cushing in the United States, both of whom stimulated the brains of conscious patients. By the first decade of the twentieth century, neurosurgery had been developed and local anaesthetics were used routinely. It became possible not only to map out the motor regions of the cerebral hemispheres in man, but also to stimulate other parts of the cortex and find out what the patient experienced during stimulation. The patient did not know when the electrode was placed on the brain or when the current was turned on or off.

It might be thought that stimulation of the living brain in conscious patients is painful and injurious. It is neither. As has been mentioned above, the brain can be touched or cut or stimulated without the subject feeling any pain or anything he can localize to the brain itself. When a part of the cerebral cortex is to be cut out because it causes fits, this part must be located accurately. From investigations by various X-radiological methods, one knows roughly what part of the cerebral hemisphere has to be cut out; but the exact region can be found best by stimulating the region electrically.

The technique of stimulation, localization, and excision was brought to a point where it became a routine neurosurgical procedure by Penfield of Montreal. He also applied Cushing's and Foerster's techniques to a systematic exploration of the cerebral cortex of man. The operations were performed for the removal of tumours, or scars, or for the cure of certain kinds of epilepsy. The brain was stimulated to enable the surgeon to reproduce the features of the patient's fits. When the patient reported having the same aura as he usually experienced with his fits, the abnormal region of the brain had been found. The surgeon then cut out this part; and this often stopped the fits.

It is rather surprising that such a crude intervention as the application of an electric current through an electrode should produce normal phenomena, normal movements, visual hallucinations, the recall of scenes from the past. One might have expected that it would produce some sort of chaos or caricature of normal phenomena. But in fact it imitates normal functioning of the brain to a surprising degree. One notes too that all the phenomena caused by electrical stimulation in these patients also occur spontaneously as a part of their epilepsy. It is apparent that the stimulation of the cortex and the discharge of neurons occurring during epileptic attacks can both teach us the functions of certain parts of the cortex of the hemispheres even though these are epileptic brains.

The regions of the hemispheres that give responses when stimulated are shown in Fig. 19.1(a) and (b). Visual hallucinations are obtained from the back of the occipital lobe and auditory hallucinations from deep in the temporal lobe. Movements are obtained from stimulating the motor strip, and bodily sensations from equivalent regions just behind the deep central fissure. The various experiences to be described later, which may all be called psychical experiences, are obtained from stimulation of the temporal lobe.

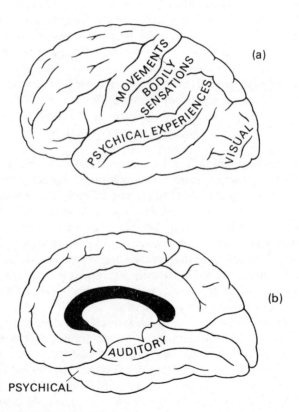

Fig. 19.1. (a) and (b). Parts of the human cerebral hemispheres which produce observable phenomena when stimulated in conscious patients.

Movement and sensation

Just as one brave man flies across the Atlantic to be followed within twenty years by a regular passenger service, so the first experiments of Foerster, Cushing, and Penfield are now repeated daily in many neurosurgical centres. When a part of the motor region of the hemispheres is stimulated, a part of the body is moved. The patient is astonished to find his arm or his leg moving of its own accord; for he does not have the feeling that he is doing the movement himself. Sometimes no movement occurs but the patient feels a strong desire to move. If a part of his body is already moving when the surgeon stimulates the motor area, the movement may be stopped and the patient is amazed to find he cannot move. The regions of the hemisphere from which movements can be obtained on electrical stimulation are shown in Fig. 19.2(a) and (b). Figure 19.2(a) shows the cerebral

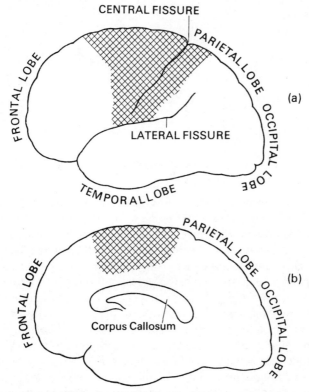

Fig. 19.2. (a) and (b). Parts of the human brain which produce movements of the body when stimulated.

hemisphere seen from the left and Fig. 19.2(b) from the medial side, which abuts against the other hemisphere. Figure 19.3 shows the same view of the left side of the brain as Fig. 19.2(a). In front of the central fissure is the motor strip. Movements of the right side of the body are most easily obtained from stimulating this part. On the figure, the points at which stimulation causes movement of the various parts of the body are marked. It will be seen that these points on the cortex are upside down: the foot is at the top and the face and mouth are at the bottom of the strip.

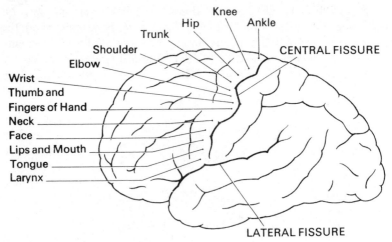

Fig. 19.3. Human brain showing the regions of the motor strip giving rise to movements of the opposite limbs.

The size of the cortical regions related to a certain part of the body is related to the importance of that part in that species. In man for instance, the cortical region related to the mouth and tongue is very large. This is because man is a great talker. Also the region related to the hands, fingers, and thumb is large—again on account of the importance of these parts in man. In the pig, the largest motor region is related to the snout, which for the pig is hands, fingers, and thumbs, as well as the organ of smell and an instrument for exploring the environment.

Stimulation of the primary receptive areas of the cortex gives the patient crude sensations characteristic of each primary area. When the somaesthetic area behind the motor strip is stimulated, the patient gets a feeling of numbness or tingling. Stimulating this region does not cause pain. When electrodes are moved away from the primary receiving areas to the surrounding parasensory area, the patient reports a sudden change from the crude sensation to a more meaningful sensation. In the case of auditory sensation, when the primary area is stimulated, the patient hears clicks, buzzing, ringing, chiming, chirping, rumbling, knocking or rushing sounds. He does not hear words or music. Stimulation of the surrounding parasensory area gives him more elaborated auditory sensations, as well as buzzing and clicks. The difference in the sensation experienced was often shown by Penfield when he moved his stimulating electrode from the primary to the surrounding parasensory area. One patient heard a buzzing when the primary auditory area was stimulated; when the electrode was moved to the surrounding association region, the patient exclaimed, 'Someone is calling'. Stimulation of this parasensory area may make the patient hear music, and he may hum what he is hearing. More than one patient has heard an orchestra playing. As long as the electrode stimulates, the orchestra continues playing. In one of Penfield's patients, whenever that particular spot on the cortex was stimulated, the patient heard the orchestra playing a certain popular song. This music was so real to her that she was convinced that a gramophone was being turned on in the operating theatre and still believed this when she spoke about the operation several days later. A boy who was being operated upon heard his mother talking on the telephone when this region of the right temporal lobe was being stimulated. Each time the current was turned on, he heard the same conversation. He said, 'My mother is telling my brother he has got his coat on backwards. I can just hear them.'

Very near the primary auditory receptive area is the primary area for vestibular sensations. Penfield found that stimulation of this area makes the patient feel dizzy; or he may get a sinking feeling or have the feeling that everything is swinging round him.

When the electrical stimulus was moved from the primary to the secondary visual area one Canadian patient of Penfield's said suddenly 'Oh, gee, gosh, robbers are coming at me with guns!' They were on his left and coming from behind him. Similar scenes were seen when the stimulating electrode was put in many places in front of the primary visual area. Stimulation in one place made the patient exclaim, 'Oh, gosh. There they are, my brother is there. He is aiming an air rifle at me.' He said his brother was walking towards him, and the gun was loaded. When he was asked where he was, he said he was at his house, in the yard.

Emotions

Electrical stimulation of certain parts of the temporal lobes in conscious patients makes the patient experience emotion. The emotion is in a pure form, a terrible fear, an intense feeling of loneliness, disgust, sorrow, or intense depression. The emotions may be strong, stronger than when felt in real life. When this part of the brain spontaneously discharges in epilepsy, these emotions may occur as the first part of the epileptic fit, or they may follow the fit. The patient finds this emotional experience very difficult to explain; it is a sort of hallucination of emotion. Hughlings Jackson first showed that strong emotions could be an epileptic attack and also that they could precede an attack; and from a correlation of the clinical manifestations of the epilepsy and the examination of the brain after the patient's death, he showed that this form of epilepsy starts in the temporal lobe. The intense fear preceding some of these attacks Jackson described as 'a fear that comes of itself'. There may be nothing the patient is frightened of; he just has fear. One patient in whom the amygdaloid nuclei were being stimulated at operation said that it was the same feeling as we would have if we looked up and found a bus just about to run us down. Another patient who was terrified as something was going to attack her would say to the doctor standing by, 'Stop them, doctor; don't let them do it'. Such a patient is still in touch with reality enough to know she is in hospital and talking to the doctor whom she knows; yet at the same time she is quite convinced that her hallucinations are real. Within one second this patient would regain a little more normal conscious awareness and then she would tell you that her hallucinations were not real but only seemed real to her when they happened, and hardly had she got these words out than the attack would return and she would say; 'There they are again', once more under the spell of her hallucinations.

In some patients, the feeling is rather one of dread than of fear; it is vague though intense, for there is no object or event that they dread. Some patients describe a transient feeling of intense anxiety, which may mount up to panic. Some have the feeling that everything is becoming dangerous. Sometimes, though this is rare, the emotional component of the fit is a strong feeling of guilt, of being guilty of having done something dreadful, though the patient has no idea what it is.

Dostoyevsky had this feeling of guilt, the feeling that he had committed some momentous crime, associated with his fits. But far more striking was a rare aura before his fits,—a feeling of ecstasy or great joy. He has described it like this.

For a few moments before the fit, I experience a feeling of happiness such as it is quite impossible to imagine in a normal state and which other people have no idea of. I feel entirely in harmony with myself and the whole world, and this feeling is so strong and so delightful that for a few seconds of such bliss, one would gladly give up ten years of one's life, if not one's whole life.

The terrible depression or despair which a few patients have during temporal lobe attacks may well have been the cause of their suicide. The patients can never say why they feel depressed. The utter misery comes on them quite suddenly, without cause or reason; and it may pass off equally quickly, so that within a few minutes it has gone. Attacks of uncontrollable rage may also occur as preludes to epileptic attacks or as the manifestation of the epilepsy itself. These are particularly common in children whose epilepsy begins in the temporal lobes. During such attacks children or adults may smash up furniture, put their fists through glass windows or attack other people.

In those patients in whom the fit starts in the part of the temporal lobe where emotion is organized, the normal experiencing of emotion may bring on a fit. This occurs commonly in childhood; and epileptic children often get much benefit from psychotherapy. Dostoyevsky, doubtless relating his own experience, wrote, 'Fright alone will bring one on'.

The part of the brain that produces these pure emotions is a region called the limbic system (from the Latin, *limbus*, an edge or border). This region includes the hypothalamus, the oldest parts of the cerebral cortex which are the under-surfaces and most internal parts of the temporal lobes, the parts of the cortex around the corpus callosum and the septal area. In Plates 10 and 11, the parts labelled temporal lobe form a part of this region; the gyrus around the corpus callosum forms another part, and the region beneath the front part of the corpus callosum is the septal area; this surrounds the anterior commissure.

Professor Heath in New Orleans has implanted electrodes in the brains of certain patients with severe and uncontrollable epilepsy or with psychotic mental disorders and left them in permanently, just as Hess originally did in small animals. In psychotic patients he found abnormal electrical brain waves in the septal area and in the part of the temporal lobes called the amygdala. When the patients got better, these electrical abnormal waves became normal. Patients who were given LSD had the same abnormal electrical waves in these regions. When the waves were excessive and abnormal, the patients were in a dream-like state and heard voices. The essential ingredient of marihuana had the same effects on these parts of the brain when it was injected into animals.

When the pleasure region is stimulated in man, the patient becomes more alert, active and brighter in mood and reactions. In one patient suffering from psychotic depression, Heath reported:

Expressions of anguish, self condemnation, and despair changed precipitously to expressions of optimism and elaborations of pleasant experiences, past and anticipated. Patients could calculate more rapidly than before stimulation. Memory and recall were enhanced. One patient on the verge of tears described his father's near-fatal illness and condemned himself as somehow responsible, but when the septal region was stimulated, he immediately terminated this conversation and within fifteen seconds exhibited a broad grin as he discussed plans to date and seduce a girl friend. When asked why he had changed the conversation so abruptly, he replied that the plans concerning the girl suddenly came to him. This phenomenon was repeated several times in the patient; stimulation was administered to the septal region when he was describing a depressive state, and almost instantly he would become gay.

Here we see clearly that one's mood and thoughts that seem to come spontaneously are due to activation of a certain part of the brain. Probably all sexual fantasy arises from the activity of this region.

Another patient, an epileptic, was one day agitated, violent and psychotic. The septal region was then stimulated without the patient knowing it. 'Almost instantly his behavioural state changed from one of disorganization, rage, and persecution to one of happiness and mild euphoria. He described the beginning of a sexual motive state.'

Immediate relief from intense physical pain and anguish has been obtained with stimulation to the septal region in patients with advanced and painful forms of cancer. Stimulation of any region of the brain that causes pleasure stops physical and emotional pain. It appears then that these regions are more powerful than those parts of the brain where pain is felt.

Many of these patients have had the electrodes left permanently in their brains so that they can stimulate the various regions when they want to. In the New Orleans group of patients, three lots of electrodes were left in, connected to three levers so that these patients could have the experience of stimulating three different structures in the brain. One of these patients would have a most pleasant feeling when he stimulated the septal region. It 'made him feel as if he were building up to a sexual orgasm. He was unable to achieve the orgastic end point, however, and explained that his frequent, sometimes frantic, pushing of the septal button was an attempt to reach a "climax" although at times this was frustrating and produced a "nervous feeling".' Another patient also found that stimulation in this region made him 'feel wonderful'; it gave him sexual thoughts. Regardless of the subject under discussion at the time, this patient 'would introduce a sexual subject, usually accompanied by a broad grin. When asked about his response, he said "I

don't know why that came to mind—I just happened to think of it".'
When he stimulated a certain part of his thalamus, he got the partial
recall of a memory, with anger and frustration. Stimulation of a
neighbouring region has made patients experience fear or rage; and
stimulation of another region close by causes a strange, unreal, dream-
like state. When the patients experienced rage, it was unmotivated and
was not directed particularly at anyone. Stimulation of parts of the
hypothalamus itself has given rise to terror, anxiety, rage, and also to 'a
good feeling'.

The disorder of schizophrenia is characterized by the patient's feeling
no emotion, his not being stimulated by the events of life and having
no energy and no initiative. Heath thought that the condition could be
treated by putting permanent electrodes into the septal region of some
schizophrenics. Stimulation of the pleasure-inducing region did give the
patients emotions of a pleasant kind. The patients felt good, they
became alert and spoke and moved faster; and like the self-stimulating
animals, they wanted to continue the stimulation. But unfortunately the
improvement in their disease was only temporary.

Strange experiences

The electrical stimulation of certain regions of the temporal lobes
produces strange feelings about the actual situation. Penfield called
them 'interpretative illusions', and Hughlings Jackson had previously
called it 'a dreamy state', as this was the name given it by one of his
patients, a doctor with epilepsy. One of Penfield's patients said: 'I had a
dream, I had a book under my arm. I was talking to a man. The man was
trying to reassure me not to worry about the book.'

Sometimes in epilepsy and during stimulation of the temporal lobes of
the brain, there may be an increased awareness of reality; the patient
says that for a brief period everything seems to be more intense and more
significant. One of Penfield's patients got this 'new awareness' both
before his fits and when Penfield stimulated his right temporal lobe; on
stimulation, he became unusually conscious of the weight of his coat and
of the weight of his feet upon the floor.

A commoner feeling is that of being out of touch with reality.
Everything has an unreal atmosphere, which the patient finds difficult to
describe. Some patients have an intense feeling of being outside
themselves and watching themselves behaving. They may feel they are
standing behind themselves, watching from a distance.

More rarely there are misinterpretations of time sense: everything
seems to be slowed down, even the movements of themselves and others

seem as if they are carried out in slow motion and very deliberately. Penfield has found that stimulation of the temporal lobes has often caused illusions of recognition or of comparison. This also occurs with fits starting in the same region. Everything may seem strange to the patient and unreal. The patient may say that everything is unlike ordinary life; suddenly the room in which the patient is sitting seems unfamiliar. Jackson reported some epileptics who described this as 'I feel in some strange place', 'A panorama of something familiar and yet strange'.

The opposite sort of feeling also occurs in epilepsy. Everything suddenly seems familiar, the patient has the feeling that it has all happened before and that he knows exactly what is going to happen next. This state is called by its French name, 'déjà vu'. Dickens mentions it in David Copperfield, like this:

We have all some experience of a feeling which comes over us occasionally, of what we are saying and doing having been said or done before, in a remote time—of our having been surrounded, dim ages ago, by the same faces, objects and circumstances—of our knowing perfectly what will be said next, as if we suddenly remembered it.

That this feeling can be a part of epilepsy had already been recognized in the last century. Hughlings Jackson first reported it and rightly associated it with lesions of the front part of the temporal lobes. The feeling that time is unrolling abnormally slowly may also accompany the déjà vu phenomenon.

During stimulation of their temporal lobes, some of Penfield's patients experienced déjà vu. One patient had the feeling that the whole operation had happened before and that she knew what the surgeon was about to do. Another patient experienced a feeling of unnecessariness, 'a strange feeling like it is unnecessary—the craziest, doggone feeling'. In two patients Penfield obtained a pure feeling of familiarity, an unattached sensation. One patient whose brain was being stimulated told him that the feeling of familiarity had already commenced before he started speaking to her, 'as though the stage or background had been set to embrace in familiarity any concomitant perception'. One patient whose temporal lobe was stimulated had the feeling of falling over, 'something which, in fact, he had not previously experienced', and yet this sensation was accompanied by the sense of familiarity.

Epileptic patients are the commonest recipients of mystical experiences. St Teresa of Avila was an epileptic. Some of the mystical experiences of saints and holy men of all religions are due to epilepsy occurring in the temporal lobes. The relation between epilepsy and mystical experiences was well-known before the arrival of Christianity; epilepsy was known as the holy or sacred malady. For before, after, or during the attack, the patient may have the feeling that he is experiencing another kind of reality, more intense and far more important than the everyday kind. What he experiences during this state is so overpowering that he continues to believe in his delusional system when he has recovered from his attack. And so, after he has seen the glory of the Lord or the power of evil, he returns to everyday life and becomes a preacher. He knows that he saw these things during an epileptic attack, but he may regard the epileptic attack as a means of experiencing religious truth. Or he may not regard the attack as epileptic but a way in which the Lord God chose to communicate with him, and that he was chosen to receive this communication from on high. Thus he must be a very special and elevated person, and he may have delusions of grandeur. If his sincerity and his emotional intensity can persuade ignorant people of the truth of his beliefs experienced during the epileptic state, then he may found a new religion.

Sometimes when epileptic patients are being examined to see if flickering light will bring on the attacks, they get the religious experience; or they may get a state of bliss or a feeling of absolute peace. This is a variant of the strong emotion of elation. When some of these patients have the psychological feeling of emotion, they may also have the feeling that they are actually elevated from the ground. Epileptic saints call this levitation, and they tell those who believe in them that they float above the earth or walk on the waves, in defiance of gravity.

Evocation of the past

Penfield classified the psychical effects of electrical stimulation of the brain in two groups, experiential hallucinations and interpretative responses. Experiential hallucinations are an evocation of the past. Penfield describes this as follows: 'The record of the stream of consciousness may be activated as though it were a strip of cinemato-graph film, recording the sight and sound, the movement, and the meaning which belonged to each successive period of time.' The emotion of the original scene is there when the scene is re-lived. Patients called these experiences flashbacks of dreams, explaining that they were similar to the flashbacks used in cinematographic techniques of story-telling.

As an example, the following case is described in some detail. This girl was operated upon by Penfield when she was aged fourteen. She suffered from terrifying epileptic fits which always started off with 'what seemed to be an hallucination. It was always the same; an experience came to her from childhood.' With this experience, she was frightened and often screamed.

The original experience was as follows. She was walking through a meadow where the grass was high. It was a lovely day, and her brothers had run on ahead of her. A man came up behind her and said that he had snakes in the bag he was carrying and how would she like to get into the bag with the snakes. She was very frightened and screamed to her brothers, and they ran home, where she told her mother about the event.

After that, she occasionally had nightmares in which the scene was re-enacted. At the age of eleven, it was recognized that she had attacks by day, in which she habitually saw the scene of her fright. She saw a little girl, whom she identified as herself, in the now familiar surroundings. She experienced the scene with such distinctness that she was filled with terror lest she should be struck or smothered from behind. . . . Sometimes this 'dream' constituted all there was of her epileptic attacks.

At operation, under local anaesthesia, I applied the stimulator to the temporal cortex. 'Wait a minute' she said, 'and I will tell you'. I removed the electrode from the cortex. After a pause, she said, 'I saw someone coming toward me, as though he was going to hit me'. It was obvious also that she was suddenly frightened. . . . In a moment she called 'Don't leave me'. Thus the stimulating electrode had recalled the familiar experience that ushered in each of her habitual attacks. But stimulation at other points had recalled to her other experiences of the past, and it had also produced the emotion of fear. Our astonishment was great, for we had produced phenomena that were neither motor nor sensory, and yet the responses seemed to be psychological, not epileptic.

By this, Penfield meant that he was observing phenomena of a normal kind and not the distorted fragments of acts and sensations that most epileptic phenomena are.

During the electrical stimulation, some of these patients no longer knew where they were; they experienced only their hallucinations. Others were aware of the situation and knew they were having a brain operation at the time. Patients explained after the current had been turned off, 'I could see the desks, and I was there'. Or 'I had a dream'. Or 'I was listening to music from *Guys and Dolls*'. These peculiar experiences had the freshness of a real experience: they were not like events remembered in the past. During the stimulation, the patients could focus attention on any chosen feature of the episode and could answer questions on it afterwards. These scenes the patients re-lived were mainly visual, but the sounds and smells accompanying the original experience were there too. All the accompanying emotions and the mood of the time were present; the patient experienced the same feeling about the event he originally had and attributed the same significance to it as he had given it at the time. What he had thought of the situation was stored with the stored experience. As soon as the stimulation of the brain was stopped, re-living the experience ceased. When the same spot was stimulated again, the same experience was usually brought up, though this was not always so. From the surrounding region of the cortex, the electrode evokes other recollections. Sometimes stimulation of the hippocampal gyrus gives rise to jumbled up fragments of memories. Indeed, it is more surprising that electrical stimulation does not always bring up a caricature of memory and that it does mainly draw out a total sensible record of a previous experience. What is also surprising is that these recollected events are insignificant in the great majority of cases; they were quite unimportant to the patients.

These records are brought up from stimulation of certain parts of the temporal lobes. Penfield realized that 'there is stored away in the ganglionic connection of the brain (i.e. the neurons and their connections) a permanent record of the stream of consciousness; a record that is much more complete and detailed than the memories that any man can recall by voluntary effort.'

Automatic behaviour

The kind of fit in which the patient lies senseless on the floor, making strong jerking movements of his limbs, is not so common. There are all sorts of fits which are not usually recognized as epileptic phenomena. One of the most disturbing of these is the kind known as automatic attacks or automatic behaviour. These were first described and studied by Jackson when in 1875 he wrote about them under the name of 'epileptic somnambulism', somnambulism being fashionable at the time. During these attacks, the patient unconsciously performs organized acts of behaviour. He is unconscious in the sense that he is not conscious of what is happening or what he is doing; and after the attack has passed he has no memory of what has happened or where he has been. During the attack the parts of the temporal lobes needed for the recording of events as they occur are not working; for this reason the patient can recall nothing. In the attack the patient goes on carrying out the routine behaviour automatically; he is not open to new suggestions; but he may be quite capable of walking down a crowded street. Quite often the patient makes chewing and swallowing movements in the attack. This is likely to be due to the epileptic discharge spreading to the insula, the part of the cortex that controls the alimentary canal. The main place where the epileptic discharge occurs during automatic behaviour is within the amygdaloid region of the temporal lobe or the region between the amygdala and the insula. As long as the epileptic discharge remains in this region, there will be no automatic behaviour. A total act of behaviour, like getting up and walking to the door, occurs only when the epileptic discharge spreads from this region to other parts of the brain.

Automatic behaviour is always to some degree abnormal behaviour. The patient may seize the telephone, examine it and then put the receiver down on his desk, or he may start tearing his clothes. He may get up, murmur something incomprehensible, walk to the window and open it. If the automatic behaviour results from stimulating the brain at operation, the patient may no longer know he is being operated on. He loses touch with the surgeon and everyone else in the operating theatre, he may try to throw off the sterile towels, get up and go off.

Sometimes, though very rarely, total acts of behaviour may be performed, carried out quite normally in all details, although the whole act is not planned and is not consciously done. The attack never lasts longer than an hour and usually not more than five minutes. In the attack, the patient may perform an act that he wants to do anyway but with full consciousness he would not do. Dr Lennox, a neurologist in America who has seen a great number of epileptic patients, has reported the case of a patient who in an automatic attack went to his boss and said 'I have to have more money or I quit'. He was amazed when at the end of the week he found his salary had been raised.

20 Sensation acquires a meaning

The general problem

I have stressed already that the input to the central nervous system and sensation are not the same. Sensation consists of what we feel, see, hear, taste or smell. It occurs only after the highest levels of the central nervous system have dealt with the mass of afferent impulses they receive. At lower levels of the central nervous system, the meaning of an input is of little importance. What matters is a correct response to the stimulation. At higher levels, the best response to the circumstances is the aim. During man's evolutionary development, it has been advantageous to have an almost complete picture of the environment at all times. This mental representation of the environment is provided by the higher levels of the nervous system.

The higher level of neural functioning is the least automatic and the most complicated; it is the most difficult to investigate, and so we know less about it than the lower levels. One of the questions neurology attempts to answer is, how do we know what a thing is, how do we collect all sensory impressions together and combine them to say: 'There is a white kitten lying curled up on that sofa;' how is it that the excitation of one lot of neurons gives us the sensation of something seen, of another lot that of something heard. The straight answer to the straight question is, we do not know.

We know a great deal about the underlying anatomy. The various kinds of sensory inputs go to different parts of the cerebral hemispheres. But this fact alone seems to be insufficient to account for our different kinds of sensation. It may be that the different neurons of various sensory inputs differ from each other in ways which at present we do not know, possibly in some physical or chemical ways. Differences in sensation might reside in the fact that the neurons have different connexions to other groups of neurons. It could be that the different sensations may be the result of the experience of groups of sensory neurons having been different. All neurons may start off the same, yet it may be that, by the time the animal has lived a portion of its life, every neuron has become different from every other one.

Or, perhaps, after all, there is no problem. One can equally well ask the question 'How can it be that nerve impulses cause the movements of my hand?' To someone who does not know any of the answers, this looks like a similar and almost insoluble problem. But because we do know most of the answers, and because we understand most of the physical and chemical steps involved, this question seems to be of a different order from those concerning sensation and perception, questions involving our consciousness. We now know what physical changes occur when a message spreads along a nerve fibre, and how the message is passed from one nerve fibre to the next nerve cell, until finally it reaches the myoneural junction. We know the biochemical and electrochemical reactions involved in passing nerve impulses on to the muscle fibres and how this electrical stimulation makes the contractile proteins of muscle fibres contract. This makes the fingers move. If we know all the essential steps for making movements out of the activity of certain neurons, it is probable that one day we shall know those for making sensation from the activity of other neurons. This seems likely as sensation is a step on the way to movements. An animal does not ask what a thing is, it wants to know what to do with it. Life consists of responding, and the response is a movement.

Inborn knowledge

For he knows that God is his Saviour.

From the work and the conceptions of the ethologists we begin to have some idea of how the world appears to animals other than ourselves. One of the most important and unexpected facts we have learned is that many or perhaps all vertebrates are born with the ability to recognize and respond to some total sensory patterns they are likely to meet. They are born with knowledge of a certain shape, a certain sequence of sounds; and when this occurs in their young lives, they react to it in a way suitable for self-preservation. Many birds already know on leaving the egg the shape and movements of the predator that may be looking for them. They know the essential outline of the hawk, planing overhead. Seeing that outline, they rush off to mother and nestle beneath her wing. The herring gull knows how to behave towards a red spot on a yellow rectangle as soon as it leaves the egg, for that is how its mother's beak will appear to it. When the little duckling breaks through the shell of the egg, it already knows the quack of a mother duck. It will follow that sound; no other sound has meaning for it. If the ducklings feel themselves deserted by her and—as Lorenz so sweetly says—peep their abandonment, then even if this is her first brood she knows the meaning of this sound. Born with this knowledge, a motor pattern of behaviour is set off by this and only this sound, and she returns to her brood. The studies of von Uexküll, Lorenz, Tinbergen, and their successors have shown as a large number of examples of inborn knowledge of visual and auditory patterns.

If we ask the question how does a newborn duckling know the sound of its mother's voice or how does it know that she is its mother, we put the question badly. If we ask how does it know what to do when it hears its mother's voice or when it sees her moving away, we are putting the question in a somewhat better way but still in a form that cannot be easily answered. When we observe a mother duck with her first brood, we see that she responds to the alarm call of her ducklings by an innate, unlearned, complex pattern of behaviour, that of defending the young. But if one of the young whose cry produced this reaction turns out when she examines it to have the wrong markings, she will attack it and drive it off. The correct markings produce mothering and sheltering response; the wrong markings make her drive off an intruder. Certain totalities of sensation automatically cause certain forms of behaviour. Whether it seems to the reacting animal that it has a free choice, that it chooses to react in that way and in no other way, we do not know. In fact there is no choice. The duckling inevitably follows the adult duck's quack. Once it has been subjected to imprinting, it follows the moving object that it saw at the sensitive period.

We come nearer the mark if we think of the animal as never asking for meanings, as not formulating such a question as 'What is it', On experiencing anything in its environment, its only questions are: 'Do I eat it, do I drink it, do I copulate with it, do I fight it or flee from it, can I bathe in it or roll in it?' For its reaction is always some sort of movement, or rarely, a freezing of all movement.

However, of course, it does not ask questions; it responds, it behaves. When the opponent squeals, it signals submission and this removes the aggression of the antagonist. Tension is reduced and peace is restored. When the ape offers itself for sexual mounting, the ape who is invited to mount knows that that the other has submitted. There are hints of this in humans. Adler is right, not Freud.

Among animals, including ourselves, there is a mutual exchange of signals. The meaning is understood not only by members of the same species but also by other mammals, by other birds. Inborn knowledge provokes behaviour, it is a part of behaviour.

As animals know what to do with things rather than know what they are, at times an animal may be said to recognize something, while at other times it does not do so; its ability to recognize depends on its needs at the time. Moreover, at different times it recognizes the same object as two different things. For the female, the male is something with which to copulate on one occasion, on another he is something to eat. To the female spider, the male is never the objectively seen male spider it is to us. What meaning an animal possesses for another of the same species depends on how it behaves, on its carrying out the right social behaviour. This is of course the same for human beings, though in our case it has to be learned. Depending on accent, on clothes, gestures, way of standing, sitting and picking the teeth, we behave to another one of our own kind in certain ways, and we do not see the other person objectively (not that there is such a thing as considering anyone objectively, anyway).

We do not know the first thing about the neural basis of these inborn perceptions and the behaviour fixed to them. We must avoid being astounded by the total phenomenon as we see it in its finished complexity. It is pleasant to stand transfixed with awe and wonder before the phenomena of nature. It is pleasant too, and more rewarding, to find out how it all works and to arrive at an understanding of what is going on around us. And this need not diminish our first feelings of wonder. When each example is finally broken down into its essential components, we may eventually find that the basic feature triggering a certain act of behaviour is quite simple. It may be that it depends on a diagonal line casting a shadow across the retina; perhaps it will be that the quacking of the mother duck will turn out to be the only frequency range of sound to which the auditory apparatus is sensitive at that stage of development.

We must avoid separating sensory from motor, the perception from the behaviour. This may be the traditional neurological and psychological way of investigation, but it may well make problems where none exist. In the examples we have been considering, what we have been noting is that certain patterns in one member of a mutually reacting pair constitute a sign; this sign-stimulus fires off an act of behaviour in the other member. Such sign-stimuli often occur in chains, each stimulus setting off an act of behaviour, constituting the new sign-stimulus to the other reacting animal. It has been found by the ethologists that many acts of behaviour are organized in this way: this is so for mating among sticklebacks and many kinds of birds, for feeding among birds, for fighting and avoiding fighting among territorial animals. This way of organizing behaviour takes us a long way from the question how we and other animals know what something is; or rather, it takes us a long way out of the psychological laboratory where such questions were investigated in traditional psychology.

The integration of many different sensory aspects of an object in the environment is unnecessary in unlearned or instinctive behaviour. A few sensory clues are enough; the rest is irrelevant. For instance, the male wasps mentioned in chapter 2 needed only to have the smell of the secretion of the female's abdominal glands to make them carry out copulation; and they would copulate with the cut out glands and not with the female wasp deprived of these glands. If man does not interfere with the natural course of events, this economic way of determining behaviour usually suffices. The proper clues are few that make the male attack, or the female present for copulation. In the case of copulation of the leopard frog, it suffices to put a rubber band round the female's chest; she will then lay her eggs. On the other hand, the sign-stimuli may be complicated and they must be correctly presented. The male may have to perform a complicated dance, each series of movements being presented in the correct order, for the female to accept him.

Work on human beings on sign-stimuli is now being done. The advertizing industry knows quite a lot about this without realizing it. They can present human figures so that they cause reactions of tenderness and a desire to give or so that they cause repulsion and avoidance. They sell little furry objects which make children and women want to cuddle them and which have no use other than that. Psychologists are now carrying out research to find out what sign-stimuli are innate in the young human and what sorts of behaviour they induce.

If we look at the whole animal kingdom, we see that every sort of sensory channel is used for signalling: emitting odours, performing dances to be looked at, making sounds, drumming on trees to cause vibration. David Lack, from his study of the behaviour of robins, has shown that it is the red breast that makes the robin attack. Whether in this case the robin is aware of other stimuli from the oncoming robin or not, one does not know. But it is clearly of no importance in the situation; it is red breast alone that determines its behaviour. The final evidence supporting this interpretation of the facts is that when the male robin sees himself in a mirror, he threatens and may attack his own reflection. Other sensory clues are not so definite. When a cock-robin hears the song of another cock-robin, he seeks further stimulation from the singer. His subsequent behaviour depends on many different factors. Some of these are the actual place where the other robin is seen. Is it within, on the boundary of, or well outside the territory of the first robin? He will respond differently in accordance with the reaction of the singing robin to his own threatening display. His behaviour is also related to the time of year, for this affects the robin's brain; the brain controls the robin's secretion of hormones; and lastly and most important, these hormones act on the brain itself and influence its behaviour.

The fact that an animal's response to the same object differs at different times indicates that our philosophical questions about perceiving the real nature of an object are the wrong ones. It seems that to many animals an object has no continuity. At one time blades of grass are something to eat, at another time, they are the wherewithal to make a nest. It would be an anthropomorphic assumption to believe that the bird knows that it is dealing with the same object on the two occasions. It is far more likely that when it eats grass, the bird sees this as pleasant tasting green stuff to be pulled out of the ground; and when it entwines it into the fabric of its nest, it sees it as green nest-building material that has to be pulled off the ground and interwined and lined with feathers from the breast. The grass is always there; but only at times do rodents and birds see it as suitable material for nest-building. Thus the meaning of sensation changes. When the season changes, the grass that was always there acquires a new meaning.

The use to which a thing is put depends on the state of the animal perceiving it. How the same object is perceived changes with the hormones secreted by the endocrine glands. When a rat is under the influence of hormones making it feel maternal, it mistakes mice for young rats and puts them in its nest, caring for them lovingly. When it is not under the influence of these hormones, it will kill them. Hormones cause the animal's needs; needs breed desires, and desires see objects in the environment that are there to satisfy them.

As the sensory clues making up a sign-stimulus may be few, mistakes are made. Man has always caught birds by decoy. Although Chaucer's birds defied the fowler and all his wiles, the fact that there are many people among us bearing the surname 'Fowler' shows us that many people used to follow this profession successfully before guns were used to shoot fowl. To a young rabbit, something moving with a hoppity motion is another rabbit to be followed. Professor Otto Koehler damaged the rear-wheel of his bicycle and rode on it while it hopped regularly over a field. He found a young rabbit persistently following him and he could not frighten it away. A fawn followed Professor Tinbergen on a bicycle with the rear-mudguard painted white. This must have been so like the white hinderparts of another deer that the young animal saw no difference. Alexander the Great thought that his sculptor was amazing because Boukephalas, his famous horse, recognized a bronze statue of itself as another horse. But we now know that this is nothing. A lifesize two-dimensional true-to-life painting is enough; a horse reacts to it as though it is a real horse and is clearly puzzled when he walks round to the other side of the canvas and finds nothing there. Throughout nature, we find examples of mimicry based on deception of predators and enemies. Caterpillars look like sticks, the hoverfly looks like the stinging wasp. Eyes may frighten animals; and so the peacock butterfly paints them on its wings and some tropical fish paint them on their dorsal fins.

Man also has inborn knowledge; though the catalogue of what we know without learning or imitation has not yet been made. We understand the meaning of aggressive, threatening, and submissive postures, and of behaviour of many kinds of animal; this is obvious for cats and dogs and equally so for their more dangerous relations, lions and tigers, and wolves. We do not need to have lessons in the subject at school nor to have this explained to us by our parents; merely seeing the posture and hearing the accompanying cries is enough. We know the squealing of an animal in pain or in terror, without having to learn it; as some would say, we know it instinctively or intuitively.

Acquired knowledge

Although this chapter is called 'Sensation acquires a meaning', we hardly ever experience a pure sensation. Almost everything we hear, feel, see or smell has meaning. We perceive things; we do not have sensory data. The elements of sensory data cause sensation; a lot more processes are required before a thing is seen and still more before it is recognized. To see something moving from one part of a room to another entails neural activity of the cerebral hemispheres that are not yet understood. We become aware of the psychological aspects of some of this activity when we recognize a melody from the separate notes spaced in time that form it. The data are the isolated notes and the sensation is what we hear; we then perceive that this is a whole, a melody, that we either know or do not know, and we put the melody into many categories, modern music, folk music, Schubert, in three-four time, in a major mode, and in the key of C. When all of this activity does not take place, a simple pure sensation occurs. We interpret what we experience as soon as we feel it. We do not think: 'There is such and such a form of green on a white background'; we say 'There is a leaf on the path'. We hear music not sound, we see objects, objects that continue in time, not light reflected from edges and angles.

Sensation is partly innate; perception has to be learned. Just as we need to go through a long period of practice to acquire the skills of walking, or of running downstairs, so it is with perception. Whatever neural processes occur when we learn, learning is as necessary for perception as it is for motor skills. It is the same for emotional development and for the acquisition of the skill of living with other members of a group.

That animals are born with knowledge of some of the things they are going to meet in their early days is a surprising fact. But such knowledge as the shape of a bird of prey in its potential victims is exceptional throughout the whole realm of perception. What is innate is only a basis. The animal has to learn to make sense of the sensory input. What the young animal has to learn has to arrive within a certain order and within a certain time range. The programme of learning is innate, it is a part of the way in which the central nervous system develops.

Some experiments on the necessity of learning for perception have been carried out in the United States. Chimpanzees were reared in total darkness from birth. When these animals are eventually brought out into the light, they behave as if they see nothing; they take no notice of their visual environment. They have certain innate visual reflexes, such as the feedback mechanism for adjusting the best amount of light to fall on to the retina; but apart from such reflexes, these young chimpanzees behave just as if they are still in complete darkness. Similarly, chimpanzees reared in an environment of universal diffuse bright light are equally blind. Some of these baby chimpanzees had their heads enclosed in a translucent plastic orb, so that all the light reaching their eyes was general diffuse light, devoid of patterns and definite colours. When these orbs were removed, these young animals behaved just like the chimpanzees reared in complete darkness. These experiments show that the animal needs to experience the varied patterns of light and the changing patterns of moving objects in order to learn to perceive.

Moreover, in order for learning to be permanent, it must come at the right time. If a baby chimpanzee is reared in a normal environment and then put into darkness for two years, it is just like a chimpanzee reared always in complete darkness. The early rearing in a normal environment did not help.

From these and other similar experiments, it becomes clear that an animal must have the proper early environment in order to develop its innate potentialities. If the right opportunities for spontaneous learning are not presented during the first two or three years of life, then the child will be unintelligent and will remain so. Freud and his successors realized that this is so for the normal development of sexuality and emotion. It is now clear that this is so for every aspect of intelligence and mental and psychological functioning. Further, the performance tests, wrongly known as intelligence tests, were designed on the premise that native or inborn intelligence is separable from what has been acquired or learned. The two are so intertwined that it is meaningless to try to separate them.

The question of how much our perception of the world depends on learning has always been one of much interest to philosophers. Locke has recorded in his *Essay Concerning Human Understanding* that in 1690 he was asked the following question by his friend Molyneux, whose wife had gone blind:

Suppose a man born blind, and now adult, and taught by his touch to distinguish between a cube and a sphere of the same metal. Suppose then the cube and sphere were placed on a table, and the blind man made to see: query, whether by his sight, before he touched them, could he distinguish and tell which was the globe and which the cube? . . . The acute and judicious proposer answers: not. For though he has obtained the experience of how the globe, how the cube affects his touch, yet he has not yet attained the experience that what affects his touch so or so, must affect his sight, so or so.

And Locke commented:

I agree with this thinking gentleman, whom I am proud to call my friend, in his answer to this his problem; and am of the opinion that the blind man, at first, would not be able to tell with certainty which was the globe and which the cube.

Diderot, too, was much interested in perception; but unlike most philosophers, he got out of his chair, went out of his room, and made some observations on the matter. He recorded in his letter on the blind that one blind man with whom he talked said that if he were offered the gift of sight by some miracle, he would prefer to have enormously long arms instead. This most perceptive man said: 'If curiosity were not to dominate my wishes, I would like to have long arms; for it seems to me that my hands would instruct me better what is happening on the moon than your eyes or your telescopes. It would be better for me to bring to a state of perfection the organ that I have than to give me the one I am lacking.'

In our time Molyneux's conditions have come true. The very cases imagined by him and by Locke have occurred. We can answer the philosophers' questions not only because the surgery of the eye has advanced but also because all the known cases have been collected together and studied by von Senden and published in his absorbing book *Space and Sight*.

Already at the end of the eighteenth century, operations had been carried out on children to remove cataracts and restore sight. When these patients came to see, it was not an unmixed blessing, as Diderot's wise informer foresaw. A lady operated upon at the age of 45 in 1826 by a surgeon, Mr Wardrop, said 'I cannot tell what I do see: I am quite stupid.' Mr Wardrop reported that 'she seemed bewildered from not being able to combine the knowledge acquired by senses of touch and sight'. All of these patients who have had sight restored have explained how they have had to learn to interpret the strange world of sight and how difficult it has been for them to acquire a visual picture of the world.

After their operations, most of these patients have been unable to see much. They cannot distinguish between shapes which appear quite different to us. They have to train for months before they have any useful vision, and some never succeed in acquiring it. They prefer to remain in a tactile world.

Those who were blind from birth till the operation have no true conception of height or distance. To those patients who are first able to see after their operations, colours are more important than shapes, and they have less difficulty in learning colours than shapes. One would probably have believed that it would have been exactly the opposite. Pictures or photographs—which are two-dimensional representations of three-dimensional objects—are at first meaningless. For a picture, like a map or a written word, is a learned symbol. In this case, the actual size of what is represented is symbolized by something much smaller (except in the opposite cases where an object is magnified in a photograph). Children, after these operations, when shown a picture or a photograph, notice the frame rather than the actual picture, for visually it is more prominent. The content of the picture is prominent only to people who know that there is one, that the picture represents someone or something. von Senden has reported that one little girl aged eight, on being shown a photograph, first noticed the wooden frame, which she called a box lid, and then added that there was something painted on it. Even when she was told it represented a human face, she could not discover any of the parts, such as the eyes or the nose. Another patient asked, when she was handed paintings or photographs: 'Why do they put those dark marks all over them?' Her mother then told her that the dark marks were shadows and if the shadows were not put in, 'many things would look flat'. 'Well, that's how things do look' the patient replied.

The first thing one patient saw when the bandages were removed from

his eyes was the face of the surgeon who performed the operation. The
patient said that he saw a blur and he knew it must be a face as a voice
was coming out of it. He thought that had he not known that voices
came out of faces, he would not have known that it was a face. At first
when he looked down from a window about 30 to 40 feet above the
ground, he thought he could easily have climbed out of the window and
lowered himself to the ground while hanging on to the window still with
his hands. He was amazed when he first saw the moon and thought it was
a reflection of something in the window.

In these patients some objects seemed to be surprisingly large and
others equally small; some objects surprised them by being too close and
others by being too far away. An American blind girl explained that to a
blind person 'a skyscraper is not thought of as towering into the
heavens, but as indefinitely higher than a blind man can reach'. All the
patients have difficulty in distinguishing two-dimensional from three-
dimensional things. One of these patients could not tell a ping-pong ball
from a white disk. At first, these patients cannot identify colours and
they have to learn to do this. They then do not see colour as we see it. The
colour does not fill out the whole extent of the coloured object.
According to Macdonald Critchley, 'In the environment there looms up
a medley of colour patches, with differing tonal qualities and with
properties of shininess or dullness.'

These rare patients who recover from blindness are quite different
from children learning to look for the first time. For the patients already
have tactile and motor experience of the world. Yet, from the difficulties
experienced by these patients in learning to see and acquire the same
perceptions and concepts of the visual world as the other people of their
culture, we get some hints of how the child learns to put meaning into
sensation, to turn sensation into perception.

Those who are born blind build up a kinaesthetic-tactile image of the
world, whereas people who can see acquire a visual image. For someone
born blind, perspective does not exist and congenitally blind people
cannot grasp what it is. Their idea of distance is very different from that
of people who see. For them, objects remain the same size wherever they
are, within touch or out of it; to us, objects appear smaller when they are
in the distance. They have never seen an object from different angles,
from above, from the side; they know the object only from feeling,
smelling or tasting it. Whereas for us, the different appearances of
objects seen from various angles teach us about perspective, distance
and space. We know that an object has a constant colour, even though
we see many shades which depend on the lighting and the shadows. We

conclude that its shape is constant too, even though our eyes don't tell us this.

The way in which our vision gives each of us our picture of the world can be learned with much pleasure by reading Trevor-Roper's *The World through Blunted Sight*. In this interesting book, Trevor-Roper discusses not only the defects of vision of many painters; he also emphasizes the results of defects of vision in forming the characters of children.

The comparable operation of restoring hearing to those born deaf has not yet been achieved. If ever it becomes possible, this will be a rewarding field of psychology to study; and it will not be all pleasure for those who have to learn to hear.

Perception always goes beyond the sensory data. What lies beyond is a guess or a prediction or a hypothesis: you may choose your word. We live in a familiar world; and perception is based on probabilities. What the child is so busy learning is the context of various inputs; it is learning probabilities, about what the sensory data in this situation probably mean.

We are not born seeing all the things that we see around us; this has to be learned. If we see a black apparently flat apparently circular object, we say we can see a gramaphone record. We still say this when we are looking at it from above, from its edge or from an angle of 45 degrees. Yet in each of these cases our retinae are receiving totally different impressions. Seeing is believing; it is believing that the dots, lines, angles and edges that we see do represent the objects we already know.

We never see a movement. We see something changing its position, we see it becoming larger or getting smaller. From visual clues such as these, we infer that a movement is taking place.

Because seeing entails guessing what things are, one can make mistakes. One sees what appears to be a mass of flowers in the distance; when one gets near, one finds that it is litter and papper. How strange that this seen material then arouses two opposite emotional reactions.

If a baby has good sight for the first two years of life and then goes blind, it is the same as if it had been born blind. If this child's sight is restored, it is found that the early ability to see has had no permanent effects. But if the child does not become blind till the age of four, all that it has learned to see remains and gives it a picture of the world. These children are quite unlike the congenitally blind. There is no doubt that the difference between the two groups—those blind by the age of three and blind by the age of five—depends on structural differences in the neurons and their connexions.

Professor Robert Fantz in the United States has studied what things young infants prefer to look at. They prefer patterned objects to plain ones and a stylized face to a face all muddled up. This preference occurs so early that it must be innate. Infants between the ages of one and six months prefer solid spheres to flat circles.

Next time we see a baby lying on its back with its beautiful big eyes wandering apparently purposelessly around, we will remember that it is fully occupied with one of its most important tasks, learning to see.

What the visual cortex receives

As we have seen above, within the retina are layers of rods and cones, bipolar, amacrine, and ganglion cells. The optic nerve fibres are the axons of the ganglion cells; the ganglion cells receive their input from the amacrine and bipolar cells, and these retinal neurons are immediately connected to the photoreceptors, the rods and cones. The retina is interested in contrast, in lines, edges, boundaries of dark and light. The optic nerve fibres proceed to a region of the midbrain where they make synapses with the next lot of neurons; and thence nerve fibres go on to the primary visual area of the cortex.

What the visual cortex receives has been investigated by Professors Hubel and Wiesel of Harvard. The receptive fields of the ganglion cells are organized on a centre-surround antagonist basis. The receptive field has an excitatory centre with an inhibitory surround, or the opposite, a central inhibitory field with an excitatory surround. Each ganglion cell is connected to one of the midbrain neurons.

This arrangement is changed in the visual cortex. Here the cortical neuron receives its input from many of the midbrain neurons, thus collecting information from a small region of the retina. These cortical neurons do not respond to spots of light but to lines in various directions, to edges and boundaries, to lines moving in one direction and not in others. For any single cortical neuron, the best stimulus might be a bright line on a dark background or else a dark line on a light background. It is likely that each cortical cell obtained its input from several retinal ganglion cells, each of which is organized on a centre-surround basis. The visual cortex combines the input from both eyes. Some of the cells respond to inputs from one eye and others to inputs from both eyes. There are cells responding only to the left eye, others to the right, and others to both eyes but they are more excited by the one eye than the other. This is the same in the auditory cortex with regard to both ears.

There are ganglion cells of the retina that are affected by a colour.

With these cells, the central field is excited by a certain colour; this colour then inhibits the surrounding retinal cells. These neurons also connect on a one to one basis with the midbrain neurons, and so they react in the same way to colour.

The visual system is not ready to use at birth. Kittens are the animal we know most about as experiments have been done on them and not on human babies. If a kitten is brought up in darkness, it will always be blind. The correct cortical connections develop as the animal practises looking and seeing. What the cat is finally able to see depends on the environment in which it lived as a kitten. Blakemore kept kittens in an environment where everything was striped vertically or horizontally. Eventually the visual cortex of these kittens responded only well to stripes and poorly to all other visual aspects of the environment.

The appreciation of colour is a complicated process. In the retina some ganglion cells are activated by a colour. Such cells have a central field excited by a certain colour. Presentation of this colour to the cell inhibits the surrounding ganglion cells. These colour-sensitive ganglion cells connect on a one-to-one basis to cells in the midbrain, which react to colours in the same way.

When there is damage to the part of the cortex in the boundary zone between the occipital and parietal lobes of the left hemisphere, the patient cannot associate colours with the coloured object, he no longer realizes that a colour is an important part of recognition of an object, such as the colour of an orange or the green colour of a leaf. When there is damage to the homologous region on the right, the person cannot match colours.

It can sometimes happen—though very rarely—that something destroys the primary visual cortex. Then there is blindness, but blindness of an extraordinary kind. The patient says he is blind and that he can see nothing; on the whole, he is right, he is blind. But when his vision is examined and he is told to touch or look at a light one puts in front of him, he can do so quite accurately. He himself says he is just guessing and that he cannot see a thing. In fact, he is able to tell horizontal from vertical bars of light; he can see the difference between Xs and Os, if they are big enough. He feels that the test is ridiculous because he can see nothing and he says that he is just looking or putting out his hand at random; yet he has the feeling that there is something there in front of him, although he sees nothing. If you try to deceive him by telling him that there is a bar of light in front of him when there isn't, he is not deceived; for then he does not have the feeling that there is something in front of him.

What is so interesting about scientific discoveries is that one never knows where the next advance is coming from. What this blind man sees is now being made clear from some experiments on the brain of the newborn hamster. This animal is born in a rather embryonic state. At this stage, there are parts of its brain that can be removed easily. In the baby hamster the midbrain region that receives the input from the retina is large and can be easily separated from the visual cortex. And so at this time two operations are possible. Either the midbrain visual region can be removed or the cortical visual region. When the visual cortex is removed, it is obvious that the hamster is blind. An analysis of the animal's visual capabilities shows that it knows where something is but it does not know what it is. It cannot recognize anything but it goes straight to an object placed in its visual field. When the midbrain visual region is removed, it knows what things are but it cannot run to them; it is incapable of finding what it sees. These are two opposite kinds of defect. These experiments on the baby hamster show us what is happening to the human being with the primary visual cortex knocked out. He is like the hamster that knows where something is but does not know what it is. That is the hamster with the primary visual cortex removed and with the midbrain region intact.

These experiments show us that there is a difference anatomically in what we see and in where we see it. This leads to the extraordinary situation of being unable to see something and yet being able to put a finger on it. On the other hand, it is possible to see something and recognize it and yet be unable to locate it and unable to put a finger on it. This is called visual disorientation. There are thus two different anatomical systems: a system for where and a system for what.

What the auditory cortex receives

The elements of sound are received by the inner ear which is sensitive to the pitch or frequency and the loudness of sounds. The two ears are able to find the source of a sound, which is of importance in the struggle for life. In the auditory cortex, neurons respond more to the changing pitch of a sound than to a note of constant pitch. Some neurons of the cat's cortex are excited by falling tones, others by rising tones and others by both. So when we listen to music it may be that what we like to hear is the changing notes and the changing loudness and softness of the sounds and not a steady tone. Apart from music, the changing pitch of a note tells us whether the source of a sound is coming or going or whether we are getting nearer or farther from it. This is owing to the Doppler effect, described in the case of echo-location of some bats.

The destruction of the primary sensory area of a sense does not cause complete loss of that sense. We have already seen how it is with the primary visual area and blindness. If the primary auditory cortex is destroyed, there is not complete deafness; there is a loss of high tones. Experiments done on cats in which the primary auditory cortex was removed also caused only a partial deafness. The animals could still hear differences in pitch and in loudness and softness. But they could not localize the source of the sound nor tell which ear it was presented to. They could not hear changes in the duration of a sound and they no longer reacted to a total sequence and pattern of sounds or tones. Bats, for whom hearing is essential, can hear far better than cats when the primary auditory cortex has been removed.

The auditory functions of the two hemispheres are different. The ability to localize the source of a sound is probably performed more by the right than the left temporal lobe. This ability is related to the appreciation of space and position in space.

Music is made up of many elements. The right cerebral hemisphere is the dominant one for musical execution and musical perception, whereas the left hemisphere is dominant for verbal language, both its understanding and its execution. Singing is done mainly with the right hemisphere whereas speaking is with the left. People with musical training use the left hemisphere more than those who are not musical and who have not been educated in music.

Combining sensory inputs

In front of the principal visual receiving area of the right hemisphere is a region essential for the recognition of people's faces. We take this ability for granted, but children of seven or eight may still find it quite difficult. If somebody comes in with a bandanna around their head or with a wig of hair of different colour, younger children may not recognize the person even though they know them quite well. In this region of the right hemisphere, the position of things in the environment in relation to ourselves is appreciated. This relation of objects to ourselves is connected with our cognisance of the relation of the parts of our own bodies, the recognition of right and left limbs, of right and left outside ourselves. With this is connected our understanding of the figures and hands of a clock, the meaning of the position of the hands, the meaning of the points of the compass, of maps, of architects' plans. If this region is severely injured, we cannot plan a journey; for we cannot visualize the route and we have no idea which road to take whenever there is a choice. Such a patient cannot draw nor construct a model of anything. He is also completely lost when it comes to getting dressed; for he cannot appreciate the difference between left and right and cannot relate the sleeves to the arms of his own body.

The ability to add and subtract needs the appreciation of space. This is quite clear to anyone who has seen someone calculating by using an abacus; for the bobbles are arranged in columns side by side. When we add and subtract using the decimal system, we are using an internalized abacus. If the relevant part of the brain has been destroyed, then the spatial aspects of adding and subtracting will be missing; and so the patient cannot take a figure from one column to the next. If he were to use Roman numerals (and one wonders how anyone could have calculated using Roman numerals), he will have no difficulty with this disruption of spatial ability; for figures are not taken from column to column.

Vestibular components are essential for our perception of space and of our own bodies in our constructed space. Both hemispheres contribute to the ability to judge distances in three dimensions and to make constructions in space, which needs an appreciation of three dimensions.

The two cerebral hemispheres are not equal and the same. It is probable that we are born with the two hemispheres having a propensity to develop differently; the differences are probably also accentuated by learning during childhood.

When we say that an ability depends on only one hemisphere, this does not mean that the hemisphere needs no contribution from the other. At first the inflow comes to one hemisphere and then it is passed to the secondary receptive area of both hemispheres; from here it is sent to the association areas. Some of the higher association areas are concerned with one kind of basic function. Although such an area of one hemisphere carries out a function related to that performed by the homologous association area of the other hemisphere, the function may be sufficiently different for us to recognize one function as being performed by one hemisphere and another function by the similar region of the other hemisphere. It is only the higher association areas that have become so specialized.

The sensory input from our own bodies, coming in via all sensory channels, is integrated in the parietal lobes; this product gives us what is called the body schema. This is the basis of our feeling that our bodies are us, that they are placed in such or such a way in the environment, and that the parts of our bodies make up a whole. With the kind of damage to the brain that occurs nowadays from wars, small circumscribed areas of the cortex of the hemisphres can be ruined without there being much damage to the rest of the brain. When a part of one parietal lobe is selectively damaged in this way, the patient no longer realizes that the limbs on the opposite side of his body to the damaged lobe are his own. He pays no attention to these parts of his body; when asked to move them, he does nothing. Often when he is told to clasp his two hands together, he merely clasps one. If one then holds up the neglected hand in front of the patient's eyes, he still does not recognize it as being a part of himself, and is unable to move it. It is in fact not paralysed, for it still moves adequately in automatic movements. When there is this inability to integrate one half of one's body, the patient usually neglects and cannot conceive the same side of the bodies of others. For example, one patient with a neglect of his own left limbs, when asked to lift my left hand, always lifted my right hand and took no notice of my left. Such a patient may show little intellectual deterioration, apart from this one sort of defect. During the last war, I saw a patient with a severe injury of the right parietal lobe. When I held up his left arm in front of his eyes, he would take no notice of it; and when I asked him whose limb it was, he answered 'Oh, that! That's the arm Sister puts the penicillin injections into'. In such cases, the patient may think that the arm on the opposite side to the brain lesion is someone else in his bed, and he may give it a name. Another of these patients I saw in the war used to say that the limbs were his brother. He strongly objected to their presence in bed with him and he would try and hurl them out of bed. Once or twice I have seen such patients throw themselves out of bed by mistake in their efforts to get rid of their right arm and leg, which they thought were somebody else in the bed.

When a patient neglects and cannot integrate half of his own body, he usually neglects the whole of surrounding space on that side of his body as well. He does not notice the half of the face of the clock, he may walk into objects in this side of space or he may even walk around in a circle, turning always to the neglected side of space. He cannot localize sounds coming from the affected side and he hears them as coming from the other side. These disturbances of perception perhaps suggest that normally our conception of the space in which we live may be arrived at as an extension of our conception of our own bodies.

The opposite kind of defect is the loss of a part of the body with retention of the part of the brain where past and present inputs are integrated. This gives rise to phantom limbs. Here the brain centres remain; the peripheral part has gone. The central integration region is intact and it tells us that the whole body is still there. One might have imagined that the loss of the part would be registered in the brain and that it would no longer be felt as being present. But this is not so. The reason probably is that there is no silence, no ceasing of impulses coming in. The nerves coming from the part that has been cut off, whether it is a limb, a breast, a finger, or the penis, are still there, though their peripheral parts have been removed. They can still function at their cut ends, and they may send off nerve impulses from their ends. This can easily be observed in anyone who has had a part amputated. If one finds one of the nerves in his stump, and then squeezes or bangs it, the person will feel some sort of sensation in the phantom limb. He may get pins and needles running down the leg to the toes; or he may get a burning pain in the ankle. For one has stimulated the very nerves which previously went to those parts of his limb.

Parts of the temporal lobes and the frontal lobes contribute mood and emotion. When parts of the temporal lobes are cut out, all emotion goes; and when the frontal lobes are cut out, there is a state of utter indifference. We have learned from the operations of leucotomy, in which bands of nerve fibres between the thalamus and the frontal lobes are cut, how these connections are needed for the person to feel involved in his own life. When this operation has been performed in patients with terribly severe pain, the pain remains but the suffering and depression is removed. How misery, anguish, loneliness, and even guilt can accompany chronic pain is shown by Tolstoy in his masterpiece *The Death of Ivan Ilyich*.

When a lesion disconnects two parts of the cortex, both of which are necessary for perception, we find some surprising abnormalities in cognition. For instance, in cases such as these, it may be that something is known and recognized when presented in one half of the visual field and unknown when it is presented to the other. If the connections between the secondary visual areas and the speech area are destroyed, the patient will know what an object is and what a visually experienced sensation means but he will be unable to say the name of the object or to explain the situation. It is clear that he still knows what the thing is, as he uses it properly. For instance he will pick up a razor and shave with it; but he no longer has the word 'razor' available to relate to the object. When the right cerebral hemisphere has become disconnected from the left, the left can still carry out certain activities if they do not need thought, conceptualization, ideas, and words. When this occurs, one can give such a patient a gardening fork, indicating that he should use it in the garden. He will then show that he knows how to do so but he will be unable to explain what he is doing or to answer a question on how to use the fork.

One part of the brain can know an object while another part does not recognize it. The left hemisphere is likely to know the object, in the sense that it can name it and put it into many different categories; the right hemisphere is likely to know it, in the sense that it knows what to do with it; but it cannot name or categorize it.

One of the difficulties we all have in discussing and understanding the functions of the brain is due to the words we use being often inappropriate; for they have been taken over from everyday speech, philosophy and even religion. Words such as 'know' or 'understand' or 'perception' are either popular or philosophic terms; they are too vague to have the clearcut meaning needed in science. Even the word 'I' is useless. If the right cerebral hemisphere knows something and the left does not, then where does 'I' come in?

21 Speech and other symbols

For he can spraggle upon waggle at the word of command.

Social animals living in groups, unsocial animals meeting for sexual intercourse, parents and offspring, all need to communicate with each other. In nature there are hundreds of ways of communicating; using the voice is only one of the ways.

The time in which we live is marvellous; for we are now reaping the harvest of a hundred years and more of the investigation of the whole universe by scientific methods. Four of man's wishes have been achieved. He is able to have sexual intercourse as often as he likes without producing children; he can fly, even better, faster and farther than the birds; he can visit other planets; and he can understand the language of the birds and some other animals and speak with them. Konrad Lorenz first learned to communicate effectively with birds; and in the United States, they have advanced considerably in learning to speak with porpoises and whales. von Frisch has decoded the dancing language of bees and now any of us can learn where to find nectar and honey. Lorenz and his colleagues now lead birds far more effectively than St Francis ever did by preaching at them.

Man is a typical social animal; he communicates by appearing to the eyes and the ears of his fellows. He makes use of signs and gestures; he uses his face and the rest of his body to communicate his emotional state; and he uses his voice to make exclamatory and other emotional sounds, to laugh, to cry, and above all, to speak. The expression of emotion and the language of gesture are innate. Speech—communication by words—is learned.

If two human beings have no language in common, they can tell each other of their needs by means of the language of gesture. We also use this language to add emphasis to our vocal speech. The degree to which we do this depends on the culture in which we were brought up. One can tell, even when standing behind someone talking, whether he is a Southern European or an inhibited man from Northern Europe. The Southerner not only uses his hands for self-expression, his whole trunk is mobilized as he swells and shrinks at the different points in the discussion.

We express our feelings in our speech whether we want to or not. There is the force and the tension heard in the voice. There are the accompanying expressions on our faces, our smiles, usually natural, sometimes put on, sometimes almost but not quite smothered, there are expressions of disgust, of disdain and all the others described in novels. Then there are the forceful communications of rage, fear and hatred, there is the involuntary pallor, blushing, the beads of sweat, the retracted upper lids with the eyes seeming to start out of the head.

Man's speech is not only a means of communication like that of all other social animals; it is really something quite new. Even if the new features are developed from elements already present in the speech of species less developed than man, they became something different, something not seen before in evolution. Propositional speech occurs only in man; and only man has developed a brain able to use symbolic speech and to think in words. Once man developed the ability to pass thought in language from one person to another and from one group to another, his way of evolution followed this trail. Any person or group who made better use of this new discovery had greater survival than others; and so natural selection in the case of man came to favour the development of propositional speech and every aspect of living that made use of speech.

Man uses speech in everything he is doing and in all he intends to do. If you pay attention to what goes on in your mind as you walk along the street, you will find that you are thinking all the time in words, something perhaps like this: 'I will go into a shop and buy a birthday card. They are on the left at the end of the shop, up at the far end. I will find one of those funny ones not one of the sentimental ones.' Then, as you enter the shop, you say to yourself: 'Ah, a glass door; smeary finger marks on it; something new at the pencil counter over there. Yes, here are the cards, pink, blue, where are the funny ones', and so on all through the day. You can observe this use of speech clearly in young children; for up to the age of 5 or 6, their speech is not wholly internal, and they keep up a running commentary to themselves about what they are doing and thinking. Then, you will hear them directing their activities by means of speech.

Using symbols

The higher levels of the cerebral hemispheres make a model of the world, based on some inborn modes of perception and on a great deal of learning. This mental world parallels the real world, with some distortions; it is a symbolic representation of reality. Man has the ability to make use of symbols to a degree vastly greater than any other animal. Indeed, it may be said that the ability to construct and use symbols is the main feature of general intelligence. According to the studies of Piaget and his colleagues, the child develops the ability to make use of symbols between the ages of seven and eleven.

Symbols provide us with a kind of shorthand; and like shorthand, they are economical of time and space. They are effective because the symbol is taken as equivalent to certain things or events of the physical world. From a first set of symbols, further symbols can be evolved. Finally, all the symbols are translated back into the things and events of the real world.

There are a great many different kinds of symbols and of ways of making use of them. One of the simplest relationships is for the symbol to be a part of the whole that it represents. Instead of the total event or the whole act of behaviour, a small part is shown, and the animal who understands the symbol assumes the whole for the part.

A symbol in which the part is taken as a token for the whole is the piece of cloth or teddy-bear that baby humans, chimpanzees, or other monkeys will accept as a substitute for their parents. They take this with them when they go to sleep and will cling to it when awake, obtaining physical comfort and psychological reassurance from physical contact with this symbol. Other examples of tokens in which the part is accepted for the whole are photographs of people we love, or the hairs of Mahomet's beard, treasured in a thousand mosques.

From the point of view of communication between human beings, an important system of symbols in which the part is taken for the whole is the natural language of gesture. This is one of the ways in which most vertebrates communicate with each other. In this case, the part is usually an imcomplete part of a total act of behaviour, and it signifies intention. Human gestures are usually a précis of the total act. When we point with outstretched arm and index finger, this is a part of following one's upper limb in the direction indicated. When we threaten someone, it is a part of the total movement of aggression and fighting. Much of this gesture-language is innate. Deaf-mutes who are not taught to speak, make use of an inborn natural sign-language, mainly based on gesture. This language is international and largely independent of the language of the speaker. Deaf-mutes of different countries have little difficulty in understanding each other. This innate sign-language has been elaborated by the Indians of North America and by some of the original tribes of Northern Queensland. Some of the evidence for the innate origin of the languages based on gesture comes from the fact that many of the signs used by the Australian aborigines, the American Indians, and deaf-mutes of all lands are the same.

This language of gesture is closely related to the intention-movement signs of many animals. When a bird makes movements preparatory to taking-off, the other birds understand that they should take wing, and do so. When a male monkey merely bares one or two of its upper teeth, the other monkeys take this initial sign of threatening behaviour for the total threat, and behave accordingly.

Man's distant cousin, the chimpanzee, is good at learning sign-language. A gesture language has been used for a long time in the United States, the American sign language; it is used by deaf-mutes and their teachers. This language can be learned by young champanzees. One of these chimpanzees had mastered a hundred and sixty signs after four years' training.

Man's speech is not essentially different from this. His verbal speech allows him to sort things and concepts into categories and to to make use of abstract entities. The chimpanzee can do this to a limited extent.

Symbols of other symbols allow us to create the universal symbols of algebra, geometry, and arithmetic. Such systems of symbols have their own existences and their own rules. We follow these rules and carry out operations on the symbols of symbols without having to visualize any objects represented during the process of working out. This allows us to arrive at solutions to problems which can then be translated back into the world of reality. This is a great saving in time and mental effort. Formal logic is another and similar system of symbols, underlying and providing us with symbols for reasoning. Musical notation is another system, similar to writing; indeed the clef signs were originally letters. The page of the score consists of various symbols representing the sounds the players should make. It is almost unbelievable that such beautiful music as that of Beethoven's quartets could come out of just a few dots, all looking much the same, printed on paper.

Another symbol developed by most of mankind is money; these tokens can also be learned by chimpanzees. This ability was studied in the 1930s in Professor Yerkes's Yale laboratories of Primate Biology in Florida by Dr John B. Wolfe and by Dr John T. Cowles. They showed that chimpanzees could learn to work for token rewards. These anthropoid apes learned to work for poker chips which they could collect and then hand in for food. Moreover, they learned the symbolic meaning of chips of different sizes and colours. They also learned that one sort of chip was useless as currency as no food was ever exchanged for it. It should be made clear that in these experiments the food was out of sight and so the animals worked for money and then stored it up to exchange it for food when the time came. They even learned to work for money on one day and give it in for food on the next day. Dr Geoffrey Bourne relates in his book *The Ape People* that 'the animals used to walk around clutching their earnings to their breasts, sleeping on them at night so that they would not be stolen, and getting very hysterical if any other animal came near their earnings or tried to take any of them away.'

These intelligent animals, then, are able to grasp that the act of pushing a lever is a symbol, that if they engage in this activity, they will eventually be rewarded. They understand that the chips, on the face of it meaningless objects, are symbols, promising that something rewarding will come their way. Moreover, they can learn that chips of different sizes and colours have different symbolic meanings: they can learn that a white one means one grape, a blue one two grapes, whereas a brass one has no exchange value. In fact, the chimpanzees understood this coinage so well that one wonders if they would be able to cope with a real monetary system.

The ability to perceive space and to relate it to one's own body depends on a region between the temporal, parietal, and occipital lobes of the right hemisphere. The ability to think spatially, to visualize a building in the three planes of space and related to its surroundings, depends on the cortex of this region. Many curious abnormalities in handling symbols associated with this kind of perception occur when this region of the brain is damaged or disconnected from other parts. Patients with lesions here may not understand the significance of the position of the hands of the clock (and note that we refer to the clock in terms of parts of the body—face, hands). If one asks them to put the hands to indicate a quarter past three for instance, either they cannot do it at all or else they do it wrong. They make mistakes in drawing maps and explaining where things are on maps. Also, in this region of the right hemisphere resides the ability to form the symbols of modelling and sculpture, the three-dimensional representation of a three-dimensional object, but in this case abstracted and generalized, and often represented on a different scale from the original. The actual object has at first to be apprehended in three dimensions, then abstracted into a generalization, and then represented again in space as a particular example of the generalization.

The ability to make use of the symbols of mathematics depends on association areas of the cortex of both hemispheres. An essential region is in the left hemisphere at the junction of the temporal and parietal lobes, in front of the occipital lobe's secondary visual area. A possible explanation of the association of mathematical symbols with this region may be that these symbols began with counting; and counting was abstracted from touching or moving the digits of the hands and perhaps the feet, this being the first and essential digital system. It is doubtless related to counting things seen; and so it is near the visual area, as well as the tactile and kinaesthetic areas.

After developing the use of his own digits for counting, man evolved the abacus, which is still used effectively in the East. With this instrument, addition, subtraction, multiplication, and division are done visually, by the manipulation of bobbles in rows. Our numeral system also depends on moving figures from column to column.

If a child is bad at mathematics but is good at most other school work, this is unlikely to be due to any defect in its brain. The reasons are undoubtedly all those factors implicated by psychotherapists and psychologists; and most important and most common of all, bad teaching.

Within the realm of mathematics, the most visual are geometry and the use of graphs. Here we see that spatial elements come into mathematical ability. This form of symbolization is related to the ability to envisage space and to locate things and ourselves in space, which depends on the right hemisphere. The region in the left hemisphere on which mathematical ability depends is between the regions for organizing speech and visual perceptions. This indicates that both verbal and visual symbolizations enter into mathematical thinking. Mathematical symbolization also needs the contribution from the auditory para-sensory area, enabling us to use inner speech, when we make concepts in our minds.

We talk about mathematical ability as though it is one entity; but it is not. It is made up of the functions of many parts of the cortex; and in different people, different regions will be used.

The ability to use symbols to represent aspects and parts of reality is one of the most advanced functions of the brain. Hughlings Jackson recognized as a general principle that when the brain atrophies, the functions most recently acquired disappear first, those longest developed during evolution remaining till the last. In accordance with this principle, we find that when the whole brain degenerates, the patient first loses the ability to grasp and to make use of symbolic thinking. The way this is usually shown up is by getting the patient to explain proverbs. For instance, when he is asked for the meaning of the proverb 'A rolling stone gathers no moss', he will explain in detail to you that a stone that keeps on moving is not able to grow moss as it is moving. When the proverb ' A burnt child dreads the fire' is read to him, he will explain that of course the child is frightened of the fire because he has been burnt. Or 'A drowning man will catch at a straw' will obtain only the response that he does this in an effort to stop himself drowning. The symbolic meaning of the proverbs, which is their whole point, escapes him, and usually he cannot grasp it even when it is explained to him.

The ability to form and use symbols depends on the working of many parts of the cerebral cortex of both hemispheres. Professor Geschwind of Harvard, considers that man's outstanding ability to use verbal symbols depends on the connections in his brain between all the parasensory association areas. Man is able to see a circle, to feel the circumference of a circle with his hands or feet, to draw a circle in the air with his hand or foot; on account of the connections between the visual, tactile and kinaesthetic areas, he can abstract a common circularity from these three senses. For this common feature, one verbal symbol is made, the word 'circle'. Had there been no connections between the secondary sensory areas, he would not have been able to recognize the one common feature. Seen circle, felt circle, and circle drawn in space would have been as different to him as the smell of a violet is to the feel of a cube. Indeed, it would be more different; for an account of these interconnections we are able to make meaningful comparisons, and from the different sensory inputs to deduce similarities and differences. I do not mean here the more obvious assimilation we make all the time when we create perceptions from all the sensory inputs, so that we know from the smell and the sight that this is a daffodil. I mean such facts as the ability to recognize a rhythm, for instance, in three different sensory modalities. We are able to recognize a rhythm of long–short–long heard as dash–dot–dash from a morse buzzer, we recognize it when it is tapped on our hands, and we recognize it again flashed in the visual field by lights.

The use of symbols is a great economy in the activity of the brain, and it saves time during thinking and remembering. Instead of nerve impulses having to make the complete circuit round the original paths, they need only make a smaller circuit. By this I mean that when we remember having a picnic last summer, we don't go through the whole experience again, taking as long as it took when it happened. The first symbol is the word 'picnic'; this separates that sort of event from every other sort of event. Then we have the symbols 'last summer'; these are two sorts of symbols, the symbols of words and the symbols of divisions of time. Again, as soon as we have thought 'last summer', we have restricted the neural activity to certain selected experiences and we do not have to recollect other experiences.

Thinking

If one asks what parts of the brain are involved in thinking, one must answer that it all depends on what you mean by thinking. One uses the word to mean remembering, for trying to recall, for imagining, for solving problems in the mind or in reality, and for any other mental activities. It is thinking that a chess-player does when he works out the possible results of moving his king. It is thinking that a dress-designer does when he imagines a new dress or when a salesman designs a plan of campaign to get the money out of peoples' pockets. Most of our thinking uses words, concepts and logic. But there is thought without words. If a painter has a stroke which takes away his ability to use speech, he may still have his mental images of things visual, forms, colours, and visual relationships and memories, and he may still be able to create paintings; his originality may be unimpaired. Similarly, sculptors can still model and carve. The parts of the cerebral hemispheres that are essential for abstract thought are in the left temporal lobe; the parts needed for painting are in both cerebral hemispheres, in the occipital, parietal, and frontal lobes. Thinking that makes use of words is organized mainly by the left hemisphere while thinking that depends on visualizing or conceiving of things set out in space is organized by the right hemisphere.

Thinking can be auditory. A composer thinks in auditory images. It is usually mixed. Thinking may be a combination of auditory and conceptual, as when a conductor plans how he will present a symphony. It may be partly auditory and partly kinaesthetic, partly tactile and partly motor, as it is for the bassoon player, remembering how to play his part in the symphony. For a ballet dancer, it is visual, auditory, kinaesthetic and very much motor. It is the same for the footballer and will then include a large element of spatial organization. All these aspects of thinking occur together; they are not sorted out, as they have been on this page.

Thinking about smells does not necessarily need words. If we try and remember the name of a smell, then we do use words; but we can bring an olfactory image into our minds of the smell of lavender, of the earth freshly rained upon or of toadstools, without using words. Though the question then comes up: would we be able to think of the smell of a toadstool without first thinking the word 'toadstool'. The answer, as usual, is not simple. The smell of toadstools might come spontaneously into our minds without us having to think the word; and in that case, we would think or imagine the smell without using the speech area of the brain. Or we might get a visual picture in our mind of the toadstool, and from there the smell of it; here again, we would not need the word. But the way I arrived at the smell of toadstools just now was via the word. I thought in fact of the word and of the visual images of various toadstools at the same time; I cannot really say which came first. That is typical of how we think. We make a shorthand conglomeration of words and visual images, secondarily auditory images, and thirdly and a long way after, kinaesthetic, tactile, and olfactory images. Needless to say, the exact mixture varies from person to person. Someone who can read and write is more attached to words than someone who is illiterate.

It may have struck some readers that we have used the word 'association' in two different ways; with an anatomical meaning and with a psychological meaning. Nerve fibres connecting two parts of the cerebral cortex are called 'association' fibres; and we speak also of the 'association' of ideas. The reason for this is that the first investigators of the anatomy of the cerebral hemispheres introduced the word 'association fibres' for this very reason: they thought that these fibres joined· or associated two areas of the cortex, and that this junction formed the basis of the psychological association of ideas and words. Now although this may be so, it was undesirable to use the same word for the two meanings; for it prejudged the whole issue of the neural basis of psychological functioning. Even though the association of ideas certainly needs association nerve fibres, the statement that two areas of cortex are joined by association fibres does not tell us anything about the mechanism of association in the psychological sense. And it may lead us to think that there is no problem here, that psychological association is explained by saying that there are association fibres between two areas of cortex. It must then be said that we really do not know what we mean when we use the psychological word 'associate' or when we say that the child learns to associate: we do not know what this means at a neural level, or what are the neural mechanisms involved.

Learning to talk

The deformed babies born without cerebral hemispheres make noises, but they never learn to shape them into the sounds of speech nor to understand that sounds have a symbolic meaning. To grasp that idea needs the cerebral hemispheres.

Human beings are learning language from birth to ninety. But the way of learning usually changes around the age of ten. Before that age, one picks it up naturally, that is to say in ways that we are just beginning to learn about; after that time, we learn it in the way we learn at school, learning grammar and spelling with conscious effort.

For the first six months of life both normal and deaf babies babble away, making the same sounds. This shows us that babbling is innate and that the baby does not need to hear its own voice in order to make these noises. After about nine months of life, a difference between the two begins to appear. The child that hears normally is listening to the sounds he hears. He makes more sounds like those of the people around him and stops making the sounds that he does not hear. The deaf child does not alter his babbling and eventually he becomes more and more silent. This ability to hear nuances is remarkable. To hear speech properly, this baby needs to hear all the frequencies used, including overtones; and he must be able to hear differences in timing and duration of sounds. He hears the melody of his mother-tongue, the right intonation.

Therefore, to speak properly, one has to hear normally. The child listens to other peoples' speech and also to its own sounds. One hears one's own speech by two routes, by air conduction through the external ear and by bone conduction through the bones of the skull. Other peoples' speech is heard only by air conduction. A child with much disturbance of hearing cannot hear correctly by either route. Yet studies of the deaf by phoneticians and linguists have revealed that a child deaf over certain frequencies can nevertheless make sounds within this frequency range. We do not fully understand how this can be. It probably is because there may be two or three cues for perceiving a phoneme. A child with normal hearing makes use of all three cues; the deaf child may still perceive the sound by appreciating only one cue; and it may be using cues that are unimportant for normally hearing people.

A child who hears speech incorrectly will model his speech on what he hears, and so he will learn to speak incorrectly. Moreover, hearing his own speech sounding just like their speech, the child cannot grasp why no one understands what he is saying. When his parents correct him, he cannot hear the differences between what they are saying and what he is saying himself. The whole problem is too difficult for him, he probably becomes discouraged, and he may give up trying to speak. He may then be regarded as mentally deficient or at any rate rather strange and stupid. When the partly deaf child goes to school, he meets a new lot of difficulties as he learns to write. He writes down the phonemes he hears. But as he does not hear what the rest of the world is hearing, he cannot learn to write what the other children are writing. If no one realizes that the child is partially deaf, then the adults again conclude that the child is mentally defective or very dull.

If a parent gets any hint that the child does not hear well, he should get him examined at a clinic specializing in deaf children; and the sooner the better. For children who start learning from specially trained teachers get on better if they start very early.

The human baby is born with the right anatomical connections. To perceive the sound first phonetically, as a total sound or phoneme, and then linguistically, the human uses the left temporal lobe. The baby can make the sounds he hears because there are connections between the speech region of the left temporal lobe and the motor regions of the frontal lobes and the kinaesthetic region of the front part of the parietal lobe.

If a baby or a young child has an accident or some malady of the brain that destroys the speech area of the left hemisphere, the child loses all the speech that he has acquired. The speech area can then be reconstituted in the right hemisphere. Yet this is done only at the cost of functions normally organized by the right hemisphere. This reorganization can take place only during the first years of life. Under the age of four, it is complete and the right hemisphere becomes the organizer of speech and thinking based on inner speech. Between the age of four and the onset of puberty, the replacement of speech is almost complete. But after puberty, the damage to the left speech area can never be completely compensated for. In adult life, a stroke affecting the left side of the brain causes aphasia, which at its worst is an inability to speak and to understand speech.

All parts of the cerebral hemispheres are not equally replaceable. There are no general rules. Experiments in baby monkeys show that lesions made in some parts of the cortex eventually cause no disability; though when the adult monkey is tired or under stress, the effect of the lesion again becomes manifest. But lesions made in other parts of the cortex cause permanent deficiencies and there is only a minimal recovery from their effects. Surprisingly enough, the rate of recovery and even the amount is different for the two sexes. This is not the effect of sex hormones; it is genetically determined.

In order to arrive at our present understanding of how parts of the cerebral cortex work together, neurology passed through various phases. At first it was believed that there was no localization of function in the cerebral hemispheres and that they worked as a totality. The next phase was a belief in very discrete localization of function. In this view, small regions of the cortex were thought of as organizing such complex kinds of behaviour as writing, mathematics, or logical thinking. Our present view is that there is localization of function; but complex behaviour such as reading, writing, adding up figures in columns, turning arithmatic into algebra, or turning algebra into geometry, requires the working together of many different local regions of the cortex of both hemispheres.

Unlearning language

The first neurologist to think that speech might depend on a special, local region of the cerebral hemispheres was F. J. Gall; this idea was a part of phrenology. Before the phrenologists, such a high level brain function would have been attributed to the activity of the whole brain, in so far as it was thought of as being an activity of the brain and not of a non-entity, the soul. Gall put 'the organ of speech' in the frontal lobes.

A stranger idea than localizing speech in the frontal lobes was that it could be in only one hemisphere. This step was taken by Marc Dax, who was a general practitioner in the southern French town of Sommieres. He concluded from the cases he had seen that all patients with a disturbance of the faculty of language had a lesion in the left cerebral hemisphere. By 1836, he had collected over forty cases. He collected others from published records; and he found no exceptions to the rule. He therefore concluded that whenever 'the memory for words is impaired', the lesion will be in the left cerebral hemisphere.

This conclusion passed unnoticed until it was rediscovered by an eminent man, Paul Broca. Broca was professor of surgery and was the founder of the science of physical anthropology. Before Broca published his evidence in 1861, Dax's son, Gustave Dax, had been collecting further evidence in support of his father's views.

Dr Macdonal Critchley has unravelled this history, and I quote the following paragraphs from his paper.

Since he had been a student, the younger Dax had been intensely interested in 'alalia' or speech loss, and applied to submit a thesis upon this subject, but he was not allowed to do so. Patiently he collected case-material and evidence from the literature. He wrote a Mémoire which he presented to his local confrères in 1858 and again in 1860, entitled: 'Observations tendant à prouver la coincidence du dérangement de la parole avec une lésion de l'hemisphere gauche du cerveau'. Later he sent it to the Académie de Médecine, where it was received in 1863. Dax *fils* was bitterly hurt by the fact that subsequent writers continued to pay no heed to his work, and failed to give the credit due to his father. . . . Lélut commenting upon the younger Dax's report to the Académie, had said that 'that mysterious organ, the brain, would be even more mysterious if its two halves were found to subserve different functions'.

Critchley has added to this history: 'Today the contributions of the two doctors Dax are no longer forgotten in the world of medicine. But even now the quiet little town of Sommières knows little of its two distinguished oppidans. No plaque adorns the wall of their dwelling in the Place du Bourguet, and though a number of eponymous streets are there, visitors will look in vain for a "rue des deux docteurs Dax".' However, that is not the end of the story; for owing to Critchley's investigations, the town has now put up a plaque to honour these two original thinkers who contributed to our knowledge of the brain.

Broca collected the brains of twenty-two patients who had had lesions that had deprived them of speech; in all cases, the lower part of the frontal lobe of the left hemisphere was damaged. He therefore drew the conclusion that this part of the brain was the essential area for speech. He supposed that the lesion in that region had deprived the patients of the memory of the procedure that had to be followed in order to articulate words. For he knew that these patients had normal hearing and that they had been able to understand speech, both heard and written. He also had one brain in which the lesion was in the same place but in the right frontal lobe. This patient had had no trouble with speech.

The next step forward in our understanding of speech and thought based on speech was made by Wernicke, who at the age of twenty four, in 1874, published his conclusions in a small book. He found that there is a region of the left temporal lobe surrounding the auditory area that is the essential area for the understanding of speech.

An account of our knowledge at present of the regions of the brain that organize speech now follows. The great majority of people are right-handed; in them, speech is organized by the left hemisphere. Ambidextrous people have speech mainly on the left with a good contribution from the right hemisphere. Of left-handed people, 70–80 per cent have speech organized by the left hemisphere, just like right-handed people; 15 per cent of them have it organized on the right, and 15 per cent in both hemispheres. Mirror-writing commonly occurs among left-handed people; this is probably their natural way of writing but it is stopped by the educators of society. If the left hemisphere is damaged in early childhood, about a half of the children organize speech in the right hemisphere, while the other half retain it on the left. If the right hemisphere is damaged, there is some disturbance of the organization of speech. The gestures that are a kind of expressive speech of the body are programmed in the same hemisphere as speech.

Sounds, including the sounds made by human beings talking, are heard in the primary auditory areas of both temporal lobes. In the left temporal lobe is the area surrounding the primary auditory area that is needed for understanding the meaning of speech. This is often called Wernicke's area; it is marked as (4) in Fig. 21.1. In the left frontal lobe is the region that is needed for articulation, the region that when electrically stimulated causes movements of the face, lips, tongue, and larynx. It is labelled (1). In front of it, labelled (2), is the region for articulation of words and joining words to make sentences; it is often called Broca's area. In the part of the brain behind and above Wernicke's area is a large region of the brain, the centre of which is an area of cortex called the angular gyrus; this is a region concerned with all aspects of language; it is marked as (5). The pattern of sound of a word is evoked in Wernicke's area. This pattern is sent to the angular gyrus and then on to Broca's area and other parts of the frontal lobe. Learned visual aspects of the sound are kept in the occipital lobe just behind the angular gyrus. These are the written symbols of the word, written in various alphabets, capitals, small letters, numerals, musical notation, and the reading and understanding of sentences and other symbols. These patterns of the visual aspect of the sound are also sent to the angular gyrus. The band labelled (3) in the figure is a large band of nerve fibres connecting Wernicke's area to the angular gyrus. Similar fibres run from the occipital lobe forwards to the angular gyrus. The band continues forwards from the angular gyrus to Broca's area. This is a two-way connection so that articulated words and sentences have meaning and bring up the sound and the visual image of the thing or relationship given by the word. In Broca's area and the area behind it,

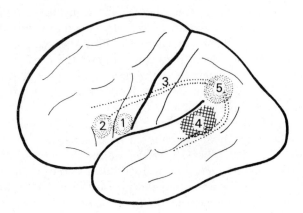

Fig. 21.1. Lateral surface of left hemisphere. (1) Face area of motor cortex; (2) Broca's area; (3) lesion involving arcuate fasiciulus (dotted lines); (4) Wernicke's area; (5) Angular gyrus.

labelled (1), the auditory and/or the visual image of the word is turned into the muscular patterns needed to emit that word.

It is clear that there is a large unknown gap in this presentation of what occurs. For what is transferred to Broca's area is a group of nerve impulses. How nerve impulses constitute a code for a known sound pattern, we do not yet know.

The commonest lesion causing a disturbance of speech is a stroke. If a stroke disturbs any part of the region labelled in Fig. 21.1 there will be some loss of the ability to use speech. What the disturbance will be depends on the site and the extent of the block of the blood vessels. If the lesion affects Wernicke's area, a sound is heard but it is not understood; it no longer has any symbolic meaning. And so a patient with this lesion cannot understand what is written; he cannot read. He can see the written words but what is seen is not interpreted in an auditory form. The patient sees the word written 'Yes' but this does not evoke the sound of yes. If the lesion affects Broca's area, the patient can understand speech and he can read it to himself; but he has much difficulty in speaking and difficulty in forming the sounds of speech. When the lesion disconnects areas (5) and (4) from areas (2) and (1), the patient tends to speak a lot but what he says is all muddled up. When Broca's area is isolated from its usual input it appears to work excessively.

In all or nearly all kinds of speech disorders due to a lesion of the hemisphere, the patient cannot remember the names of many things. This may be slight and the same as may happen to any of us; or it may be so bad as to make speech very difficult.

Understanding the sounds of speech is not only auditory; we also may make use of our own articulation. This becomes clear to us when we have difficulty in understanding someones indistinct speech. We repeat what we have heard, pronouncing it correctly. If we cannot silently articulate to ourselves the sounds of speech that we are hearing, we probably do not understand them. This is one of the ways in which we make corrections for mispronounciations due to speech defects, foreign, or dialect accents. Thus to some extent, the understanding of speech depends on the production of speech. This is so for the sounds recognized as speech sound; but the perception of all other sounds is not done in this repetitive manner. We recognize the sound of thunder without being able to make it; and we comprehend the undeniable statements of music without necessarily being able to produce them.

When in a patient being operated upon under local anesthesia an electrode is made to stimulate the cortex of the speech region, the patient finds that he cannot speak. If he had been just about to say something, he cannot say it. Afterwards when he is asked what happened, he says that he stopped speaking as he could not find the words; he could not remember the words he wanted to say. As soon as the electrode stops stimulating, the patient knows the name of the object which a second before he could not remember.

Reading and writing

Writing enables man to make use of what has been learned. Thus man has at his disposal not only what he has learned during his own brief life, but also the whole of culture, all that his species has acquired during its progress in and out of various epochs of civilization and savagery. It is thus that each generation, though no more intelligent, can start by standing on the shoulders of the previous generation.

We take writing for granted, except when we are laboriously learning it at school. And yet, as the Lady Sei Shonagon wrote in *The Pillow-book* in Japan at the beginning of the eleventh century (translated by Arthur Waley);

Writing is an ordinary enough thing; yet how precious it is! When someone is in a far corner of the world and one is terribly anxious about him, suddenly there comes a letter, and one feels as though the person were actually in the room. It is really very amazing. And, strangely enough, to put down one's thoughts in a letter, even if one knows that it will probably never reach its destination, is an immense comfort. If writing did not exist, what terrible depressions we should suffer from!

A simple kind of reading and writing can be taught to young chimpanzees. A psychologist of the University of California, Dr Premack, has had an amazing success in teaching one of three young chimpanzees to read and write. In the language he made up for his animals, different coloured and shaped plastic labels were used to symbolize objects. The animal learned to read these symbols and to put them on a board when it wanted the objects the symbols represented. With time and patience, he and his colleagues taught this chimpanzee not only to read and write the names of objects, but also abstract conceptions, such as sameness and difference. This animal could manipulate the agreed symbols of 'the same as' and 'different from'. It could classify the objects it knew as the same or as different. It understood that objects had common attributes, such as shape, colour, and size. It could read, write, and understand the different signs 'red on green' and 'green on red'. The young animal enjoyed the game, and would put out questions for itself which it then answered. It was able to answer such a complicated question as 'apple red, banana yellow, implies that apples and bananas have different colours: true or false?' It understood prepositions such as 'above' and 'below'. It even learned the meaning of a conditional 'If . . . , then. . . .' After two and a half years Dr Premack's chimpanzee Sarah constructs sentences in plastic signs. Another American chimpanzee that had been trained to communicate using these plastic signs, on first seeing a duck, spontaneously brought out the two signs 'water' and 'bird' and put them together to name the duck 'water-bird'. Another chimpanzee learned both the English spoken word, an auditory sign for an object, and the visual sign for the object. Thus this animal knew both the auditory and the visual signs for an object. This is reading.

One cannot conclude that, because a chimpanzee can be taught a kind of reading and writing, these skills are easily acquired. The conclusion is how amazingly intelligent the young chimpanzee is. There are children who have specific reading and writing disabilities. They have defects in the functioning of cerebrally based abilities that cause difficulty in learning to read and write, though they are fully intelligent in other ways. This is called dyslexia or congenital alexia. Like many other congenital defects, it runs in families. One finds that other members of the family stammer or are slow in learning to speak; and in these families there is a large proportion of left-handed and ambidextrous people. It is far commoner in boys than girls. These children are often slow in learning to talk and they are poor at learning new words. A part of the difficulty is due to these children having poor memory for words. When they are tested by being shown written words and are asked later to remember these words, they do far less well than normal children. Tests show that normal forgetting which occurs over a few minutes does so more quickly in these children; they cannot remember a list of numbers. Some psychologists have obtained evidence that in many of these children there is difficulty in learning to scan from left to right. This also accounts for these children often muddling up and reversing letters such as 'p' and 'q' and 'b' and 'd', and also for doing mirror-writing, reversing whole syllables, and writing for instance 'dab' for 'bad'. Most of the children have difficulty in categorizing sounds; and this makes spelling very difficult for them.

Reading entails seeing the written word, realizing that it is writing, a graphic code, having meaning. The grapheme is then turned into a phoneme, a sound. One then has to decide whether the sound is a word or not, whether it has meaning; psychologists call this the lexical address. Writing is doing this in the reverse direction. The child usually makes the sound of speech to himself, then he substitutes the graphemes for the phonemes. A child who speaks a dialect and not the standard language will have similar difficulties to a partially deaf child. For instance, if the aspirate 'h' is dropped in his dialect, the child will write 'come ere' for 'come here'. The partially deaf child cannot hear the phoneme correctly, and so it cannot chose the right grapheme. The Chinese child does not have this obstacle; if he cannot hear normally, he can still appreciate the ideogram.

When it comes to shaping the letters or the ideograms, the child has to have a spatial sense, adequate vision, and good control of the movements of hands and fingers.

Different parts of the cerebral cortex are used by a child copying letters and by one writing to dictation. When the child copies letters, he is really drawing; he does not have to hear the phonemes in his mind's ear and he does not have to think of the meaning of the phonemes or graphemes. When he writes to dictation, he has to go through the whole process of writing alphabetically, understanding the meaning of the words, hearing the phonemes and remembering the graphemes that in his language stand for these phonemes.

Japanese writing has three sources, two syllabaries called hirogana and katakana, and ideographs, called kanji. What is interesting is that ideographs, kanji, are treated by the brain like pictures and images and are kept in the right cerebral hemisphere; the syllabaries like our alphabet, are treated like signs and symbols and are kept in the left hemisphere.

This example of writing shows us that the ideas of the phrenologists on the localization of our abilities were naïve; it is only in the last few years that we have begun to understand that functions are localized in the cortex and that it is no simple matter to know what functions underlie our various abilities.

When the child learns to read, it has to repeat the amazing feat of its ancestors: to change an auditory symbol into a visual symbol. It first has to learn that certain seen, heard, and remembered objects have to be associated with a certain sound or group of sounds. Then it has to change these sounds into visual signs. If it is blind, it has to change them into tactile signs. When the child writes, it has to change the visual signs into a set of movements. These very difficult tasks make use of several regions of the cortex. It is not surprising that mentally defective children may not be able to achieve them; it is far more amazing to me that ordinary people do learn to read and write.

Nearly all we know about how the brain organizes reading and writing has been learned from patients who have had strokes. What is needed is to study the patient and his disabilities while he is alive and then to find out the extent and the position of the damaged part of the brain after death. This necessitates, needless to say, removal of the brain in a post mortem. Often the relatives refuse permission for this. Religion, ignorance, and low intelligence remain the enemies of scientific investigation and the acquisition of knowledge.

From the brains of patients, it was deduced that the ability to read depends on laying down connections between the visual region of the occipital lobes and the large speech area of the occipital, temporal, and parietal lobes of the left hemisphere. There is no doubt a best time to establish these connections. In some children it is earlier than others; these children generally show other evidence of high intelligence. It is probable that it is much harder to do it after puberty. Once the relevant nerve cells are connected, then the seen symbol of a word immediately calls out the word for the object. And so as we read 'table' we immediately hear 'table' in our mind's ear.

A long time before congenital alexia was recognized, patients were seen who had acquired alexia. Following a stroke, the patient is able to speak and understand speech normally. He understands the meaning of pictures. But he cannot read. He can usually write, but he cannot read what he has just written. Interestingly enough, these patients can usually read the numerals used in Western culture but cannot read or make use of Roman numerals; these of course are combinations of letters. In such a patient, the part of the brain that has been destroyed is the posterior part of the corpus callosum, the large bridge of nerve fibres connecting the two hemispheres together. The nerve impulses can no longer get from the visual region of the right hemisphere across to the speech region of the left hemisphere. The artery that had been blocked and had caused the stroke had also supplied the visual part of the left hemisphere. The patient thus cannot see the right visual field with the left hemisphere. He is left with the speech area in the left hemisphere intact and the right visual area intact. But what he sees with the right visual area cannot get across the corpus callosum to inform the speech area what it is seeing. It sees the letters on the page, but they are just dark lines on a white background, strokes and curves without meaning.

This deficiency may not be as complete as has just been described; there are curious cases in which some signs are no longer recognized and others are. For instance, a patient may lose the meaning of arithmetical signs, such as plus and minus. He can do the calculations in his head but cannot do them when they are written down. If you ask him what twice eight is, he tells you it is sixteen; but if you write down $2 \times 8 = ?$, he may write 10 or 6.

Learning braille is learning a sensory tactile skill. One has to learn that palpable spots set out in space can provide a verbal meaning. A blind child learning to read by braille is using its left hemisphere for the symbolic understanding that we call reading and its right hemisphere for the estimation and remembering of the position of the dots. It has been found that blind children read more efficiently with the left fingers than the right, the left hand being organized by the right cerebral hemisphere.

Making the sounds of speech

For his tongue is exceedingly pure so that it has in purity what it wants in music.

Among most mammals, the parts of the body used for talking and singing are the lungs, the trachea or windpipe, the larynx with the vocal cords, the mouth, tongue, teeth and lips, the nose and the nasal sinuses. This vocal apparatus is like a musical instrument, a wind instrument such as the bagpipes. The lungs are the bag of air, ready to be squeezed; the windpipe is the conduit-pipe; the vocal cords are the reed; and the rest of the apparatus is a complicated and variable resonance box.

The differences in the sounds made by various mammals largely depend on differences in the resonance boxes used. The South American howler monkey has a resonance chamber developed from its hyoid bones, the two little bones beneath the lower jaw on which part of the tongue is rooted. In this small monkey, this chamber is larger than the brain; it is connected to the windpipe and the animal's throat. If one takes this vocal apparatus out of the dead monkey and blows up the windpipe, one can make the howling noise the monkey makes.

We make the sounds of singing and speaking by breathing in and then blowing the air out through a narrow opening between the vocal cords. The sound is made just as it is when a child makes a noise with a toy balloon. The narrow neck is the space between the two vocal folds in the larynx. These folds are made to vibrate by small muscles inside them; the frequency of vibration is controlled by the nervous system. The noise that comes out of the larynx is incomprehensible; it has to be shaped by the resonance chambers of the pharynx, nose, and mouth to be turned into speech.

Speaking is subsidiary to breathing; the body's needs for air come first, and speaking has to be fitted in with these necessities. We sing and talk while we breathe out; and so we have to breathe in enough air both to oxygenate the blood and to last to the end of the sentence. The messenger in *Alice Through The Looking-Glass* 'was far too much out of breath to say a word, and could only wave his hands about, and make the most fearful faces at the poor King'. The reason was that, after running, he needed all the breathing he could do to get rid of the carbon dioxide from his lungs and get more oxygen in; and the body considers this to be much more important than speaking to a King. A singer or a wind-instrument player has to train to keep constant both the volume and the force of air coming up the windpipe so as to keep the note constant throughout its length. In their cases the other requirements of the body have to take second place to the emission of a pure note. When singers take in a deep breath, they must do it quickly so as to go on with the music, and quietly too. When they record or broadcast and are near the microphone, we may hear them taking their breath in, which is inaudible at a concert.

To make the movements of speech and control the length of syllables, to put stress on them, to emit the proper volume of sound, we have to control our breathing. This comes down essentially to controlling our intercostal muscles. Contrary to what singers believe, we have little conscious control of the movements of the diaphragm. When they think they are working their diaphragms, they are actually working and controlling their abdominal muscles.

The air comes up the larynx with a slight pressure. The stream of air is then interrupted by the vocal folds. When we are not speaking, the pressure is low, between zero and 2 cm of water. The pressure goes up to about 12 cm of water during speaking, and during singing very loudly it goes up to 50 cm. A trained singer can maintain a steady tone for a maximum of 40 seconds.

The pitch of the note depends on the frequency of vibration, the mass, and the tension of the vocal folds. The resonating chambers of the pharynx, nose, mouth, and facial sinuses make the voice deeper and more resonant.

The fundamental frequency of the male adult voice is between 130 and 145 cycles and of the female between 230 and 255 cycles a second; thus the female voice is around middle C. The lowest note made by basses of cathedral choirs is about 66 cycles a second, and the highest notes of sopranos are about 1056 cycles a second, some four octaves higher. If one includes the overtones, the male voice makes use of frequencies up to 7500 cycles and the female voice up to about 10 000 cycles a second. In terms of octaves, most singers have a range of from $2\frac{1}{2}$ to 3 octaves.

The reason why male voices are deeper than female voices is that the vocal folds and the resonance chambers are larger. This increase in size occurs with growth and in both sexes at puberty. In boys, the lower limit of the voice drops by about an octave and in girls, by about a sixth. If puberty never comes, the voice remains that of a child, but the volume is that of a man. Alessandro Moreschi, the last of the castrati, who died in 1922, fortunately made nine records. The sound is neither like the voice of a woman nor a boy. If castration happens after puberty, the voice is unaffected.

When we play a wind instrument—and that includes singing and even speaking—we have to keep the sound at constant pitch for set lengths of time. To maintain the note constant, both in pitch and intensity, we use our ears; we are monitoring the sound all the time by auditory feedback. It is of course well-known that good hearing is a fundamental requirement of musicians. To hear onself emitting a note and to change it if it is not quite right takes a certain time, in fact about 140 ms. Thus the correcting of a note while it is being held can cause a wobble in the voice; 140 ms causes a wobble of about 7 cycles a second. This is the rate of vibrato in singing that sounds pleasant to our ears.

The child learns to make the right sound by listening to the sounds of speech made by those around it. Interestingly enough, the child also looks at lip movements, just as the deaf are taught to do. All the time the child is imitating the sounds it hears. The delicate movements of the larynx, tongue, and lips that are needed for talking are developed earlier than the movements of the trunk and limbs. This is surprising and indicates how fundamental speech is for human beings. How a child knows to turn the sounds it hears into contractions and relaxations of small muscles of the larynx, we do not know.

Eventually sounds that the child never hears are no longer heard properly. One difficulty in learning to speak a language like a native-born speaker is that the sounds, rhythms and cadences are not heard. When I asked a Chinese waiter in a restaurant why some prawns were called butterfly prawns, he replied 'Because they are flied in butter, I suppose'. He could not hear any difference between l's and r's.

Saints and other psychotics who hear voices or hear people talking about them are actually saying the words they hear but enunciating them without forcing any air through the vocal cords. Microphones placed over the larynxes of such patients detect the words enunciated though they detect no sound. These otherwise inaudible sounds have been recorded on tape, amplified, and then played back to the patient. The patients then recognize them as the voices they hear.

22 Learning

For he is docile and can learn certain things.

Learning, retaining, and reproducing

Learning is the process by which experience changes behaviour. We use the word 'learning' only when this change is long-lasting or permanent. In general, we speak of learning and remembering when these activities are performed with consciousness, and when we use these words, we are thinking of psychological activities. In neurology these terms are used more generally. We talk of learning when even a part of the nervous system changes its behaviour permanently owing to experience and not as the result of fatigue or disease. This way of using the word anchors it in the physiology of the nervous system. For learning is one of the manifestations of neural activity. It occurs in simple single-celled animals. Gelber has shown that paramoecia learn to look for food in association with a wire. He put suitable food for them on a platinum wire and they congregated round the wire. Then he removed the wire and washed it clean. When he put the wire back, the paramoecia continued to congregate round it.

Professor Horridge in Aberdeen has done some experiments that show that the lower parts of the nervous system of locusts and cockroaches learn. He cuts the head off the insect and then suspends the rear end above a dish of saline. When a leg is extended and touches the saline, it gets an electric shock. After about ten minutes, this rear end, consisting of a ventral nerve cord and the trunk and the legs, learns that it must avoid extending the leg to avoid getting a shock. It keeps the limb out of the saline. This lesson is retained. For if the animal without a head is re-tested ten minutes later, it learns to avoid the shock much more quickly; clearly, some of the previous lesson has been retained.

Professor Yerkes showed that earthworms could learn which way to go at a T-junction. When the earthworms went along one limb of the T, they were given an electric shock; they learned to avoid that limb and always to take the opposite direction. Even when the top twelve segments of the worm had been cut off and thrown away, the rest of the worm still avoided the wrong limb of the T.

This experiment with the earthworm implies something about worms and other animals that is not usually noticed in such experiments: the animal explores. It is interested in its surroundings and always notices anything new and strange. If a rat explores a similar T-maze every day, it may choose either limb to visit. If you make a change in one limb, say paint it a new colour, the rat immediately notices this and goes into this limb to explore. But if you first frighten the animal, then it will always go into the familiar limb and will leave the strange one until a time when it is feeling more confident.

The amount of knowledge that is inborn and the amount that has to be learned varies from species to species. It used to be thought that insects whose organization is obviously based on inborn knowledge were incapable of learning. But experiments with ants learning mazes show that these animals can learn and that some individuals are much better at learning to find the way through a maze than others.

As the scale of vertebrates is ascended, the proportion of what has to be learned to what is innate becomes greater. Conversely, among the animals lowest in the scale, learning is unimportant. Just how important it is among vertebrates we have only begun to find out during the last twenty years.

We realize now that behaviour is not innate *or* learned; it is innate *and* learned. And, what is innate is not necessarily there when the animal is born. Its seeds are present within the central nervous system, and it will come to fruition at some time when the development of the central nervous system and the rest of the body has reached the appropriate state. What is inherited is the potential. This has to be developed. If the circumstances and environment are not right for developing the potential at the correct time, then the potential is wasted and a potential form of behaviour is never used. In the nervous system, there is always an interaction between what is inherited and what is acquired from living.

Further, learning is selective. The young animal is born with the propensity to learn some things and not others, just as we saw in the example of the baby's interest in the human face.

Whatever the neural process of learning is, it is an active process. It seems that mere repetition can reinforce what has been learned but something more active has to take place on the first occasion when anything is learned. We have to make efforts to learn, we have to concentrate. This is so whether we are learning a poem by heart, learning to ride a bicycle, or learning Greek.

Facts and hypotheses of learning

Rats brought up in a stimulating environment with lots of things to do have heavier brains than those brought up in boring conditions. The cortex of the cerebral hemispheres is thicker. Under the microscope one sees that the rats from the interesting environment have neurons with more dendrites on them, the dendrites have more branches and on the dendrites are more spines. It only needs a few hours a day in a challenging environment to produce these changes in the cerebral hemispheres. In the brains of the rats brought up in a stimulating environment there is more protein and more RNA in the nuclei of the neurons. The learning by experience does not include the social learning of being with other young rats. That makes no difference. It means learning by exploring everything in the environment. Being in such an environment is so important that it can overcome the adverse effects of removing much of the thyroid or of malnutrition.

Longer and more branched dendrites with more spines on them provide greater surface area for receiving connections from other neurons. Learning has an anatomical basis; and that is forming connections.

It is thought that frequent use allows impulses to pass more easily and so they follow a well-used path rather than other routes. Eccles concluded from some of his work on this problem: 'Activation of synapses increases their efficacy; . . . some regression of synaptic function occurs with disuse.' How this mechanism seems to work is that use makes the cell-body and the dendrites enlarge; and a large neuron provides a larger surface for connections with other neurons. With disuse, neurons shrink and the spines on the dendrites disappear. Thus their surface area diminishes and they provide a smaller area of connecting nerve fibres.

It is a general principle in the nervous system that if connections are not used, they are no longer able to work. A clear-cut experiment showing this was carried out by Professors Hubel and Wiesel. They kept one eye of a newborn kitten closed by sewing the eyelids together. After three months they removed the stitches and examined the working of the neurons of the fourth layer of the primary visual cortex. They found that almost none of the neurons connected to the covered eye could be excited into activity. They then examined the connecting neurons of the midbrain that linked these visual cortical neurons to the retinae. These midbrain neurons were working normally. They obtained exactly the same result if, instead of closing the kittens eye, they covered it with an opaque shield so that diffuse light without any patterning got to the retina. Thus what had stopped the cortical neurons working normally had been the deprivation of stimulation by contours, edges, moving light, and patterns of dark and shade. After the eye had been uncovered, some recovery of a few neurons occurred; some then responded to stimulation by light and dark. The time in the life of the kitten when this deprivation of visual stimulation is most damaging is from 4 weeks to 4 months. Examination of the neurons after the animal's death by microscopy shows that the neural structures connected to the covered eye are not normal. The neurons are small and the dendrites and spines on them are much smaller than in normal kittens. These are structures laid down before the animal's birth; disuse had made them deteriorate. Covering eyes in a series of experiments has shown that merely covering an eye for three days is enough to damage the neurons connected to that retina.

When we ask what these physiological and anatomical findings mean in terms of everyday life, we find that three month's closure of a kitten's eye makes it blind or almost blind in that eye. At best, it can just tell light from dark. Hubel and Wiesel found that if they sewed up the lid of the other eye after opening the first covered eye, the previously blind eye recovered within one or two years. But if they did not close the good eye, the previously covered eye never recovered. The cat used the normal eye, continuing to neglect the uncovered blind eye.

The same thing can happen with human beings. A young child develops what is called a lazy eye. It may be that the refraction of this eye is abnormal; more commonly we cannot find anything wrong with the eye or its connections. If the child suppresses the visual input from that eye continually up to the age of five, the eye becomes almost blind. The good eye has to be kept covered up to make the child use the lazy eye; otherwise the lazy eye will end up useless.

When rats or mice are raised in the dark, the whole visual system fails to develop normally. The electron microscope shows abnormalities in the rods of the retina, at the synapses between the rods and the neurons connecting to them, in the ganglion cells of the retina, and in the cells of the primary visual area of the cortex. The essential abnormality is that the pathway from the retina to the primary visual area is simplified: only a very few connections are made.

These are examples of use and disuse affecting connections between neurons. When no impulses pass along a nerve fibre, the number of vesicles in the nerve-ending diminishes. The opposite condition is that the spines on dendrites increases with use; they provide areas for synaptic connections.

Connections that are made when an animal learns should be thought of too in terms of large bands of nerve fibres as well as in terms of synapses. One supposes that when something is learned by the cerebral hemispheres, connections are made between two parts of the brain.

When a blind person learns braille, we presume that connections are made between the secondary tactile area for the index finger and the speech area. When he feels a certain configuration of dots, they automatically bring first the letter, and later the word, to his consciousness.

Much learning of this type also demands connections between the cortex and structures deeper in the cerebral hemispheres, such as the thalamus and the large motor centres in the middle of the hemispheres between cortex and hypothalamus. Many of these connections could not be made in babyhood or even during early childhood. For when mammals are born, many of the nerve fibres within the brain are rudimentary and cannot yet carry nerve impulses. The nerve fibres that will become myelinated may not have a myelin sheath at birth or even for years after birth. If learning depends on these fibres making connections between two regions of the brain, it cannot occur till these fibres have completed their development and are ready to conduct impulses. One reason why certain things can be learned only at certain times is that the neural structures needed for this learning may not yet be adequately matured. For instance, if puppies two weeks old are put on a table, they crawl around and keep falling off and hurt themselves. At this age, they cannot profit from this experience and learn. The reason for this is that the parts of the brain needed for acquiring knowledge about edges and ledges is not yet developed, nor is the part of the brain that corrects tendencies to fall when the feet are not placed firmly on a surface. But at this age, when they are placed on their backs, they can turn round and right themselves, for these reflexes are active already at this time.

The first step in learning is the sensory input. There must be stimulation from the environment; something has to be experienced, to be seen, smelt, or felt. For learning to take place, this stimulation needs to come at the right time. We now know, from much experimental work on young animals deprived of their normal psychological environments and the usual stimuli, that once the right time for acquiring a skill or a certain behaviour has passed, this skill or behaviour can never be properly learned.

The invention of the technique of sensory deprivation has made it clear to us how important the usual environmental stimulation is for normal development. In this technique, from the time of weaning or earlier, various aspects of the usual environment are removed and the young animal is brought up bereft of them. Such animals never become normal. The sensory deprivation occurring in infancy and during their early months ruins their ability to learn anything and they never adapt to many of the features of their environment. Puppies reared in isolation from puppyhood to maturity are always unable to respond intelligently even to dangerous features of their surroundings. What is very surprising is that they do not respond adequately to painful stimulation and they cannot localize painful stimuli accurately on their bodies. Such puppies would put their noses into flames and never learned not to do this. They seemed to be indifferent to being pricked with a needle and they often damaged themselves by bumping into things or falling off heights. When they did fall or even if someone accidentally trod on one of their paws or on their tails, they never yelped; they did not seem to feel the pain. And when they were obviously hurt, they did not learn to avoid the painful stimulus.

It is obvious that if the needed stimulation comes before the nervous system is sufficiently developed to receive it, it can have no effect. But also if the stimulation comes too late, learning cannot take place. The critical period for learning is particularly short in the case of imprinting in young birds and mammals. It may be as short as hours, according to some investigators, or days, according to others. In birds, this period starts a few hours after hatching and it never lasts for more than ten days.

Normal social and emotional development probably also needs the correct stimulation at the right time. We can observe evidence of this in those fortunately rare cases of children who have been completely neglected from birth. Sometimes illegitimate children in the country are put away in haylofts or barns to conceal their existence from the neighbours. They are taught nothing, not even to be house-trained or to speak. These children then grow up mentally defective. Even if they are found and rescued by the age of four or five, it is too late; though they can be taught a lot, their speech is always inadequate and their brains never reach the standards of their siblings. To a lesser degree, the same thing sometimes happen in orphanges. Rows of beds of illegitimate children fill these institutions. The children never have the love normally given by parents and they get nothing more than rudimentary care of the body. They usually grow up unintelligent or even mentally defective, and they are equally defective in social and emotional development.

That we speak our own language perfectly and the languageṡ we learn later imperfectly also depends on learning this skill at the right time. The brain develops in such a way that it is ready to learn to speak between the ages of about ten months and ten years. Languages learned later are not spoken perfectly. The ability to speak a language is a mixed motor and sensory skill, as in fact, all skills are. It is necessary to hear all the sounds, the subtle differences between similar but not identical sounds, the rhythm and lilt of the language, where the voice goes up or down, where the accent on a word falls. One has also to work tongue, throat, and lips, to control breathing, so that the right amount of force in expelling the air is used, the amount of air taken in must be controlled so that it takes one along to the end of the sentence. And all this has to be managed at one and the same time. From some time after birth until the age of six or seven, normal children can learn all this perfectly; and without much difficulty they can learn two or even three languages at the same time, without muddling them up. But later, most of us cannot acquire this skill. We may learn to write and read the new language perfectly; but to acquire the right inflexion and the accent and the ability to speak so that no one can detect that the language is not our mother-tongue hardly ever occurs.

But those of us who still want to learn foreign languages after these early milestones have been passed need not worry; for though we may not learn to speak a new language like the natives, we know from thousands of examples that we can go on learning languages beyond the age of eighty. There are so many activities adding up to the simple word 'learning' that although some of the processes become less efficient with ageing of the brain, our actual experience of learning helps us in learning new material.

The critical period during which a language can be learned perfectly is a few years in humans; in most birds, it is a few weeks or months. Thorpe of Cambridge University found, for instance, that the chaffinch has to learn most of its song, and that this learning has to occur during the early weeks of the bird's life and also during the first spring. If the bird is hand-reared and isolated from other birds from the time of hatching, it sings only very simple songs and it never learns the song of its species correctly. Its song will be elaborated if it hears another chaffinch singing, even though the other chaffinch has also been hand-reared and isolated and has never heard another bird sing. The singing of these birds is so dependent on learning that chaffinches from different parts of the country sing differently. Just like the human inhabitants of these islands, they have regional accents; though the birds do not base their pecking order on them.

Birds listen to their own singing and they practise. If a bird is made deaf, its song deteriorates; the earlier in its life the bird's hearing is destroyed, the poorer its song will be.

If necessary connections are destroyed, learning cannot occur. When monkeys have had their temporal lobes removed in experimental operations, they can no longer learn what objects are. They can see them alright, but they cannot recognize their meaning. They keep picking up everything, smell it and examine it by mouth to see if it is edible and then put it down. A minute later they may pick up the same object without any signs of recognizing it, treating it as though it is something strange and new. They cannot retain anything they may have learned about the object. When certain tracts of nerve fibres are divided in the frontal lobes of dogs or rats, these animals are unable to learn essential social relationships. They treat their fellows as objects, walking on them and taking food even from animals larger and stronger than themselves. Although they get bitten repeatedly, they are unable to learn from this punishment and keep on doing it.

Learning is made far more effective if strong emotion accompanies it. Indeed it seems to be that the stronger the emotion, the more firmly fixed the knowledge will be. A child or a chimpanzee will have learned after receiving one prick from a needle on a syringe to fear the needle. When something is learned with strong emotion, it is likely to be retained for years.

Something happening only once may be fixed in the memory for ever. Professor Yerkes has recorded that once one of their chimpanzees escaped from its cage and wandered around the colony, making a nuisance of itself, refusing to go back. One of Yerkes's assistants got a revolver intending to fire a bullet near the animal's legs and frighten it back into its cage. The chimpanzee who had been born and bred in the colony had never seen a revolver before. Unfortunately when the man fired, he hit the animal by mistake in its leg. The terrified chimpanzee immediately rushed back to its cage and stayed there. From that moment the chimpanzee was terrified of the revolver. The staff of the colony could always make the chimpanzee do as they wanted merely by showing it the muzzle of the revolver. As Yerkes points out, the chimpanzee saw the revolver only once and very briefly. Yet the traumatic experience of being shot in the leg fixed the memory of the object for ever. This kind of learning when something that happened once is retained for ever is usually, perhaps always, associated with fear.

Rats will learn and retain for months an experience that has occurred only once, if it is painful and unpleasant. A rat put in a hammock in a cage, the floor of which is electrified, so that it gets a shock every time its foot touches the floor, will learn after only one shock never to touch the floor of the cage again. In other experiments, it was shown that when rats learn something to the accompaniment of fear, this will be remembered even after both cerebral hemispheres have been removed. The cortex is needed for learning; but once the task has been learned in association with fear, the knowledge is passed on to deeper levels of the brain. This passing on of acquired knowledge from one set of neurons to another is a feature of neural organization.

Undoubtedly the same thing happens with the young human. An experience fixed with emotion is firmly fixed and it may remain for life. It can influence the child's behaviour always, forming the basis of certain aspects of its character. Such emotions are terror, disappointment, great interest, happiness at being rewarded or appreciated.

One of the main theories of Adler's school of psychology is the importance of early childhood memories in the formation of character. Adler considered that the person's first memory is a clue to that person's whole personality. Whatever the person remembers longest has been fixed with a great deal of emotion and remains a fundamental influence in his character. Looked at from the outside, such an experience may not seem very interesting or important. But seen with the eyes of the small child, it may have a deep and important meaning.

Emotions such as love, the arousal of interest and enthusiasm are effective in helping children and adults learn; though few professional teachers are capable apparently of making use of these adjuvants to remembering. The one method they make most use of is boredom; this deters remembering and learning. But rote memory is helped by frequent repetition even though this is inevitably accompanied by boredom.

Physical or psychological pain is effective in fixing things in the memory. For thousands of years teachers and parents have made ample use of physical pain; now that many people disapprove of whipping children, only psychological pain is used.

A great deal of learning is naturally rewarded by pleasure or pain. When a young animal learns a skill or the parts of a skill, it experiences pleasure: this reinforces what it has learned and makes it want to do it again. But if the animal makes a wrong response, it is not rewarded or it may even be hurt. The pleasure could be that accompanying satiety from eating or drinking enough, or it could be the feeling of contentment from being in a correctly adjusted environment, correct in terms of humidity, temperature, flow of air, and other physical factors. The punishment could be the mounting hunger felt with the failure to find food or the mounting frustration and discomfort from failing to find a partner for sexual activity.

Punishment may be more forceful than this. If rats are given poison and they survive, they will always avoid that particular food in the future. In this case there is a long time between the taking of the poisoned food and experiencing its effects; yet these intelligent animals learn straightaway to connect the two.

In the simplest organisms, the reward or punishment must follow the activity quickly for the animal to learn. For such animals do not have memories long enough to connect what they have just done with success or failure, with pleasure or pain, if there is much delay between the act and its reward. For this kind of learning, what psychologists called 'temporal contiguity' is necessary.

Learning induced by being rewarded by something desired or by punishment is called instrumental learning or operant conditioning. The kinds of behaviour that can be taught in this way are very surprising. Professor N. E. Miller of New York has taught dogs to alter autonomic nervous responses which are usually regarded as unconscious. He has taught rats to control the rate of their hearts, increasing or decreasing it by 20 per cent. They have been taught to increase or decrease their intestinal activity, the movements of their stomachs, to increase or decrease the amount of urine secreted by the kidney, even to dilate the blood-vessels of one ear. He has taught cats to alter certain waves of their electroencephalograms. This work not only shows us that activities that we regard as quite unconscious and outside our control can be controlled; it suggests to us that the animal normally learns to make those glandular and visceral reactions that give it comfort and to avoid those that bring it disease.

But not all learning is accompanied by the reward of pleasure. The kinds of learning occurring at the lowest levels of the nervous system occur merely with frequent repetition. Imprinting occurs automatically provided it comes at the correct time.

For an animal to learn something it need not make an immediate response. The learning may be all internal; there is no movement, nothing to be seen.

As learning causes changes in our central nervous systems and as we are learning all the time, we see that every brain must be different from every other one, apart from the fact that each one starts off with a different inherited constitution. Every brain is different according to what its possessor has put into it. One person has learned a new language, another has learned tea-tasting. These differences in the brain cannot yet be detected by the histological and biochemical methods of investigation now available.

Making two brains into one

Weber, who early in the nineteenth century was the first scientific investigator of sensation and perception, observed that children taught to write with one hand could then produce mirror-writing with the other hand, without any further practice. Psychologists later found that this transfer of training occurs for a great many kinds of learning. In all of them, the untrained side of the brain learns more quickly than it would have done had there been no training at all, though it performs less well than the trained side. In the last decade this kind of learning has been investigated in detail by two research workers in the United States, R. S. Myers and R. W. Sperry.

We assume that when something has been learned, a change takes place in the brain. In the case of learning to write, the changes, whatever they are, occur mainly in the left cerebral hemisphere. Without any further training or reinforcement, these unknown physical changes are transferred to the right hemisphere. When the changes are long-lasting, we speak of memory. Realizing that something physical is conducted from one hemisphere to the other, we can look for the anatomical pathways along which these changes could pass.

The main bridge between the hemispheres is the corpus callosum; this bridge or commissure is shown in Plate 13. In this photograph of a human brain, the middle parts of both hemispheres have been cut away to show the corpus callosum. At both ends it curves round and continues downwards for a short distance, out of sight. On the right side, a part of the frontal lobe has been pulled away so as to show the thickness of the grey matter covering the white matter.

The corpus callosum is by far the biggest of all the commissures joining the two halves of the brain. It is the most recent one, having evolved in company with the two cerebral hemispheres, which it links together. The first parts of the hemispheres to evolve were linked by a small structure called the anterior commissure, and by the hippocampal commissure, linking the two hippocampi.

Some functions of the corpus callosum can now be explained with the help of Fig. 22.1. It will be seen in this figure that each half of the retina receives light from the part of the world opposite it. The right half of both retinae receives from the left visual field, and the left half of both retinae from the right visual field. Each occipital lobe of each hemisphere receives nerve impulses from the half of the retina on its own side; the right occipital lobe receives from the right half of the retina of both eyes and the left occipital lobe from the left half of both. Thus what

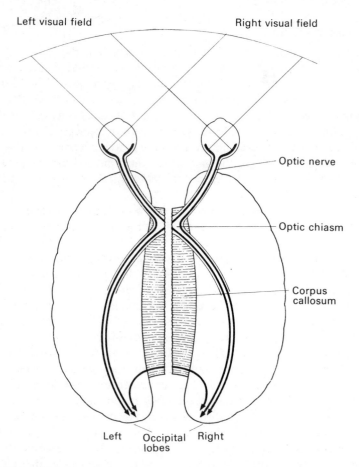

Fig. 22.1. Diagram to illustrate experiments in which the optic chiasm and the corpus callosum are divided.

is seen in the right field goes to the left cerebral hemisphere and what is seen on the left to the right hemisphere. Between these two areas of the hemispheres there are nerve fibres running through the corpus callosum, connecting one point with another of the two occipital lobes.

In order to find out the role of the corpus callosum in visual learning, Myers in 1955 cut through the corpus callosum and the optic chiasm in cats. When this is done, all the nerve fibres from the left eye go to the left hemisphere and all those from the right eye go to the right hemisphere; for the operation divides those fibres that normally cross. And so after the operation, the left eye and the left cerebral hemisphere form one visual system and the right eye with its hemisphere form another. These cats were then taught two different solutions of a problem. One solution was taught to the left hemisphere via its eye and the other solution was taught to the right hemisphere via its eye. For instance, one cerebral hemisphere was taught to make the animal press a lever for a food reward when it saw a white circle, and the other hemisphere to do so when it saw a white square. After the corpus callosum had been cut through, transfer of training did not occur. Each hemisphere then learned independently and neither knew what the other hemisphere had learned. Each system, consisting of one eye and its hemisphere, functioned well and behaved as was expected; it acted as if it had no cognizance of the existence of the other hemisphere.

Myers and his colleagues in further experiments found that it is possible to teach each hemisphere an absolutely opposite and contrary solution to one problem. At first, they cut through the corpus callosum in some monkeys. Then they trained one hemisphere to make the monkey depress the lever when it saw the outline of a square, and the other hemisphere to make the monkey depress the lever when it saw the outline of a circle. The first hemisphere was also taught that it must not allow the monkey to touch the lever when the circle appears, and the second hemisphere that the lever must not be touched when the square appears. Thus each hemisphere learns exactly contrary things, the one that the circle is bad and the square is good, and the other that the circle is good and the square is bad. The monkeys with corpus callosum divided had no difficulty in learning this task. The animals had no emotional problems and showed no evidence of mental conflict. Intact monkeys would have had severe and intense symptoms of neurosis if they had tried to learn these contrary solutions to problems.

Each hemisphere of an animal with the corpus callosum divided can be taught the contrary solutions to a problem at the same time. In each teaching session, first one hemisphere is taught something via its eye and then the other one is taught the opposite information via its eye; then for the next five minutes the first eye is trained again, and so on throughout the session. A cat or monkey with division of the commissures and the optic chiasm ends up by learning its two different solutions to a problem in the same time it takes the normal animal to learn one solution; and it achieves this without any mental or emotional conflict.

The solution to a food-obtaining problem can also be based on tactile clues instead of visual ones. In this case, the one hemisphere is taught to press a lever when the forepaw examines and feels a certain tactile sensation and the other hemisphere is taught to press it when exactly the opposite sort of tactile sensation is felt. Again, each sensory cortex learns an opposite solution to the problem and there is no conflict between the two solutions, as they never meet.

What each hemisphere learns via its own sensory input coming from the opposite side of the body is learned better and retained longer than what it learns by transfer across the corpus callosum. What has been learned, for instance, by the left hemisphere coming from the left halves of both retinae (things seen on the right) is well retained, whereas what has been learned in the right hemisphere (things seen on the left) from transfer from the left hemisphere is poorly retained and soon forgotten.

We presume that under normal conditions, what is learned by one hemisphere is automatically transferred to the other via the corpus callosum. It is first learned by one hemisphere, and then a weaker carbon copy, so to speak, is kept in the other hemisphere. We do not yet know how this transfer is done nor what mechanisms are entailed in the word 'automatically' used in the above statement.

The experimental situation of dividing the corpus callosum has been used in the treatment of certain epileptic patients. The idea has been to stop the severe fits from spreading from one hemisphere to the other and hence from one side of the body to the other. The effects of the operation were similar to those produced in cats and monkeys. After the operation, each cerebral hemisphere acted independently, as if it were ignorant of the existence of the other. There were no obvious intellectual defects and with superficial observation nothing abnormal might be noticed. Any activity usually performed exclusively by one hemisphere could still be performed. Each hand could work separately. The patient could move each finger; he could use a spoon and fork and he could hammer in a nail with either hand. But the left hemisphere did not know what the right hemisphere was doing or what it had just done. Any activity needing the two hemispheres to work together could not be done well.

However, there was one essential difference between the patients and the animals in which the corpus callosum was divided. In man, speech is mainly in the left hemisphere. The right hemisphere had lost its connections with the speech area. There were many consequences of this disconnection. The patient could do some things using only his right hemisphere but he could not then explain what he was doing. The independent activities of the right hemisphere had lost their connections with the speech area, and so the patient could not explain. He could not write at all with his left hand. Right-handed people of course cannot write well with the left hand; but these patients had not even the slightest idea how to write with their left hands, this hand had no knowledge of the shapes of letters and words.

The anatomical situation is illustrated in Fig. 22.2. This represents a section through the two cerebral hemispheres, made from side to side through the frontal and temporal lobes. The corpus callosum has been divided. This cut separates the right hemisphere from the region of the left hemisphere that organizes speech, reading, writing and all thinking depending on speech. As the speech region is cut off from the right hemisphere, this hemisphere cannot direct the left hand to do things related to speech, such as writing letters, words, or numbers.

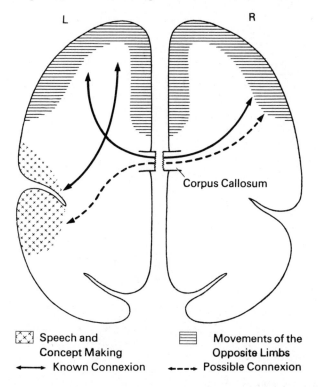

Fig. 22.2. Connexions between the speech area of the left cerebral hemisphere and motor regions of both hemispheres.

When the pathways through the corpus callosum are cut, there are similar disorders with vision. If we present something to such a patient in his left field of vision, he can see it but he cannot explain it or write about it. He cannot read anything presented in this field, though he can read it when it is shown him in the right field. This situation is explained by Fig. 22.3. The left hemisphere sees what is in the right visual field and the right what is in the left. When the corpus callosum is divided, although the right hemisphere can still see what is in the left field, it cannot communicate it to the left hemisphere. As reading is organized in the left hemisphere, the patient sees the printed page shown him on the left; but it no longer makes any sense; the letters are meaningless lines of black on a white page. As soon as the page is shown him in the right field, he not only sees it, it makes sense and he can read it. For the connections between the reading areas and the visual areas of the left hemisphere are intact.

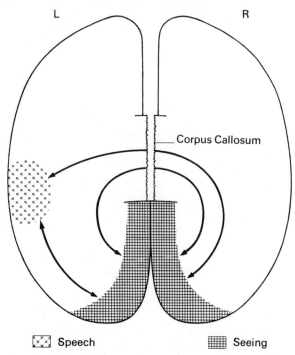

Fig. 22.3. Connexions between the two visual areas and the region of the left hemisphere for reading and writing.

If such a patient is blindfolded and something is put in his left hand, he knows what it is, but he can neither say what it is nor describe it in writing. That he knows what it is is shown by the fact that he knows what to do with it. If it is a comb, he combs his hair, if it is a toothbrush, he brushes his teeth. Yet he cannot explain what he is doing. The right hemisphere not only knows what to do with the object, it remembers seeing it and recognizes it among a lot of other objects. As Professor Sperry says, 'While all this is going on the other hemisphere meanwhile has no conception of what the object is and, if asked, says so.' However, the right hemisphere is not, as Sperry puts it, 'entirely illiterate; it reads a word like cup, fork, or apple flashed to the left visual field, and then picks up the corresponding object with the left hand'.

This work on the corpus callosum shows us that the environment we see is a product of the organization of the two hemispheres. For all nerve fibres from the left half of both retinae go to the left cerebral hemisphere and all those from the right half of both retinae go to the right hemisphere. In order for whole objects to be seen, the two hemisphere inputs have to be joined. This is done instantaneously by fibres crossing in the occipital end of the corpus callosum. Similar fibres in the middle regions of the corpus callosum are used for the integration of sensation acquired through paired limbs. When we feel something with both hands, we make the sensations into a whole; we don't have to think 'On the left hand it feels rough, on the right hand it feels rough too; and so it must be rough all over'. Before we realize what something is, this information from the two sides of the body has been integrated; and the main pathway for this is the corpus callosum.

When we examine patients with lesions cutting off a part of either hemisphere from the speech area, the patient cannot tell us about his defect. Indeed most of these patients are ignorant of having a defect. This is because 'I'—if we have to use such a philosophical concept—resides somewhere within the speech area on the left. In such a case, 'I' honestly does not know what the right cerebral hemisphere is doing. These patients are difficult to understand, for there is another problem for the neurologist. In most of these patients, the gap left by the sensory deficiency is filled by confabulation. When a sensory input is suddenly cut off, the result is not usually a state of blankness or nothingness; the patient does not say he feels or knows nothing. Spontaneous input or hallucinations fill the gap. The patient does not say, for example, that his left arm is lacking in all sensibility; he says that that limb is not his and that it should be thrown away. This has nothing to do with intelligence. The person with the corpus callosum cut through really has a split mind.

From Myers's investigations on cats and monkeys and from Sperry's work on man, we can draw the following conclusions about the functions of the corpus callosum. It is needed for transferring what one hemisphere learns and making it a common possession of the brain. It is essential for keeping each hemisphere informed about what is happening in the other one. It is necessary for learning any skill that is bilateral, using both sides of the body. The co-ordination of movements, apart from the reflex part of movements laid down at lower neural levels, depends on the passage of impulses across the corpus callosum between the motor regions of the two hemispheres. It is needed when any motor skill depends on vision. It is also necessary for us to make our visual conceptions of the world, our concept of distance and space, in the world around us.

23 Remembering

The word 'memory' is used in neurology to include many activities that have in common the retention of an experience. The word is used when the retention is of any duration, from a few seconds to many years. We know that the experience has been retained when it later affects behaviour or when it is reproduced. When we speak of memory in everyday life, we either mean recalling an event that we have experienced or something we have heard of or learned. In neurology this kind of memory is often called highest level memory.

Memory used in skilled movements and perception

A sequence of learned movements is a memory. In dancing, you have to remember previous gyrations in order that the whole series should be made into a satisfactory pattern. In drawing, you have to remember how the previous lines were arranged in order to complete the picture. You must also remember the total shape of an object you are drawing from memory. In listening to music, we must remember the first part of a melody for the later part to make sense. One could not appreciate the simplest musical form—a canon, for instance—if one did not remember the phrase that has just been played or sung; and a fugue would be meaningless without great attention being paid and a trained memory for musical forms. It is the same with speech. One has to remember the words of the beginning of the sentence for the whole sentence to make sense. Sometimes when we are speaking, we may be distracted in the middle; then the short-term memory may fail, and we have to admit that we have forgotten what we were talking about.

Memory is necessary in perception, in the recognition of what you see and hear. A rose is a rose only when you compare what you see with the memory of previous roses. You know the national anthem because it sounds the same as your stored version of previously played national anthems. If you have no previous version in your memory, then you know that this is an unfamiliar object, something new. This recognition of the familiar based on stored perceptions takes place so quickly that we do not know we are doing anything. We are just seeing a rose.

Lower level memory

All essential features of memory occur at the lower levels of the central nervous system. In two examples that follow, the experience has been fixed and retained by neural mechanisms at spinal level.

The first example comes from a patient with cancer. To stop the pain, which was most severe in her case, she had an operation on the spinal cord. This operation makes the whole of the body below the level of the operation on the spinal cord insensitive to pain. It does not interfere with the tactile forms of sensation, and so the patient can still feel the ground he walks on and knows where to put his feet. This particular patient had had a car accident six years earlier which had caused a severe and painful fracture of the right knee-cap. The knee-cap had been removed, the pain went, and the patient had forgotten all about it. But after the operation on her spinal cord, she found to her amazement that any painful stimulus applied to her right lower limb produced the identical pain she had had in the right knee six years before. The stimulus did not merely produce the pain in her knee; it caused all the sensations which she had had six years previously when her knee-cap had been fractured.

The second case shows the same thing. At one time I was studying the problems of the relief of pain sometimes experienced by patients after amputations of limbs. One of these patients was a young man, who had lost his leg during the Korean War. During the course of a day, I carried out various procedures to the stump of his lower limb, many of which were painful and all of which had the effect of sending into the spinal cord a barrage of nerve impulses from that limb. On the night after these tests, the patient was suddenly woken from his sleep with severe pain in his absent leg. He immediately knew what this pain was. For five years previously, before he had had his leg amputated, he had been playing ice hockey, had fallen, and had had the outside of his leg cut open by a skate. On the present night he re-experienced the identical sensations in his phantom leg that he had had at that time. It was not that he remembered having had this injury; he felt all the sensations again in his absent leg that he had previously felt.

In these two patients, the pattern of activity of certain neurons within the spinal cord has undergone some permanent change as a result of the pain in the lower limb. What this actual change is, we do not know; but the presence of some change was shown by stimulating the same neurons again on another occasion, several years later.

This is really the same phenomenon as memory, though we do not think of this sort of thing when we use the term. This same sort of memory has also been seen occurring within the neurons of the sensory nerve of the face. During the last war, a dentist and a doctor in the United States became interested in the pain in the face that pilots sometimes got during high-altitude flying. This was before planes were pressurized. They found that many of the pilots got pain in the teeth as well as pain located in the facial sinuses, where it might be expected to occur. In going into the dental histories of these pilots, they found out that the pain was felt in those teeth that had sometime before been subjected to some trauma, such as dental treatment. This trauma could have been extraction of the tooth or simply a filling. To reproduce these results once more and to investigate this phenomenon further, one of the two, the dentist, did some routine fillings. Ten to sixteen days later, the other one, the physician, applied a painful stimulus to the inside of the nose. The pain caused by this stimulus was felt not only at the place where the needle pricked the inside of the nose; it was felt also in the tooth that a few days before had been treated. In a further investigation, they divided the patients into two groups. In one group the dental fillings were carried out under general anaesthesia, so that the patient was unconscious at the time. In the other group the dental fillings were carried out with local anaesthesia, so that the nerve carrying impulses from the tooth to the central nervous system was blocked. They found that the phenomenon still occurred in the group of patients in whom the fillings had been done under general anaesthesia; stimulation of the nose still caused pain in the treated tooth. But it no longer occurred in the patients in whom the fillings had been done with a local anaesthetic. This showed that if the nerve impulses were prevented from reaching the brain, the recording and retention of this experience did not occur.

What has happened here is that the painful stimulation has caused some change in the lower level of the brain, in the part to which the nerve from the face goes. It is a permanent or a long-lasting change. This is memory occurring at a low neural level. There is the registration of an experience, its storage and then its recall. When the material is recalled, it returns with the stamp of the past upon it, and also the sense of familiarity. The experience has become a part of this region of the sensory system, and it alters subsequent behaviour. We presume that the neurons concerned have been altered in some way. When they are stimulated (but not with every sort of stimulation), they work together and in the same way in which they worked on the previous occasion.

The change in the next case must have taken place among the neurons of the thalamus within the cerebral hemisphere. A builder's labourer had a painful ingrowing toe-nail. He fell off the scaffolding and broke his back cutting the spinal cord in two. From then on, he was completely paralysed in the lower part of his body and he could feel no sensation. If he was pricked, pinched, moved or touched anywhere in the lower part of his body, he could not feel it. If the toe-nail were squeezed or banged, he felt nothing. And yet after this injury to the spinal cord, he still continued to be aware of the painful toe-nail. This means that certain neurons at a higher neural level than the spinal cord had been changed by the pain. They continued to register pain in the toe-nail, even though all impulses from the foot had been cut off.

Two facts need emphasis here. The first is that these phenomena occur only very rarely. The second is that they exist, whether they are rare or not; and their existence shows that this sort of memory occurs at these lower levels of the nervous system. It is important to realize this, for it appears that all the functions of the higher levels of the nervous system are elaborations of functions already present at lower levels.

The same sort of retention of change due to experience occurs at higher levels of the nervous system. At this level it involves that thalamus and the neurons of the cerebral cortex; but this is not the remembering of psychology. In some patients when there has been a severe pain going on continually for a long time, the neurons related to this sensation and this part of the body became altered in some way. This is shown up this way. In normal people, all parts of the cerebral cortex can be stimulated electrically at operation and the patient does not experience pain. When the sensory regions of the cortex are stimulated, the person feels tingling, a feeling of numbness or a sensation of the part being moved or about to be moved. But in patients with persistent pain, the electrical stimulation of large regions of the cortex does cause pain, and it causes the identical pain from which the patient suffers. One sees here that the cortex has become altered; areas that normally have nothing to do with pain now subserve the conscious perception of pain. The pain has changed these neurons, and they now make their owner suffer pain when they are excited.

Highest level memory

When we speak of having a good memory or of trying to remember something, we are thinking of the highest neural level of remembering. For this kind of remembering, the event has to be registered; then it is retained or stored; and then it is retrieved so as to be reproduced. This highest level memory includes a sense of familiarity; what is retained is familiar when it is reproduced. Inherent in this kind of memory is a sense of pastness; what is remembered is localized in the past. This remembering needs consciousness. It is needed for registering the experience and for its recall.

The terms 'consciousness' and 'being conscious' are unsatisfactory. When we are conscious, much of our mental and psychological activity is in fact not conscious. We make use of conscious effort only in the small and last parts of our mental activities. An intriguing example of this can be seen in the very short-term remembering, called by psychologists 'memory span'. If we are partly listening to what someone is saying, and he then accuses us of not paying attention, we find that we can prove him wrong by repeating to him his entire last sentence or more. It has all been recorded for us, just as on tape; but until his accusation we were paying no attention to it. It was being recorded but not thought about, probably not even understood. Then when we play it back we take in its meaning. This is a remarkable mechanism and really a most useful one. We can make use of it to take in two conversations at once. We listen to one of them and understand it as we hear it; and we let our short-term memory take the other one down and then attend to it later.

A remembered scene is not the same as the original scene. It is pale and weak in all respects. The accompanying emotion is far less, much of what was first experienced has dropped out of the remembered scene, much else has become changed or distorted and a great deal has been forgotten. How vivid the remembered scene is depends on its importance for the person. If it was important, it will have originally had, or later acquired, much emotional accompaniment. And so the intensity of a remembered scene or event usually depends on the amount of emotion associated with it. It is the same with the intensity and the reality of hallucinations.

As the memory of an event is not exactly the same as the experience of the event, all the neural pathways and neurons activated during the original event cannot have been activated during the remembering of the scene. As the remembered event or scene has additions as well as omissions, it is clear that other neurons are working in producing what has been remembered. Some neurons may be the same; but the original pathway used when the entire event was experienced is not used when the event is recalled. What is recollected is a shortened and compressed version; it arrives in consciousness with memories of emotions rather than the emotions themselves in their original intensity. Remembering is similar to imagining a scene; in some respects, remembering is re-imagining. The memory is a reconstruction, based on the original experience.

As our memories give us a sort of symbolic representation of the previous event, it was surprising to learn that Penfield evoked such real pictures of the patients' past lives when he stimulated regions of their temporal lobes. For what Penfield obtained was, as he wrote: 'not a memory, as we usually use the word, although it may have some relation to it. No man can recall by voluntary effort such a wealth of detail. . . . Many a patient has told me that the experience brought back by the electrode is much more real than remembering.' Whole scenes from the past were thrust into the patients' consciousness. The patients always recognized the scenes as having happened to them, although till the electrode has been applied to their brains, they had no idea that they had retained these memories.

One might have guessed that memories aroused so unnaturally as by the electrical stimulation of a small part of the brain would appear distorted and jumbled up. But this was not so. The scene would appear like a film: in the proper order and at the proper pace. As long as the electrode was kept on the same point of the cortex, the remembered event continued to appear. When stimulation was stopped, the internal film stopped, and the patient no longer remembered the scene from his past; when stimulation was started again, the story went on from where it had been let off, or it began again at the beginning.

The actual reminiscences in most cases were trivial. It seemed most unlikely that they had any special significance for the patient. They were not usually the sort of material that is repressed. Penfield has recounted that one of his patients said to him: 'You forced me to live things again that I'd forgotten. What were you doing? Were you stimulating my subconscious mind?' As Penfield wrote, 'Her question seemed naïve. And then I stopped to consider. Wasn't that exactly what my electrode had done?'

The stimulating electrode breaks into the storehouse of memories and taps the store. The patient does not have to do the work of recalling. Suddenly, there is a familiar episode out of his past before his eyes. And with that experience there is the emotion recorded at the time; not a memory of the emotion; the patient feels that same emotion in its original intensity. He experiences the same interpretations of the event that he had at the time. Penfield expalins it: 'Thus evoked recollection is not the exact photographic or phonographic reproduction of past scenes and events. It is reproduction of what the patient saw and heard and felt and understood.' And what is obtained from raiding the patient's store in this way is far more detailed than anything the patient can summon to memory in the normal way.

Had Penfield not shown us this evidence of the existence of these remembered experiences, we would probably not have thought that this sort of record exists. One would have thought that only the symbolic representation of it is in the brain. For the normal process of recall does not reproduce these realistic scenes, unrolling before one's eyes.

Penfield and some other workers in this field have concluded from their observations when stimulating the temporal lobes that the record of all we have experienced remains in the central nervous system. Nothing is forgotten. Penfield writes:

Since the electrode may activate a random sample of this strip from the distant past, and since the most unimportant and completely forgotten periods of time may appear in this sampling, it seems reasonable to suppose that the record is complete and that it really does include all periods of each individual's waking conscious life. . . . The stream of consciousness flows inexorably onward, as described in the words of William James. But, unlike a river, it leaves behind it a permanent record that seems to be complete for the waking moments of a man's life, a record that runs, no doubt, like a thread along a pathway of ganglionic and synaptic facilitations in the brain. This pathway is located partly or wholly in the temporal lobes.

There is evidence from psychology that older memories tend to be retained better than recent ones, and that the longer something has been remembered, the more likely it will be retained in the future. Fixation of what has been retained improves with time, and conversely, the more recent memories are the more vulnerable. This holds throughout the time scale: something registered for a few seconds is more vulnerable than something registered for five minutes, and something retained for a day is more likely to disappear than something retained for a year. If we keep recalling something, it is less likely to be forgotten. Whatever memory is, it improves with repetition.

One naïvely thinks that forgetting is due to the event not being retained. One supposes that it is soon discarded, perhaps leaving no trace, no change in the brain. But the little knowledge we have of this subject indicates that this is not always so. Certainly a great deal of what we have experienced is still there. A lot of evidence shows that forgetting is often due to an inability to recall.

Apart from Penfield's striking physiological evidence from stimulating the brains of subjects undergoing operations, there has always been good psychological evidence that far more is retained than might seem possible. Merely carrying out free association shows that one has stored a lot of material one had never realized. We need merely to rest and relax (while remaining vigilant and avoiding falling asleep, which is easier said than done) and all sorts of things come to mind that we did not know we knew or thought we had forgotten. We suddenly see a face and we realize we saw that face yesterday in front of the British Museum. It is the same with our dreams. A strange episode appears to be the product of fantasy. But if we let ourselves associate to that episode, we recognize it as a distortion of an insignificant event which happened the previous day. It was so unimportant that we would not have imagined that it could have been recorded, stored, and recollected.

One or two curious cases have been reported of patients with Parkinsonism who become mentally excited with the drug L-dopa. During the excitement memories of their earlier lives crowd into their minds. As they relive their previous experiences, these patients use the slang and fashionable expressions of the time. Until that moment they had no idea they still retained the memories of forty or fifty years ago. When the amount of the drug is reduced, the recollections pass away with the excitement, and the patient once again is no longer aware that the memories are hidden in his mind.

During psychotherapy, similar memories from the past roll up, though they had not been recalled before. Often they return with full emotion; and the adult will be raging at the way one of his parents was treating him at the age of four. This again surprises us, for we did not know we had retained the memory of these experiences.

Nevertheless psychologists regard forgetting as a normal and probably necessary process. They think that it is normal to forget the large accumulation of trivialities that are at first committed to short-term memory. We choose to retain some of this material and not to commit all of it to long-term memory. There is a process of selection and filing going on somewhere along the line. How the content of memory is sorted out so that certain experiences are forgotten and others retained and how it is divided so that some will be retained for days and others for years, we do not know. One imagines that some sort of review goes on; but this is merely a verbal simile and brings us no nearer knowing what is happening in the nervous system.

The ability to recall is not the only criterion there is of the retention of something experienced. This can be deduced also from the ease of re-learning. If one knew a language at the age of five, had never spoken it since that time, and had apparently forgotten it completely, one will learn this language far more quickly at the age of twenty than someone who had never known it at all. Something, then, must have remained.

The ability to recognize also shows us that something has been retained. When we fail to remember something and somebody else reminds us of it, we then recognize that what he has remembered for us is correct. This shows us that we had registered and stored it; the failure was only in recall. Recognition is sometimes used as a test for memory. Objects are shown to the patient and then removed. A few minutes later some of these objects are shown him again, this time together with new objects he did not see before. If some memory traces remain, the patient will be able to divide the material into two groups, the part that is familiar and the part that is new.

Recognition depends on retention. It is a more complicated mechanism than at first sight appears. For what is remembered is never identical with the experience that gave rise to the memory. Recognition starts one step away, so to speak, from the perception of the re-presented material.

An example of failure to recognize a retained experience as a memory was recorded by Claparède, the founder of the Geneva school of psychologists. He had a patient who had the typical disturbances of memory due to years of alcoholism. To test her memory, he concealed a pin in his hand and stuck it into her fingers while shaking hands. Some minutes later, as he was leaving her, he proffered his hand to shake hands with her again. She pulled her hand away, but she apparently had no idea why she did so. When he asked her why, she said 'But hasn't one the right to withdraw one's hand?' And when she was questioned further, she said that he might have a pin hidden in his hand. When Claparède asked 'What makes you think I want to prick you?' she replied that it was an idea that came into her head. Then when she was asked to explain this surprising idea, she said 'Sometimes people do have pins hidden in their hands'. But she never remembered that she had been pricked a few minutes before, and she did not recognize these ideas as being based on memory.

Recognition has many degrees; one can recognize something completely, or one may merely recognize it as being vaguely known. There are also degrees in the amount of forgetting. If the material is almost completely forgotten, its buried presence is shown only by the saving of time in re-learning. If it is more easily available, this is indicated by recognition. When it is least buried, it can be mustered by the usual processes of recall.

When something is remembered, it comes back correctly ordered in time. This ordering in time may be a separate function. For where there are defects in remembering, this function alone may be disturbed. The person remembers that he was on the way to Scotland but he does not remember if the event occurred on his 1975 or 1977 visit. He may remember an event but cannot relate it in time to other events.

When something is recognized, it evokes a feeling or emotion of familiarity. In fact, familiarity is a necessary part of recognition. Whether this emotion of familiarity is the same as the strong sense of familiarity discussed in chapter 16, is not known. Certainly the sense of familiarity occurring before an epileptic fit or that occurring during stimulation of the temporal lobe at operation feels different to the patient from merely recognizing a familiar object or event. But under these abnormal conditions, the emotion is pure and isolated; and so one might well expect it to feel different.

Familiarity is a basic part of recognition. It is not only an essential part, it is also essential in all behaviour. Animals behave differently to something familiar than to something new. What is familiar evokes the previous pattern of behaviour. One knows it and one knows how to behave towards it. Something new brings out exploratory behaviour, it may cause a startle reaction, it evokes vigilance. Familiar and not dangerous brings out one kind of behaviour; familiar and dangerous brings out another. But unfamiliar brings out quite different behaviour: careful, vigilant, exploratory, a mixture of curiosity and fear.

Recognition being a part of remembering, and familiarity being an essential part of recognition, we see that familiarity is an essential part of remembering. In a more simple form, familiarity is present too at the lower neural levels of remembering. In its reactions, it is as if the spinal cord also says 'Has this happened before or is it totally new?' Its reactions are different in the two cases.

In certain disturbances of the brain, such as may occur with chronic and prolonged alcoholism or after severe head injuries, material may be registered and retained, yet when it is reproduced the sense of familiarity is lacking, and the subject does not recognize it.

The failure to recognize one's own thoughts as coming from something one has read leads to literary plagiarism. The sense of familiarity and the localization in the past does not accompany the thought as it arrives in consciousness. That is why, if one wants to write one's own thoughts, it is essential not to read what other people have written on the subject; one cannot trust one's memory. The mechanisms of recognition may be dormant; and what has been taken in from reading or hearing may appear to be one's own marvellous contribution.

A blow to the head temporarily stops the higher levels of brain function; this is well-known and is the condition of concussion. During this time the patient does not always lie pallid on the ground. As many footballers know, he may go on with what he was doing at the time. This state was first described in 1501 by the first great Mogul Emperor, Babur. He wrote in his Memoirs:

As I turned round on my seat to see how far I had left them behind, my saddle-girth being slack, the saddle turned round, and I came to the ground right on my head. Although I immediately sprang up and mounted, yet I did not recover the full possession of my faculties till the evening and the world, and all that occurred at the time, passed before my eyes and apprehension like a dream, or a fantasy, and disappeared.

During this time, mental functioning is apparently normal; it is only the continual registration and storage of experience that is not working. Mental testing during this time may reveal that the person is not working at his most efficient intellectual level, or it may not show anything abnormal. The case of one patient has been recorded in which the patient's mental functioning was so good that he learned to type; yet this period was included in the patient's period of absence of memory. Although he always remembered how to type, he never remembered learning the skill. Cases such as this show us that memory for recent events can be normal while complete memory during that period is deranged.

The reproduction of retained material without knowledge that it belongs to oneself may cause some strange abnormalities of memory in patients after head injuries. One patient who was seen in the Hospital for Head Injuries at Oxford during the war had a vision of a horse in a cloud as he recovered consciousness. He had a clear view of the horse. He said it was a brown cob, galloping with its head up, coming from right to left. This vision soon passed, and he then became conscious that he was in bed and that two nurses were making his bed. He asked them what had happened. They told him he had had an accident. He then asked whether it was anything to do with a horse, and they replied that they did not know, but that he had already told them that it was due to a horse. He himself had no recollection of having spoken to them before and no knowledge that he had had an accident and no memory of the horse. Later it was confirmed by the police that a runaway horse was the cause of his accident and that it must have passed by the patient from right to left. Even when the story of the accident was pieced together and told to the patient, he could not remember anything about it; nor could he remember the horse as he saw it in the vision.

Sometimes a vision of what had actually happened occurs suddenly, and the patient does not know why he is seeing this vision. Something, perhaps an episode in a film or the sight of a car, brings the whole event back to his mind, even though he did not know that he had retained any recollection of the event. Professor Ritchie Russell, who studied thousands of cases of head injury over the past forty years, has reported the case of a patient who was injured while standing on a tramway island. He recovered consciousness twelve hours after the head injury. On several occasions in the ensuing weeks he would suddenly have a vision of the huge tyre of a motor lorry bearing down on him, while he threw up his arms unable to escape. In fact this was exactly what had occurred. But the patient could never remember these details of the accident. The vision that spontaneously came into his mind might just as well have happened to someone else.

In cases such as these material has been retained. It is unaccompanied by the usual sense of familiarity or by the feeling of my-ness, and the patient cannot recall it by voluntary effort.

A patient who has had a severe head injury may come to the doctor two weeks later and say that for the past two weeks he does not know what has happened, that he has no memory of anything that happened since a minute before his accident. During most of this time he may have been normally reading, writing letters, playing cards, as patients do. Although he has been behaving normally, in the true sense of the word he has been unconscious; he recovered consciousness only when he started to have continuous memory. During the period between his head injury and the day when he came to, he remembers either nothing or a few scattered isolated events.

From cases of head injury, we have learned that the first part of memory, the fixation of the experience, takes time. The time varies from a split second to about a minute. During this period what was happening to the patient can never be recollected. If the head injury is very severe, this period of permanent absence of memories is longer. The more severe the damage to the brain, the longer this period can be. There may be obliteration of all memories for months or even years: what was normally registered and stored has disappeared. The most recent memories go with less severe head injuries, the older memories go with the more severe damage to the brain. Although we usually consider memory as short-term and long-term, these divisions are really matters of degree, the one merging into the other. The longer a memory has been established, the more firmly it is fixed. As time fixes memories, those things that have been retained for a short time may disappear for ever. The result of this for young children is that a severe head injury can sometimes obliterate the child's memories of its entire life before the injury. The child's mental state is then reduced to that for babyhood. Everything he ever learned, he has to learn all over again.

We understand very little of the neural processes underlying the retroactive effects of trauma to the brain; we understand still less about the recovery of some of the forgotten material. For sometimes, months after the head injury when the patient's cerebral processes are again normal, the period of absence of recollections before the head injury shrinks, so that in the end the patient can recall a large period of the time that he had previously forgotten, and he ends up with a short period of absence of memories just before the injury.

Experimental studies of this obliteration of what has already been registered have been undertaken in cases of head injury and in electroshock treatment of psychiatric disorders; for in this case too the patient does not remember what occurred for a brief moment before the shock to the brain. Here also it proves impossible to bring back memories for the split second or few seconds immediately before the trauma to the brain, although we can be sure that this material was taken in.

When we recall something from the past, we may have to make some mental effort. We search for what we hope we have retained. Exactly what parts of the brain are used for this activity and what we are doing in terms of the physiology of neurons and synapses, we do not yet know.

Whatever the physiology of this recalling ability is, a conscious effort to look for the past experience is not always the best way of finding it. The retained experience may come to mind spontaneously. After we have suspended control, suddenly what we were trying to remember is there before our eyes. This may also happen when we are asleep; on waking up, we find we have remembered it. Whether the process of searching goes on when we are asleep, we do not know. Certainly memories may return during dreams, under hypnosis, and during various states of dimmed consciousness. More automatic and less controlled thinking can be more effective for recall than conscious control. And so one should have confidence in unconscious processes of thought to fulfil one's needs. They mostly do so, though they sometimes arrive too late. Only after one has written a paper or given a lecture does one suddenly know how one should have done it.

Memories can be brought to mind by the psychological process of free association. When we do this, we relax and let one memory bring up another. Sometimes an event reminds us of a similar event that occurred before or a sensation brings to mind another occasion when the same sensation was experienced. The sense of smell as is well-known to us all is particularly evocative of memories.

Memory is an important ingredient of creative thinking. Strange as it may seem, creation comes from pouring a great mass of ill-assorted things into the mind, leaving them to ferment, and then getting something new out of it. The mechanism of getting something out is an ability that depends on character as well as on intelligence. It is done with effort, with searching concentration, with merely sitting and waiting, or with sleeping, lying around or doing other things. A lot has to be put in and all of it has to be stored. For memory consists of experiencing, retaining the shadow of the experience and recalling; they are also the essentials of creation.

As the biological purpose of memory would seem to be the organization of present behaviour in the light of previous experience, it is obvious that some sort of classification is necessary. It seems likely that the contents of the mind are classified and cross-indexed in many different ways. When we try to remember something, we can seek it via many different routes. If, for instance, I try to remember the name of a particularly beautiful East African starling, I first remember that the name was that of a German, then that it probably ended in 'dt'. I also know that it is in J. G. Williams's book on *Birds of East and Central Africa*, and that in this book, the colour plate of the starling and the description of the bird are on different pages. And I also remember that this starling has an orange eye. Thus I find that in my mind Hildebrandt's starling is classified under the heading of foreign names of birds, sub-heading German, birds in Williams's book, sub-heading starlings, and most important of all, I have in my filing system a visual picture of the bird, so that I can match a proffered picture of it against my visual memory of it, and then recognize the bird.

It is probable that the more cross-indexing there is, the better. Material is probably classified in accordance to its effect, pleasant or unpleasant, as usual or unusual, as what happens on holidays, as games to be played at silly parties, as nursery rhymes, as jokes to amuse ten-year-old children, and so on.

But this is all armchair psychology, and tells us nothing about how the brain organizes these psychological mechanisms. Penfield has reported the case of an epileptic patient who shows us other aspects of this mechanism of classification. The patient was a young man who would get fits when he saw someone grab something from someone else. On one occasion he saw someone snatching a rifle away from a cadet on parade, on another a man snatching his hat away from the cloakroom attendant; on both occasions he had a fit. Seeing someone grab or snatch something 'would immediately produce a vivid recollection of an occasion when he was thirteen years old. At this time he was playing with a dog, grabbing a stick from its mouth and throwing it. The patient would associate the two events, become confused, and have a seizure.' As Penfield was operating on the left temporal lobe, he stimulated one point, and the patient suddenly cried out: 'There he is!' When Penfield questioned him, he said: 'It was like a spell, he was doing that thing: grabbing something from somebody.' As any sort of grabbing of something from somebody precipitated his fits, this brain must have classified experience to include a category of grabbing something from somebody.

The anatomy of highest level memory

When we think about the highest level memory, we have to separate the different kinds of memory that are covered by this one word. There is memory for the events that occurred to one in the distant past, memory for what happened yesterday, and memory for what you read in the sentence before this one.

We have already related how Penfield found that when he stimulated certain parts of the temporal lobes, he brought back memories that the patients did not know they still had. Penfield made many other important contributions to this subject by studying the effects of cutting out parts of the temporal lobes in the treatment of brain tumours and of epilepsy. When certain parts of the temporal lobes are cut out, the record of a life is cut out with them. It is as if one's memory is in a filing cabinet and someone has taken it away. In principle, just like a tape-recorder, what is stored in a person's memory could be consulted by anyone. We have two ways of doing this. We have the psychological way of asking its owner to tell us what is there; and we have the physiological way of electrically stimulating certain parts of the brain. This aspect of one's memory should perhaps be emphasized, as we regard our memories as so personal, so much a part of ourselves, almost as ourselves. Yet in fact once the registered experience is stored, it is there to be tapped, almost regardless of us.

When all the front parts of both temporal lobes are cut out, the faculty of memory is destroyed. But each neuron or each circuit of neurons within this region of the brain is not the repository of something experienced; it is not a kind of pigeon-hole in which a memory is stored. Penfield has emphasized that when he stimulates a little spot of the cortex and this stimulation produces a flashback, cutting out that little spot does not remove the flashback. After it has been cut out, the patient can still remember the whole episode by using his memory in the ordinary way; the remembered event has not gone. It is only when a very large area of the temporal lobes of both hemispheres is destroyed that the entire memory is ruined.

In chapter 24, certain aspects of a case will be related in which this operation was done. The disastrous results were that the patient could not recognize anybody. He treated his own mother, to whom he had been very attached before the operation, in the same manner as he treated the nurses in hospital, calling her 'Madam', and he no longer showed any emotional attachment for her. Here we see that his sensory input is normal, and that he makes a perception from what he receives. He can recognize the moving object as a woman. But the significance of that particular woman depends on previous experience of her; that is to say, it depends on memory. With no remembrance of her, there is no accompanying emotion, such as one is used to having in relation to one's mother. He perceives a woman and behaves to her as he would to any unknown woman. He 'not only could not remember anything that had happened recently, he could not remember anything of his past'. When the doctors tried to get him to talk about the town he lived in, his own house, his family, he could not answer the questions and did not seem to understand them, 'as if their object was entirely unknown to him'. The patient lived without a past and without a future.

Scoville, a neurosurgeon working in the United States, tried to help patients with most severe epilepsy and mental disorders by removing or disconnecting parts of the temporal lobe; the important parts were the uncus and amygdala and anterior part of the hippocampus and the hippocampal gyrus. One of his patients was extensively studied by Dr Brenda Milner over a period of years. This patient had the most severe loss of recent memory. After the operation, he had completely forgotten everyone in the hospital and could not recognize any of them. He could not find his way about. He did not remember that he had been in hospital before the operation and had no memory of the previous two years. But he remembered his life before that.

Ten months ago the family moved from their old house to a new one a few blocks away on the same street; the patient still has not learned the new address, though remembering the old one perfectly, nor can he be trusted to find his way home alone. Moreover, he does not know where objects in continual use are kept; for example, his mother still has to tell him where to find the lawn mower, even though he may have been using it only the day before. She also states that he will do the same jigsaw puzzles day after day without showing any practice effect and that he will read the same magazines over and over again, without finding their contents familiar. This patient has even eaten lunches in front of us without being able to name, a mere half-hour later, a single item of food he had eaten; in fact, he could not remember having eaten luncheon at all. Yet to a causal observer this man seems like a relatively normal individual, since his understanding and reasoning are undiminished.

Patients who have had the anterior parts of the hippocampal regions cut out or damaged on both sides of the brain cannot remember what happened one to two years before the operation. But they can remember the more distant past. They cannot learn anything new as they are unable to commit events to memory. Provided they are paying attention to what they are doing, they can retain it for a minute or two; but as soon as anything else comes along, what they have just been doing and recording all disappears. Each new event washes away all trace of the things that had just happened before.

The same inability to store what has just occurred is seen when the lower part of the hypothalamus and a large mass of cells in the thalamus are damaged in a certain phase of alcoholism. The condition is called Wernicke's encephalopathy, after the neuropsychiatrist who described it; encephalopathy merely means something wrong with the brain. Some of these cases used to be called delirium tremens, or D.T.s for short. These patients are suddenly very ill; they are confused and a few of them do see frightening hallucinations such as the classical pink elephants; they walk around as if they are drunk; and they have paralyses of the eye muscles, so that they squint and see double. When this condition is cured or alleviated by the injection of vitamin B, the patients are usually left with confusion, apathy and indifference to everything. Their outstanding symptom is a severe defect of memory.

These facts show that the recording of new experience is done by parts of the temporal lobes. Essential for memory is the passing of messages onto certain regions of the hypothalamus and from there onto a large part of the thalamus. In addition to these regions, long-term memory needs the more lateral parts of the temporal lobes.

Total remembering, the storage of what has been experienced, is one kind of memory. There are also localized functions of memory. There is verbal memory, that is memory for what you heard spoken; a variation of this is memory for what you see written. There is visual memory, memory for what you have seen. Verbal memory is a function of a part of the left fronto-temporal region. The memories of things seen are stored around the visual areas of the occipital lobes, the memories of things smelt around the olfactory area, and so on for the other sensations. The memory of location—the ability to find your own bed in a ward in hospital or to find your way home in the town—depends mainly on the right parieto-occipital region of the cortex; though patients with bilateral temporal lobe lesions also have difficulty in remembering the places they know and how to get about.

There are other kinds of memories which probably depend on connections between various parts of the cerebral cortex. There is the kind of memory needed in playing cards: you have to remember the cards played by yourself and other people or the cards that are now lying face downwards on the table. The chess-player has to remember the moves he and his opponent have already made.

In such examples of remembering, people remember in different ways. Some people remember more verbally, others more visually. The verbal person says it silently to himself, then repeats this when he recalls it. The visual person sees the situation in his mind's eye and has a picture of it in his memory.

Some people's ability to remember is just amazing. Blindfolded chess champions can play twenty games of chess simultaneously. They are told the various moves, announce their own moves, and remember the strategy of twenty games at the same time so well that they win them all. Stanley Spenser said that he never made sketches when he was out walking. For those detailed and realist paintings of his, such as the magnolias or the path through a field, he had remembered everything he had seen when he was out. He remembered the exact appearance of every ear of wheat, of the curls of the petals of the magnolias, of the way the light and shade was laid on every leaf. There are some musicians who go to a concert or an opera, come back and play the entire thing on the piano, an extraordinary and effortless feat of auditory memory.

What we have learned in the last thirty years is that the intellectual faculty of memory is localized. Before, it had been assumed that so general a function would make use of the whole brain. We now know that the ability to commit something to memory and later to retrieve it from one's store depends on the temporal lobes and the connections they have with deeper structures of the brain, the hypothalamus and thalamus, the septal region and the midbrain.

As has been mentioned above, chronic alcoholism damages the hypothalamus and parts of the thalamus. When these patients make some recovery from the acute illness of severe confusion, hallucinations and paralysis of the movements of the eyes, they go into a condition called Korsakoff's psychosis. High level memory is ruined. The patients have lost recent memory although they still retain what happened up to a few years before the final damage to the brain. They can no longer learn as they cannot remember for more than a few minutes. But one of the patients described by Korsakoff in 1889 could still play a good game of chess. He could not remember all the moves that had brought about the position of the pieces on the board, but he could still work out the probabilities of moves yet to be made. These patients fill out the gaps in their memories by confabulating, and the likely stories they make up are often quite convincing.

Cases such as these show that disorders of memory affecting the whole personality can be due to damage to a small region of the hypothalamus and thalamus and not only to damage to the temporal lobes.

It seems that we must envisage something like this. When something happens to us, this affects the neurons of all sensory parts of the brain. Something has been seen and heard. Messages are also sent to the association areas of the cortex, to the speech area, and to areas concerned with emotion. And messages are sent to the parts of the temporal lobes particularly concerned with memory. From here they are sent to lower parts of the brain, to the septal region, to the hypothalamus, to the thalamus and to the midbrain.

The experiments on dividing the corpus callosum that were explained in chapter 22 show that what is learned can be transferred from one part of the brain to another. This goes on after we have learned something, without our being aware that it is happening.

We do not know what is happening in the brain when we have a memory of an event. We imagine that the regions of cortex that were active when the original external stimulation occurred are re-activated, that there is activation of the relevant association areas and that the parts of the hemisphere necessary for memory that we have been examining are also active. To provide us with such mental images is one of the main functions of the higher levels of the brain; and it is the same for other mammals. This is one of the neural activities labelled mental. It is customary to say that when one evokes such images or models of the world, one has the picture in ones mind.

24 Personality and the brain

For he is a mixture of gravity and waggery.

It is only during the last thirty years that research workers in the many branches of neurology have come to investigate the physiology and anatomy of personality. Before then, the subject of character and personality had been left to psychologists and psychiatrists. It may have been reckoned that ultimately this subject would have to be related to the physiology and anatomy of the brain. But it appeared as if everyone had agreed that the time when this correlation would be made would always lie in the future. Freud, who was a neurologist before he invented psychoanalysis, always thought of psychoanalysis as being based on the physiology and anatomy of the nervous system. Yet, as it turned out, psychoanalysis and Jung's contributions increased the distance between a scientific study of the neural aspects of personality and psychology and psychiatry. Those influenced by Freud, Groddeck and Jung, and their successors, seem to have known nothing of the scientific method. Such psychotherapists established schools, behaving more like priests than scientists.

That the frontal lobes are somehow related to personality could have been deduced during the past eighty years or so. But this did not happen. Most neurological text-books merely stated that the frontal lobes have to do with man's intellectual attainments. There was no evidence for this belief. It seems to have arisen merely because the frontal lobes are large and well-developed in man and man is an intellectual animal.

Scattered throughout the pages of medical literature are the names of certain famous patients. We have already mentioned two of these, Dr Beaumont's Alexis St Martin, and Wolf and Wolff's Tom. More incredible is the case of Phineas Gage, reported in the Boston Medical and Surgical Journal of 1848 by Dr J. M. Harlow.

Phineas Gage was a capable and efficient foreman who in 1848 suffered an amazing accident. During some rock-blasting operations, an iron bar four feet long was blown through the front part of his head. The iron bar entered the left side of his face below his eye and passed out through the top of his skull. Gage was taken in an ox-cart a distance of three quarters of a mile, and then about one hour after the injury got out of the cart by himself and walked from the cart to the surgery. While the doctor examined the hole in his head, Gage 'related the manner in which he was injured to the bystanders'. From the position of the bar it may be deduced that the greater part of the left frontal lobe and the front part of the corpus callosum were destroyed.

This damage to the brain brought about a great change in Gage's personality. Dr Harlow reported that

The equilibrium or balance, so to speak, between his intellectual faculties and animal propensities, seems to have been destroyed. He is fitful, irreverent, indulging in the grossest profanity (which was not previously his custom), manifesting but little deference for his fellows, impatient of restraint or advice when it conflicts with his desires, at times pertinaciously obstinate, yet capricious and vacillating, devising many plans for future operation, which are no sooner arranged than they are abandoned in turn for others appearing more feasible. . . . His mind has radically changed, so decidedly that his friends and acquaintances say he is 'no longer Gage'.

He died, in the words of Dr Harlow 'twelve years, six months and eight days after the date of his injury.' The skull of Phineas Gage is now in the museum of the Medical School of Harvard University.

Until that time, it was generally held that the entire cerebral hemispheres worked as a totality to produce thinking and all intellectual activities. But here was a case in which a large amount of the hemispheres had been destroyed and yet purely intellectual activities had not suffered. Also till that time, it had not been appreciated that the brain had anything to do with personality and character. It was true that this was indeed claimed by the phrenologists, but they had been relegated to the realms of quackery. Here was a case in which the personality and character had been disastrously altered by a lesion of the frontal lobes.

Although the case of Phineas Gage became famous in medical literature, all the implications were not fully grasped. Doctors were amazed that such a large amount of the brain could be damaged and that the patient could walk and talk immediately after the injury and that he could go on living for years. They were also amazed that so much of the frontal lobes could be damaged without causing a great defect in speech, in calculation and thinking ability. That character and personality could be changed so disastrously came as a striking fact to all who knew about the case; but still no one seems to have drawn conclusions about the frontal lobes being related to personality and social relationships.

For a hundred years or so, no more cases like this were reported, but now there are others. In the second world war, two officers were playing Russian roulette, a game in which a revolver with one bullet in it is put to the temple and fired. The idea is that the single bullet in one of six chambers will fall to the bottom, this chamber being the heaviest, and that the chamber fired will contain no bullet. An officer put the revolver to his temple and fired; and was surprised to see the face of his friend turn ashen grey. He then put his hand to his temples on both sides and found they were wet and sticky, and the cause was blood. Realizing that he had shot himself, he fell to the ground. But then he thought that there was no need to fall, that he had done so only because it seemed the correct thing to do, so he got up again and walked off to see a doctor.

A similar case was reported in March 1977 at Troyes in France. A workman had a quarrel with his wife, told her he was going to put an end to his life, left the room, and returned in a few minutes, saying 'Ça y est, je me suis suicidé.' His wife took no notice of this histrionic remark. She did notice a few drops of blood on his pillow in the morning but did not think anything of it. But her husband seemed a little odd all day and could not remember that it was Friday, although he was repeatedly told what day it was. The wife and son thought they had better go and see the doctor owing to his defective memory and odd behaviour. They all walked to the doctor next day. An X-ray examination of his head showed two bullets from a rifle in the front of his brain. The man had never said anything about it, apart from his first announcement, as he could not remember what he had done.

So we see that the front part of the brain is not necessary for living; one can pass in a crowd without it. Not only the frontal lobes are important for character and general behaviour; parts of the temporal lobes are also of fundamental importance. In 1939, Klüver and Bucy reported experiments in which they had removed parts of the temporal lobes in monkeys. These were the phylogenetically oldest parts, the parts that evolved in relation to the hypothalamus and septal area. They are shown in Fig. 24.1. In this figure a good slice of the cerebral hemisphere has been cut off so that the amygdala and hippocampus are revealed, although they are really buried deep inside the temporal lobe. The large band of nerve fibres connecting these regions of the temporal lobe to the septal area and the hypothalamus can be seen, encircling the thalamus.

When the amygdala and hippocampus were removed from both cerebral hemispheres of the macaque monkey, some amazing changes in the animals' personalities occurred. Normally these monkeys hate men and bravely attack them or else they hide away from them. But these animals showed no emotion of any sort when they were handled by humans. They were neither aggressive nor fearful; they had become

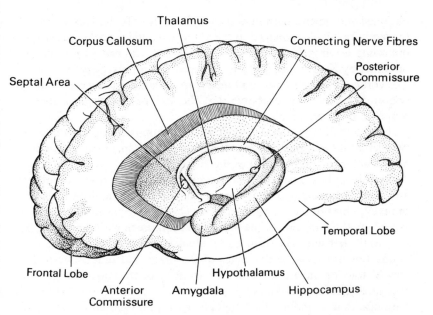

Fig. 24.1. The amygdala and the hippocampus in the depth of the opposite temporal lobe. The three commissures, anterior, posterior and corpus callosum are shown.

docile and indifferent. Even if they were hit or bitten by other monkeys, they did not seem to mind. They showed no fear of or affection towards other monkeys. After the operation, one mother macaque became indifferent to her own baby. When the baby continued to demand attention, she did eventually react and bit it. Such behaviour is totally unlike the normal behaviour of monkey mothers, who go on carrying around the body of their baby for days if it dies.

Another abnormality of behaviour shown by these animals was continual eating. They would pick up anything and try to eat it; they even chewed sticks and ate meat, which macaques never do. They also had the same voracious appetite for sexual activities. They masturbated the whole time and regarded both female and male monkeys and even cats and cushions as legitimate sexual objects.

Other research workers then did the same experiments in many other species of animals, including other kinds of monkey, dogs, rats and agoutis, lynxes and cats. They obtained the same results. The next step was to make smaller lesions within this region of the brain, to find out which are the crucial regions the removal of which causes the various parts of the total picture. It now appears that the increased sexuality is obtained only when a particular part of the cortex of this oldest region of the temporal lobe is damaged. If the amygdala and hippocampus are cut out while leaving this region of cortex intact, the rest of the picture obtained by Klüver and Bucy is obtained but not excessive sexuality. The voracious appetite for food results from damage to a neighbouring region of cortex. It is probable that the lack of aggression is due to removal of the amygdala.

In chapter 22, the effects of dividing the commissures connecting the two cerebral hemispheres were described. These operations have now been combined with removal of the amygdala on one side of the brain. At first the optic chiasm, the corpus callosum, the anterior commissure and the hippocampal commissure are divided in a ferocious macaque monkey. This produces a monkey in which things seen with the right eye go only to the right side of the brain and things seen with the left eye go only to the left side. The situtation is illustrated in Fig. 24.2. There is no connection between the two sides of the brain; but unless one makes special tests on such abilities as the transfer of training, one will not recognize that this monkey's brain is abnormal. Now the tip of the right temporal lobe including the amygdala is cut out. Normally cutting out one amygdala has no effect; one has to remove both to get the results described by Klüver and Bucy. An amazing thing is now found. If the right eye of the monkey is covered with an eye-shield, it sees people with its left eye and this eye is connected to the amygdala in a normal manner. The monkey reacts to people in its usual way, emotionally and aggressively. Now the left eye is covered, and the monkey sees people with its right eye; but this eye has no connections with the amygdala, for it has been removed. The animal is now quite indifferent and docile when he sees human beings. As Downer, who did these remarkable experiments, wrote: 'One can in effect "remove" and "replace" the amygdala, and thereby change the animal's emotional state, merely by opening and closing the appropriate eye.' We are seeing two totally different personalities in one monkey. One half of the brain makes the monkey behave in its usual aggressive way towards people. The other half makes it behave in a docile manner to the very same people.

Similar operations have occasionally been carried out in humans. The patients who have effectively had the amygdaloid nuclei removed on both sides of the brain show a similar increase in sexual bahaviour, combined with a lack of the conventional social inhibitions. They also show a voracious appetite for food. One of these patients ate as much as four normal people. They tend to eat anything, with no preference for any particular kind of food. One patient was observed 'to look for a

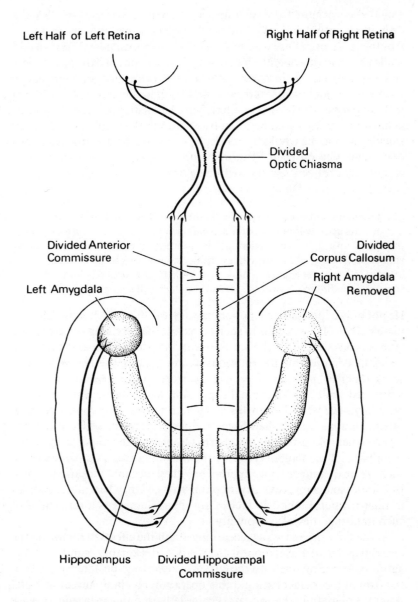

Left Half of Left Retina

Right Half of Right Retina

Divided
Optic Chiasma

Divided Anterior
Commissure

Divided
Corpus Callosum

Left Amygdala

Right Amygdala
Removed

Hippocampus

Divided Hippocampal
Commissure

Fig. 24.2. Diagram to illustrate experiment in which the corpus callosum, other commissures and the optic chiasm are cut through; in addition the right amygdala has been cut out.

secluded corner far from anyone, eat everything voraciously, lick the dish incessantly, and after fifteeen minutes asked for more food'. Another patient, whose case has been well documented by Terzian and Dalle Ore, had this operation performed on account of extremely severe epilepsy originating in these parts of the brain and uncontrollable outbreaks of aggression and rage, making him dangerous to everyone including himself. He also had terrifying hallucinations and automatic behaviour during which he often tried to strangle people or to commit suicide; at times he would fly at people, including the doctors. After two operations one on each temporal lobe, the patient's personality was completely changed. He showed no aggression and no emotion of any sort. Terzian and Dalle Ore reported:

The patient no longer manifested the slightest rage reactions towards the nurses and doctors upon whom before the second operation he used to rush as soon as they came into sight. The patient on the contrary now assumed an extremely childish and meek behaviour with everyone and was absolutely resistant to any attempt to arouse aggressiveness and violent reactions in him. He was completely indifferent towards everyone, including his parents.

He not only expressed no emotion, it was clear that he felt none. He was unable to display emotion to such an extent that even his voice became monotonous, losing all the variations in intensity, pitch and tone that normally demonstrate the emotions we are feeling, whether we want to show them or not. His face usually wore 'a conventional and un-motivated smile. An emotional expression was noticed in the patient's face only once when he saw his image in a mirror, betraying a childish satisfaction because he had found human features in a lifeless object.'

When neurologists and psychiatrists learned of the importance of the front parts of the temporal lobes for controlling and organizing drives, such as sex, hunger, and aggression, they began to examine some psychotics and aggressive psychopaths to see if they had abnormalities in their temporal lobes. In fact, brain tissue damage is a rare cause of such abnormalities of personality.

At the same time as we were learning about the effects of removing the anterior parts of the temporal lobes upon personality, similar obser-vations were being made on the effects of removing the anterior parts of the frontal lobes. Jacobsen did this operation on chimpanzees at Yale. After the operation, the animals became lethargic and apathetic; they no longer took any interest in life. And, what turned out to be more important, Jacobsen noticed that these animals no longer became worked up or upset about things. If, before the operation, a chimpanzee had been upset by failure to do a psychological test, after the operation, it no longer cared.

Damage of the same sort as that caused by this operation to both frontal lobes may occur in man. It often results from people trying to shoot themselves without knowing how to do it. They usually put the barrel of the revolver against the right temple and fire. If this does not kill them, and it may well not do so, it usually causes what is called a through-and-through gunshot wound; the bullet goes through one side of the head and comes out of the other. It commonly damages one or both optic nerves, making the person blind in one or both eyes. What may happen in such patients is that after this damage to the frontal lobes of the brain, the depression is gone. This is not only because they have made their gesture; it is that their personalities are now different. They are more like Jacobsen's chimpanzees; they are indifferent to everything.

In the wars and the everyday violence that characterize the present century, damage to the frontal lobes occurs. The strange kind of indifference that is a feature of damage to the front parts of the frontal lobes is made clear if I quote from the notes I made on a patient I saw in Italy during the war in 1944. The patient was a lieutenant in the New Zealand army. He was picked up soon after being wounded, and it was then noted that his brain was oozing out of the wound in the front of his head. When he was operated upon twenty-four hours later, the roofs of both his orbits were found to be shattered and the front of the brain on both sides was reduced to pulp. Twenty-one days after the injury, his state was as follows:

His condition is best described as one of apathy. He lies in bed doing nothing and responds to nothing, except that sometimes he follows with his eyes anything that is happening. He leaves his lit cigarette on the bed; he holds up the paper in front of him as if he is reading it, when it is put in his hand. Recently I observed him lying on his back with the paper held up in front of him; on his chest was the feeding cup where someone had put it, and the spout was between his lips; but he was making no attempt to drink from it, nor did he put it down; he just lay there with the feeding cup full of tea touching his lips, his paper in his hand; and he did nothing. The greater part of the day he spends sleeping or lying on his bed with a paper held in front of him, pretending to read it, but never turning over the pages; however when I handed it to him upside down, he did turn it the right way up.

But this is not the whole picture, for he does sometimes get up and put on some of his clothes, go to the table to eat or look out of the window. Such activities are done with an intense preoccupation with what he is doing at the moment and an equal indifference to any circumstances relating to other people. What he does, he carries out perfectly, as he puts on his shoes and laces them, eats his food with the other officers with correct manners; he spreads jam on his bread and cuts it and makes a sandwich of it, all neatly. While I was talking to him and trying to take a medical history from him, he got up, put on the top of his pyjamas and went and looked out of the window, all while I was asking him questions and attempting to examine him; he went through these activities just as if I were not there. As I talked to him and examined him, he repeatedly stretched out to get a cigarette and light it, although I kept moving them away from him. I had the impression that each time he began again, he did not realize that he was not to do it. Once, as he walked about the ward, he defaecated while walking, showing no interest in this act whatsoever.

His speech is entirely normal and he seems to understand everything or at least everything simple. But he is unwilling to speak. It seems to need much effort for him to speak, and he does not make this effort.

This picture of apathy and total indifference to social relations does not last, though the amount of recovery varies from case to case. Actually, that young man's father wrote to me from New Zealand eight years later and told me that his son had eventually made a good recovery and satisfactory adjustment. However, after such lesions the patients are usually left with some degree of apathy or restlessness, tactlessness and lack of self-control, difficulty in maintaining attention and thus difficulty in learning and in planning, easy fatigability and a lack of interest in things and other people.

In 1935, Moniz, a neurologist working in Portugal, came to the conclusion that if the operation of dividing the frontal lobes from the rest of the brain reduces the excitement and the frustration of the chimpanzees, it would probably do the same in patients. He therefore invented the operation of prefrontal leucotomy for the treatment of certain psychiatric patients, an operation that is no longer done.

The first results obtained with prefrontal leucotomy were the same as those obtained in the chimpanzee. When much of the frontal lobe was divided from the rest of the brain, the patients had no energy and there was little spontaneous activity arising from internal motivation. In the most severely afflicted patients, the lack of initiative was such that the patient would stay in bed until he was got out of it. If food was put in his mouth, he may have done nothing about it, merely leaving it there without chewing or swallowing it. When the effects of the operation were less severe, the patients were just placid: whatever they did, they did slowly and without much interest. They lacked emotion, or rather, they lacked any persistence in emotion. They often had sufficient insight to explain that since the operation they had no feelings. As one previously hypomanic and intelligent patient put it: 'I am dull, a bore, and I know it.' These patients did not have enough initiative to start doing anything and they could not concentrate for long. The patients who were less damaged could carry on a routine, doing the things that they knew well how to do. But they undertook no new projects, made no plans and lived without enthusiasm.

They were uninhibited. Some of them were sexually disinhibited; others ate excessively. Although they were not aggressive, some of them easily lost their tempers. They could not resist the first impulse that occurred to them; and their impulsive actions were not curbed by the reactions of other people, as they had lost much of their feeling for others and also the ordinary social inhibition. A patient who had had a leucotomy would start undressing and going to bed in front of his guests because he was sleepy.

Patients who returned to the same job after this operation were less good at their work; these included a judge with powers to condemn people to death and life-imprisonment. The more intellectual the work was, the more their capabilities were affected. Freeman and Watts put the matter well by saying that one would not call on a patient who had had a leucotomy 'for advice on any important matter. His reactions to situations are direct, hasty, and dependent upon his emotional state at the moment.'

This operation became obsolete by the sixties, as it was superseded by effective drugs.

From observations on neurotic or psychotic patients it is hazardous to draw conclusions concerning how these various parts of the brain contribute to our personalities. Yet if we do not try to make use of material such as this we may be discarding the only large body of data we have.

It certainly appears that the frontal lobes and their deeper connections are important in giving us our general energy and our interest in living. Perhaps related to this motivating energy or perhaps something different is the ability to respond to the environment in a long-term way. The frontal lobes allow us to deliberate and to consider the consequences of possible courses of action. This foresight enables us to plan intelligently and adjust ourselves to future probabilities. The ability to stop and think is a characteristic of man. Pleasure as a delayed and not an immediate reward illumines many aspects of man's way of living, such as planning and following a career, saving money for the future, building for unborn generations.

The frontal lobes are not the region of the brain concerned with intellectual attainments. The social feelings and relationships that we learn appear to be laid down in the frontal lobes with their connections to the other parts of the brain. The control necessary for living in a community depends on the frontal lobes. They have been affected by the experience of living and by years of upbringing and by our knowledge of how to relate ourselves to other human beings.

Not the whole of the frontal lobes are devoted to these general activities. The parts in front of the primary motor region are also concerned with movements, with turning, with speaking and swallowing, with all the skills we have learned. The parts nearest the mid-line are also related to the hypothalamus. These are the parts of the brain used for the control of the bowels and the bladder and they are also concerned with sexual activity. When this part of the brain is removed, none of these activities are controlled; they are no longer fitted into the rest of the patient's living, they tend to lead an independent existence, the bowel and bladder emptying when they are full, and sexual urges demanding immediate gratification.

When the changes and deteriorations of old age affect the brain, the results vary according to what parts are chiefly affected. It is common for the memory to go, as we all know. When the memory becomes severely impaired, learning is no longer possible. Commonly when intellectual capacities are much diminished, the senile person confabulates. Perhaps the ability to recollect if an event is a part of one's own past or is something one has heard about becomes disturbed; and this may contribute to apparent confabulation.

Similar changes are seen in the realms of personality, of emotion, of social relationships. The senile person is less able to control his emotion, or rather, the manifestations of emotion; yet most of such people will say that the emotions they are showing are not deep. They may cry if they see anything sentimental or are reminded of an emotional occasion. Patients relate that they cry when they hear 'God Save the Queen' played in a crowd.

When the oldest parts of the temporal lobes degenerate, the effects are similar to those produced by removal of these parts at operation. One such patient would stuff everything into her mouth, which included her flowers and handkerchiefs, and would chew and try to swallow them.

When the front parts of the frontal lobes become atrophic, the patient loses finer sensibilities and may become indifferent to the feelings of others. As the lobes become more atrophic behaviour becomes more ruled by the needs of the moment and less cognizant of social requirements. One patient I saw threw a chamber pot out of the window of a top floor of the house; she explained that as she had finished with it, she threw it away. These old people become indifferent to personal appearance; the preening instinct ceases to be important. Then certain

basic features of their personalities come out. The obsessional personality becomes more marked; rituals and compulsions dominate their
lives, the patient worries about the few things he has to do, and cannot
think of anything else. The choleric person loses his temper even more
readily. The jovial person becomes fatuous. The ability to make use of
symbols deteriorates. The patient still understands the concrete and no
longer understands abstractions.

When intelligence decreases, the patient can no longer read a book,
but can still read the newspaper. For he cannot remember enough of the
book to keep the general scheme in mind or to remember the plot of a
novel; but he may still have enough memory to remember the theme of
an article or an essay. He has difficulty in composing letters, in thinking
what to write, though he still retains the mechanical part of writing.
When the right parieto-occipital region of the cortex atrophies, the old
person has great difficulty in finding his way about. This may not be
noticed as long as he remains at home; but it becomes clear if he is taken
away. When these patients come to hospital, they cannot find their way
to the bathroom, and on returning to the ward, they do not remember
which is their bed. This difficulty in getting their bearings is always worse
at night, in the dark. In the daytime, there are numbers of sensory clues,
everything is clearly seen. At night, they may have to feel their way
about, the light being inadequate to show up the total environment.

Eventually their exhibition of facile emotions goes off, and they
become indifferent to everything. This indifference of senility may
perhaps be a further stage in the contentment of later middle age that
comes when desires have become less urgent and demanding. Between
the indifference of age and the urgency of youth, there may be a period of
serenity—or is that saying too much?

What we are seeing when the cortex becomes atrophic is the decay of
the functions organized by this part of the cerebral hemispheres.
According to the principle deduced by Hughlings Jackson, the most
recently acquired functions disintegrate first, leaving the oldest established to the end. He also pointed out that when the higher level of
function goes, the lower level one is released and manifested in an
exaggerated form. The higher functions are often related to lower
functions by exerting an inhibition on them, and this inhibition is
removed when the higher functions go off.

One cannot sum up in a few well-chosen words the relation between
the cerebral hemispheres and the hypothalamus and the thalamus—
mainly because we do not really know what it is. It is not simply, as the
early psychoanalysts conjectured, that there are lower parts which are a

pool of instinctual urges, controlled by the educated and trained cerebral hemispheres above. The relationship between the two levels of the brain is a reciprocal one. Each part can bring the other part into activity and then the two parts of the brain work together.

It is on account of the reciprocal and intimate relation between the cerebral hemispheres and the hypothalamus and thalamus that psychotherapy is possible. The whole of our nervous systems and secondarily of our bodies can be influenced by all we experience, all we hear. Frequently repeated persuasion and explanation, the awakening of emotion, the reliving of experience, and re-awakening of memories, all of this can have effects on our personalities and behaviour because the cerebral hemispheres influence the rest of the brain. The hypothalamus controls the autonomic nervous system and the endocrine system of the body, and in turn they affect many parts of the brain. Patients find it very difficult to understand how 'just talk' can help them or even cure their ills. But everything we have ever experienced and which made us what we are has entered our brains through some sensory channel, through the skin, the nose, the eyes or the ears. For us humans, a good deal of it has entered via the ears, in the form of speech. And so there is no reason why further talking should not continue to affect us and influence our personalities.

The pioneering work of Hess is only thirty years old, and the investigations of the parts of the cerebral hemispheres related to the hypothalamus have been undertaken only in the last ten years. Operations on the frontal and temporal lobes designed to affect human personality and behaviour have been done only since the last war. Our knowledge of the nervous system has grown so rapidly in the last fifty years that we can be sure that many of the present problems in animal psychology and in our understanding of the function of living cells will soon be solved. Lest we should have illusions about what science can do we should be clear about one thing. Science brings knowledge and this knowledge brings the ability to make new things and to change the world. But science does not bring happiness, except perhaps to those whose lives are dedicated to its service.

Glossary

Weights and measures are now expressed in SI units (Système International d'Unités)

$Å$ = Ångstrom unit = 0.1 nanometre = 10^{-10} metre

acetylcholine: the transmitter used by vertebrate motoneurons, parasympathetic neurons and by some sympathetic neurons.

adrenal glands: a pair of endocrine glands resting on the kidneys. They consist of two parts, the adrenal cortex and the adrenal medulla. The cortex forms hormones playing a part in metabolism of carbohydrates, fats and minerals, in sex, growth and response to all sorts of stress. The medulla supplies the body with adrenalin and noradrenalin, which are needed for activity.

adrenalin: one of the two hormones secreted by the adrenal gland and also emitted by neurons as a transmitter.

adrenocorticotrophin (ACTH): a hormone secreted by the pituitary gland that stimulates the adrenal cortex to release its hormones.

afferent nerves: nerves taking impulses to the central nervous system.

amino acids: chemical substances containing an amino group (NH_2), a carboxyl group (COOH), a hydrogen atom, and another group, attached to a central carbon atom. Amino acids are the components of proteins.

amygdala or amygdaloid nuclei: large groups of neurons in the front part of the temporal lobe.

anion: a negative ion.

anterior horn: the anterior part of the grey matter of the spinal cord in which the motoneurons lie.

anthropoids: a sub-order of the primates. Living forms of anthropoids are the chimpanzee, gibbon, gorilla, man, and orang-utan.

aphasia: a difficulty in organizing language, there being no paralysis of the muscles needed for making the sounds of speech.

arthropod: a member of the largest division of the animal kingdom, which includes insects, spiders and crustaceans; animals characterized by having an exoskeleton and externally jointed limbs.

axon: the central part of the nerve fibre. It is an elongated process of a neuron, usually single, sometimes double or triple, which conducts nerve impulses over long distances in the central and peripheral nervous systems.

brain stem: the parts of the brain between the cerebral hemispheres and the spinal cord, including the medulla oblongata, pons and midbrain.

cation: a positive ion.

cerebellum: part of the brain superficially resembling the cerebrum, hence its name of little cerebrum. It is usually considered to be part of the brain, but W. S. Gilbert (1882) established another convention, thus;

> When in that House M.P.'s divide,
> If they've a brain and cerebellum, too,
> They've got to leave that brain outside,
> And vote just as their leaders tell'em to.

cerebral cortex: grey matter of the cerebral hemispheres, forming the outermost part of the hemispheres.

cerebral hemispheres: the largest and most recently evolved part of the brain.

cerebrospinal fluid: liquid circulating throughout the ventricles of the brain and surrounding the whole of the central nervous system. When a patient has a lumbar puncture, some of this fluid is taken by means of a needle introduced between two vertebrae in the lower back.

cerebrum: the two cerebral hemispheres.

cholinergic: nerve fibres emitting acetylcholine as transmitter substance.

cholinesterase: enzyme that breaks down acetylcholine into inert choline and acetic acid.

cilia: fine motile hairs that are outgrowths of cells. Their arrangement is the same in all organisms, there being a ring of nine with two in the centre.

code: a system of signals used to convey information.

commissure: a transversely running band of nerve fibres connecting homologous parts of the central nervous system across the mid-line.

confabulate: to recount made-up experiences glibly, mostly about oneself; it is done to fill in gaps in the memory or to try and put sense into a state of confusion.

convergence: the principle according to which many neurons send their axons to a few neurons, thus bringing much information to a few channels.

corpus callosum: large commissure joining the two cerebral hemispheres together.

cortex: Latin for the bark of a tree; used in anatomy to mean the outer layers of any structure.

cutaneous: adjective pertaining to the skin.

cytoplasm: the living components of plant or animal cells, apart from the nucleus. Together with the nucleus, it forms the protoplasm.

DNA: deoxyribonucleic acid. This long threadlike molecule is the hereditary material of the cell; it reproduces itself and it codes the production of proteins. It is within the chromosomes.

dendrite: a branching process of a neuron, specialized for receiving nerve impulses from other neurons.

divergence: the principle according to which one or a few neurons send branching axons far and wide to many neurons, thus sending information to many parts of the nervous system.

dopamine: a monoaminergic transmitter substance.

echo-location: echo-ranging: a method for finding objects and measuring distances utilizing the time taken for sound waves to travel.

efferent nerves: nerves taking impulses away from the central nervous system.

electroencephalogram: recording of the electrical activity of the cerebral hemispheres by means of electrodes fixed to the scalp.

electrolyte: a chemical substance that can form ions.

encephalopathy: disease of the brain. Wernicke's encephalopathy is a disorder affecting particularly the hypothalamus due to lack of vitamin B and chronic alcoholism.

endocrine gland: a gland which passes its secretion into the bloodstream directly and not through a duct or pipe.

enzyme: a protein which speeds up metabolic activities.

epilepsy: a disease characterized by the spontaneous or induced discharge of groups of neurons of the forebrain.

ethology: the scientific study of the behaviour of animals in their normal environment.

excitability: a characteristic of cells that allows them to respond to irritation; very marked in neurons and receptors.

excitation: the process of arousing a cell or a group of cells or an organism into activity.

extensor muscles: the muscles that straighten out the back and the limbs.

feedback: a term borrowed from radio technicians to mean the diversion of a small part of the output to control the input. It occurs both in natural and in man-made systems.

firing: the neuron is said to fire when it sends off a nerve impulse.

flexor muscles: the muscles that bend the trunk and limbs.

forebrain: the part of the brain in front of the midbrain.

fovea: a small area of the retina composed of cones; light rays are automatically focused here for greatest visual resolution.

fusimotor: the name for motoneurons or nerves going to the small muscle fibres within the muscle spindle.

GABA: inhibitory transmitter.

ganglion or ganglion cells: a group of nerve cells collected together having a common function.

grey matter: the parts of the central nervous system made up mainly of neurons.

gyrus: smooth folds of the cerebral hemispheres and cerebellum.

hair-follicle: a little sac in the skin from which a hair grows. It is supplied by several nerve fibres.

hallucination: perception of a non-existent object.

hippocampus: a part of the temporal lobe of the cerebral hemisphere of great importance for memory.

homeostasis: the capacity of animals to preserve a constant composition in the face of a changing environment.

hormone: chemical substance secreted by endocrine glands or neurons.

horseshoe crab: an ancient and primitive arthropod.

hypothalamus: the central and basal parts of the brain.

inertia: a fundamental property of matter, making it resist change in its motion.

inhibition: the opposite of excitation.

ion: an electrically charged particle of an electrolyte carrying either a positive or a negative charge.

kinaesthesis or kinaesthesia: the sense of the movements and/or position of parts of the body.

lsd: lysergic acid diethylamide. It causes hallucinations and abnormal behaviour.

lesion: damage to tissues by trauma or disease; may be made surgically as treatment or for experiments on animals kept in laboratories.

limbic lobe or limbic system: A group of nuclei within the brain that are essential for feeling and expressing emotion and instinctual drives, such as sex, aggression, fear, eating, drinking, micturition, and defaecation.

mammals: vertebrates with mammary glands and hair.

medulla: the marrow or inner part of any structure.

medulla oblongata: the lowest part of the brain situated immediately above the spinal cord.

membrane: a boundary layer forming the walls of cells or tissues.

membrane, basilar: a layer within the inner ear which is thrown into folds when sound waves are transmitted to the inner ear.

membrane, tectorial: a layer within the inner ear covering the receptor cells.

metabolism: the life process of cells and organisms, comprising the building of tissues, anabolism, and the breaking down of tissues, catabolism.

midbrain: the part of the brain above the pons and below the hypothalamus and thalamus.

migraine: a particular sort of headache, characteristically restricted to one side of the head: hence the name, which is a contraction of hemicrania.

millisecond: ms: 10^{-3} second.

molecule: smallest particle of a substance that retains all the properties of a larger mass of the same material.

monoamines: the chemical substances used for monoaminergic transmission in the central and the peripheral sympathetic nervous systems.

motor end-plate: the special end-organ where the nerve fibre terminates in the muscle.

muscle: a tissue of animal bodies consisting of protein fibres which contract when they are stimulated. Organs such as the heart and the bladder are made almost entirely of muscle. Limbs consist essentially of muscles attached to bones which are hinged at joints.

muscle spindle: receptors of the muscles.

myelin sheath: lipid sheath surrounding axons of myelinated nerve fibres.

myelinated nerve fibres: nerve fibres surrounded by myelin sheaths.

myo-neural junction: another word for neuro-muscular junction.

μ **m:** micrometre: 10^{-6} m.

nerve cell: neuron.

nerve fibre: the long process of a neuron consisting of the axon surrounded by supporting cells.

nerve impulse: the brief activity passing along nerve fibres that constitutes the message. It is usually detected in experimental investigations by the electrical phenomena; but there are other aspects of it, such as visual and thermal phenomena, chemical events.

neuroglia: cells needed for the nutrition and support of neurons in the central nervous system.

neuron: nerve cell: the essential conducting unit of the nervous system. It consists of cell-body, dendrites and one or more axons.

neuro-muscular junction: the modified synapse where nerve impulses are transmitted to the muscle.

noradrenalin: the main transmitter of the sympathetic nervous system; also used in the central nervous system

oestrogen: any compound which acts as a female sex hormone.

olive: a structure in the medulla oblongata consisting of neurons and making an eminence on the surface, which recalled an olive to earlier anatomists.

ommatidium: the unit of the compound eye of arthropods.

optic chiasm: the point of crossing of the optic nerves behind the two orbits.

optical isomers: chemical substances having the same composition and the same molecular weight but different properties with regard to the transmission of light.

oval window: small membrane-covered opening between middle and inner ear.

ovary: egg-producing organ in the female animal or plant.

parasympathetic nerves: a system of motor nerves going to viscera; their main neurotransmitter is acetylcholine. In general, the action of these nerves is the opposite of the sympathetic nerves.

peptides: a class of chemical compounds formed of two or more amino acids; they are linked together as follows $-NH = CO =$. Depending on the number of amino acids in the molecule, they are called di-, tri-, tetra-peptides and so on. Proteins are made up of many peptides.

perception: the interpretation of sensation.

piezoelectric effect: when certain crystals are subjected to mechanical stress, they produce an electric charge. Conversely when a charge is applied to such a crystal, the crystal shows a slight change in dimensions. This principle is used in making high-frequency loud speakers, microphones, and gramophone pick-ups.

polarity: a field or circuit in which ions and electrons are flowing between positive and negative poles.

pons: the part of the brain situated immediately above the medulla oblongata.

posterior horn: the posterior part of the grey matter of the spinal cord in which afferent neurons lie.

potential, electric: the work done on or by a unit positive charge as it moves from infinity to some point in an electric field or as it moves from one point to another in an electric field.

primates: order of mammals characterized by having nails on some of the digits. Living forms of primates are the tree-shrews, lemurs, tarsiers, monkeys, and anthropoids.

progesterone: hormone concerned with pregnancy, produced by the ovary.

proteins: a class of compounds made up of 100 to 1 000 000 molecules of 20 amino acids, joined together as peptides.

RNA: ribonucleic acid; it has a long thread-like molecule consisting of a single polynucleotide chain. Messenger RNA carries the information encoded in DNA to the sites of protein synthesis outside the nucleus of the cell.

receptor: a neuron or a non-nervous cell specialized to respond to stimuli from the external or internal environment. If the receptor is not itself a neuron, it converts forms of energy into nerve impulses.

reciprocal innervation: organization making a muscle relax when the muscle with an opposing action contracts.

reflex: rapid, simple, innate reaction to stimulation. The reaction starts in a receptor or sensory organ and it finally causes contraction of muscles, a muscle, or a part of a muscle, or the secretion of a gland.

reflex, scratch: reflexly organized scratching movements of vertebrates in which the hindlimb is brought forward to scratch the forelimb, trunk or head and neck.

round window: small membrane-covered opening between middle and inner ear.

Schwann cells: cells surrounding and nourishing nerve fibres of the peripheral nervous system. They form the myelin sheaths of peripheral myelinated nerve fibres.

serotonin: a monoaminergic neurotransmitter.

servo-mechanism: automatic mechanism in which the output is partly controlled by feeding back a part of the output to the controlling elements.

sex hormones: masculinizing or feminizing hormones produced in the testes and ovaries. These steroid chemicals cause the secondary sexual characteristics. Their production and release into the bloodstream is controlled by the pituitary.

sign or signal: the element in a communication system that carries the information.

somatic: having to do with the skeletal part of the body, being opposed to visceral, having to do with the internal organs. Often used as the adjective for body, as in somatotrophic, making the body grow.

species: a basic unit of classification of all living organisms. Usually, organisms belong to the same species if they can mate and produce living offspring. But there are exceptions to this as lions and tigers, horses and asses produce living offspring; and it is reported occasionally that dogs and cats can do so.

steroids: chemical substances with the characteristics of lipids. They have a particular chemical configuration, with at least 17 carbon atoms and four rings.

swim-bladder: a thin-walled sac lying in the body cavity in front of the vertebral column in fish, filled with gas, and used in helping the fish live at various depths with their different pressures.

sympathetic nerves: a system of motor nerves going to blood-vessels, sweat glands and viscera; their main neurotransmitter in mammals is noradrenalin. In general, the action of these nerves is the opposite of the parasympathetic nerves.

synapse: the region where two or more neurons meet and where impulses are passed from one to the others (divergence) or from others to one (convergence).

testosterone: a steroid hormone produced by the interstitial cells of the testis, causing masculinization.

thalamus: a large ovoid mass of nuclei in the centre of the cerebral hemisphere, consisting chiefly of relays between the cerebral cortex and lower level structures of the central nervous system.

tissue: a group of cells with the same structure and with the same or similar function. The body of a plant or animal is considered to be made up of many kinds of tissues.

vertebrate: an animal having a backbone.

vertigo: sensation of rotation in which either the surroundings seem to rotate around the subject or the subject seems to rotate.

white matter: the parts of the central nervous system made up mainly of nerve fibres.

Index